Practitioner's Guide to Empirically Supported Measures of Anger, Aggression, and Violence

ABCT Clinical Assessment Series

Series Edited by Association for Behavioral and Cognitive Therapies

For further volumes:
http://www.springer.com/series/5553

George F. Ronan • Laura Dreer
Kimberly Maurelli
Donna Wollerman Ronan
James Gerhart

Practitioner's Guide to Empirically Supported Measures of Anger, Aggression, and Violence

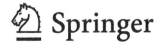

George F. Ronan
Department of Psychology
Central Michigan University
Mount Pleasant, MI, USA

Kimberly Maurelli
Department of Psychology
Central Michigan University
Mount Pleasant, MI, USA

James Gerhart
Department of Behavioral Sciences
Rush University Medical Center
Chicago, IL, USA

Laura Dreer
Department of Ophthalmology
University of Alabama at Birmingham
Birmingham, AL, USA

Donna Wollerman Ronan
Psychological Training
    and Consultation Center
Central Michigan University
Mount Pleasant, MI, USA

ISSN 1869-2281   ISSN 1869-229X (electronic)
ISBN 978-3-319-00244-6   ISBN 978-3-319-00245-3 (eBook)
DOI 10.1007/978-3-319-00245-3
Springer Cham Heidelberg New York Dordrecht London

Library of Congress Control Number: 2013938486

Printed on acid-free paper

Springer is part of Springer Science+Business Media (www.springer.com)

Preface

Anger, aggression, and violence continue to present salient concerns for society in general and mental health providers in particular. Unfortunately, there is no text that has systematically reviewed measures for assessing these constructs. This book reviews over 130 measures of anger, aggression, or violence. This book contains two parts. Part I includes an introductory chapter and an applied chapter on conducting a risk assessment. Part II provides a description of how the measures are organized and quick-view tables that provide easy access to measures with enough information to allow for an estimate of the likelihood that reading additional information about a particular measure would prove fruitful. Measures are organized alphabetically into tables for measures of anger, aggression, or violence. Each of the tables provides the name of the measure, the purpose for which the measure was developed, and the targeted population. The tables also provide information on the method of assessment, the amount of time required to use the measure, and the page number where additional information is available. Part II also contains the review of each measure. The Appendix provides examples of measures that can be copied for research or clinical purposes.

I want to thank a number of people who helped with this text. In particular, we wish to thank students and colleagues who helped with the review of measures in Part II. We also thank the authors of the measures we reviewed. Without their work this text would not be possible. Finally, we extend a heartfelt thanks and profound respect to the authors who allowed us to reproduce their measures in the Appendix. Sharing their work in this manner is likely to have a significant impact on advancing the assessment of anger, aggression, and violence.

Mount Pleasant, MI, USA	George F. Ronan
Birmingham, AL, USA	Laura Dreer
Mount Pleasant, MI, USA	Kimberly Maurelli
Mount Pleasant, MI, USA	Donna Wollerman Ronan
Chicago, IL, USA	James Gerhart

Contents

Part I

General Issues in Assessing Anger, Aggression, and Violence

Introduction

Human anger, aggression, and violence are interrelated concepts, all associated with verbal or physical actions which inflict discomfort or pain. They are commonly observed in clinical settings; however, delineating the exact boundary conditions for these constructs is difficult. That is, the point in which anger becomes aggression and aggression becomes violence is difficult to determine. To further complicate things, anger, aggression, and violence occur across syndrome types and severity levels. For instance, anger, aggression, and violence can become the central focus of a referral for treatment of an individual initially presenting with mood disorder, personality disorder, or many other currently popular diagnostic categories. Some have argued that the clinical impact of these constructs is so common in clinical settings that new diagnostic taxonomies should be developed that directly classify these concerns (e.g., DiGiuseppe & Tafrate, 2007).

Despite the difficulty inherent in differentiating interrelated concepts, attempts have been made to define anger, aggression, and violence. Anger is generally defined as an uncomfortable emotion characterized by antagonism toward someone or something, and it is frequently implicated as a precursor to aggressive or violent behavior (e.g., Kassinove & Sukhodolsky, 1995). Although anger often serves to motivate behavior, the resulting responses are malleable and a function of an interaction between a variety of personal and situation variables (Anderson & Bushman, 2002). For instance, as a result of being unfairly treated by a supervisor, one person might choose to work harder to demonstrate clear signs of competence, another person might choose to assert his/her right to be treated equally and fairly, and still another person might lash out and risk incurring additional problems. For purposes of this text, we have operationally defined anger as a commonly experienced emotional state that often results from the perception of a personally meaningful injustice.

In contrast to anger, aggression has overt behavioral referents that should allow it to be more easily identified. Aggression can be broadly defined as hostile, injurious, or destructive behavior. However, this process is qualified by ongoing debates regarding the most appropriate way to classify aggressive behaviors. Some have attempted to classify aggression using the underlying motivation for engaging in aggressive behavior. As an example, aggression that appears to arise from frustration or a lack of emotional control has been labeled as reactive or emotional aggression (e.g., Berkowitz, 1993; Hubbard, McAuliffe, Morrow, & Romano, 2010; Vitaro & Brendgen, 2005). Alternately, aggression that appears to arise from a planned attempt to obtain a desired object or outcome has been labeled as proactive or instrumental aggression (e.g., Berkowitz, 1993; Hubbard, McAuliffe, Morrow, & Romano, 2010; Vitaro & Brengden,

G.F. Ronan et al., *Practitioner's Guide to Empirically Supported Measures of Anger, Aggression, and Violence*, ABCT Clinical Assessment Series, DOI 10.1007/978-3-319-00245-3_1, © Springer International Publishing Switzerland 2014

2005). Other taxonomies classify behavior based on a qualitative analysis of the emitted behaviors such as direct versus indirect displays of aggression (e.g., Verona, Sadeh, Case, Reed, & Bhattacharjee, 2008), or verbal versus emotional displays of aggression (e.g., Vickerman & Margolin, 2008). Each of these approaches has evinced some popularity, however, coding behaviors into one class or another is difficult and there is a lack of support for the stability and specificity of these categories (see Bushman & Anderson, 2001). For instance, the same person can display reactive, proactive, indirect, direct, verbal, emotional, and physical aggression within different or similar contexts across time. For the purpose of this volume, we have strayed from these classification schemes and have broadly defined aggression as behavior emitted with the intent to psychologically harm an animal or person.

In contrast to aggression which seeks to cause psychological harm, violence refers to the exertion of physical force so as to injure or abuse. There is general agreement that violent behaviors occur at a lower frequency than anger or aggression, and that violent behaviors contain qualitatively distinct features that often generate considerable attention (e.g., Natarajan & Caramaschi, 2010). Except under controlled contexts such as criminal sentencing (e.g., death penalty) and war, behaviors categorized as violent are often illegal actions. Violent behaviors encompass a fairly large group of behaviors including assault and battery, bullying, child maltreatment, destruction of property, elder abuse, gang-related violence, genocide, homicide, intimate partner violence, sexual assault, suicide, terrorism, and vigilantism (World Health Organization, 2002). Although some researchers have attempted to organize violent behavior by the targets and types of violence (e.g., Krug, Dahlber, Mercy, Zwi, & Lozano, 2002; World Health Organization, 2002), there currently is no agreed upon classification. For the purpose of this volume, we have defined violence as behavior that is committed with the intent of causing physical harm to an object or person.

Background

It is well accepted that anger, aggression, and violence have been significant sources of human suffering throughout history and remain a problem in society today. The impact of such destructive human behavior has been assessed through epidemiological studies, statistics collected through the criminal justice system, evidence provided by authorities including the World Health Organization, and experts representing particularly vulnerable populations such as children and teens, women, minorities, and the elderly.

Problematic expressions of anger, aggression, and violence occur across a variety of contexts. The ramifications of such behaviors are detrimental to society and have contributed to aggression and violence being classified as serious health concerns by the Centers for Disease Control and Prevention. A considerable amount of aggression and violence observed in the USA occurs during the commission of a crime. The US Department of Justice Federal Bureau of Investigation (FBI) defines a violent crime as any criminal offense that uses force or threats of force and includes murder, rape and sexual assault, robbery, and assault (2010). The FBI estimated that a violent crime occurs every 23.9 seconds (2009). Due to underreporting of violent offenses (Hart & Rennison, 2003), the actual number of violent crimes committed might be higher than the reported numbers. Data collected within the US correction systems during 2008 suggests 52 % of state prison inmates and 8.4 % of federal prison inmates were serving time for crimes involving aggression and/or violence (West, Sabol, & Greenman, 2010). Despite a notable drop in violent crime over the past decade, according to the FBI over 1.2 million violent crimes were reported to law enforcement agencies in the USA in 2009 (Federal Bureau of Investigation, 2010). Data from the National Crime Victimization Survey collected during 2010 revealed that an estimated 3.8 million violent victimizations occurred in the USA that year, with

1.4 million of those victimizations characterized as "serious violent" (Truman, 2011).

Workplace aggression and violence is another area that has received the attention of professionals and researchers in recent years. A substantial literature has addressed issues regarding negative personal and business outcomes related to violence in the workplace (e.g., Chang & Lyons, 2012; Glomb & Cortina, 2006), as well as factors which mitigate the negative impact of workplace violence (Mueller & Tschan, 2011). Workplace aggression or violence appears to be a common phenomenon and cannot be attributed to the behavior of a few "disgruntled employees" (Barling, Dupré, & Kelloway, 2009). Workplace aggression can take a multitude of forms (e.g., physical, verbal, emotional, psychological). It can be perpetrated by men or women and can take the form of covert or overt behavior, with men more likely to engage in overt aggressive behavior and men and women equally likely to engage in covert aggressive behavior (Arnold, Dupré, Hershcovis, & Turner, 2011). The perpetrators of workplace aggression can be supervisors, coworkers, or organizational outsiders such as customers or significant others (Barling et al., 2009; Chang & Lyons, 2012). There is no prototype of an aggressive employee and attempts at profiling employees who are at risk of behaving aggressively have met with limited empirical support (Barling et al., 2009). The consequences of workplace aggression or violence are significant (e.g., emotional strain, lower morale, higher rates of employee turnover) and there is a consensus that violence at work is a serious health concern (Chang & Lyons, 2012; Mueller & Tschan, 2011). However, research suggests that workplace aggression is predictable and, similar to aggressive behavior in other contexts, often follows some form of provocation (Barling et al., 2009). This suggests it might also be preventable by implementing effective assessment and organizational practices (Barling et al., 2009).

Clinicians working in medical and mental health settings report frequently dealing with incidents of anger, aggression, and violence. The frequency of aggression and violence observed in these settings is at least partially responsible for all

50 of the states within the USA passing "mandated reporting" laws within the past two decades. These laws require physicians, psychologists, other healthcare workers, and professionals in education to report suspected incidents of aggression or violence emitted toward vulnerable persons (e.g., children, elderly, disabled persons) to social service agencies. The concern over incidents of child abuse has remained high in recent years as the prevalence of child abuse continues to be estimated at alarming levels. For instance, in 2010 it was estimated that 695,000 children in the USA experienced some form of maltreatment (U.S. Department of Health & Human Services, 2011). This suggests approximately 9 out of every 1,000 children were reported to experience abuse in 2010. More concerning is the fact that this estimate is likely an underrepresentation of the true prevalence of child abuse as this report only included incidents of reported abuse or neglect that were substantiated by government authorities (U.S. Department of Health & Human Services, 2011).

Over the past decade there has also been a rise in the concern over abuse of the elderly, a group which may include individuals who are just as vulnerable and dependent on caretakers as children. The Centers for Disease Control identify elder mistreatment as a specific concern on their webpage devoted to public health problems associated with violence. Supporting the increased concern regarding elder abuse are alarming statistics indicating the prevalence of such forms of aggression and violence. The National Elder Mistreatment Study found that 11 % of respondents (aged 60 or older) reported experiencing some form of maltreatment in the previous year, with most victimized by family members or caretakers (Acierno, Hernandez-Tejada, Muzzy, & Steve, 2009). This is consistent with estimates from the National Center on Elder Abuse (2005) that suggest rates of elder mistreatment may be as high as 10 % with two million victims in the USA alone. Mandated reporting laws have been minimally effective in bringing perpetrators of abusive behavior to the attention of law enforcement, but considerable work remains in identifying characteristics which predispose some to abuse vulnerable individuals.

Intimate partner violence and sexual violence are also a source of concern. Lifetime prevalence estimates for incidents of intimate partner violence in the USA tend to hover around 26 % for females and 16 % for males (e.g., Breiding, Black, & Ryan, 2008). The National Intimate Partner and Sexual Violence Survey (NISVS) was conducted in 2010 and revealed that more than one million women are raped in a year and over six million women and men are victims of stalking in a year (Black et al., 2011). Based on the results of the survey, these researchers estimated that on average 24 people per minute are victims of rape, physical violence, or stalking by an intimate partner in the USA (Black et al., 2011). These high estimates are consistent with the view of the Centers for Disease Control and Prevention, which identifies violence as a serious public health problem and recognizes intimate partner violence and sexual violence as specific areas of concern (Centers for Disease Control, 2012). Violence against women also represents a global problem. Amnesty International released a report based on statistics from the United Nations and World Health Organization that indicated violence against women and girls is one of the world's most widespread human rights violations (2004). Violence cuts across the boundaries of age, race, culture, wealth, and geography. Aggression and violence take place in multiple settings: at home or at work, on the streets and in schools, during times of peace, and times of conflict. Up to 33 % of women and girls will be beaten, coerced into sex, or otherwise abused in their lifetime (2004).

In addition to recognizing the high prevalence and serious negative consequences of intimate partner and sexual violence, the Centers for Disease Control and Prevention (CDC) identifies violence in general as a serious public health problem and reports that in 2007 more than 18,000 people in the USA were victims of homicide. The CDC further recognizes child maltreatment, elder maltreatment, youth violence, and global violence as specific areas of concern (Centers for Disease Control, 2012). As the above illustrates, the effect of violence in the USA is substantial. The impact of violence on a global level is even more staggering.

In a World Health Organization report, aggression and violence were described as the leading causes of death in all parts of the world for people ages 15–44 (Krug et al., 2002).

Purpose of This Text

All told, anger, violence, and aggression are ubiquitous in Western culture and within human civilization. Multiple theories have been expounded to explain this destructive strain in human interactions. The first contemporary students of human nature viewed aggression as a basic force in human interactions (Brierley, 1934) and a primary component of personality. More recent scholars have propounded evolutionary (Sell, 2010), genetic (Haberstick, Schmitz, Young, & Hewitt, 2006), psychosocial (Anderson, Buckley, & Carnagey, 2008), and neurobiological (Siever, 2008) explanations of the human propensity toward anger, aggression, and violence. There has been considerable progress made toward a multidimensional framework for understanding anger, aggression, and violence; however, there remains considerable work to do in terms of defining the constructs, assessing risk, and predicting anger, aggression, and violent behavior.

The purpose of this text is to address some of these issues by providing professionals with a compendium of information on over 130 measures developed to assess anger, aggression, and violence. Measures collected for inclusion in this book were identified using a variety of strategies. We searched through hundreds of publications that were available through popular search engines (e.g., PsycINFO, PubMED, and MEDLINE). In addition, e-mail requests were sent out across relevant professional listservs that described the project and solicited measures to include. Finally, we contacted researchers and asked them to recommend measures they had either used or developed. Although we made an honest effort to conduct an exhaustive search, we recognize that some worthy measures may have eluded our attention.

Organization of Measures and Information

Measures are organized according to whether they reflect anger, aggression, or violence. More specifically, we categorized 40 measures as assessing anger, 38 measures as assessing aggression, and 55 measures as assessing violence. Measures that assessed more than one construct are classified based on the primary focus of the measure. A standard outline was used to describe each instrument. The overall goal was to provide enough information to screen whether a measure might be useful for a given purpose. We also provide at least one reference for readers interested in obtaining additional information. The standard outline used for each measure is described below.

Title

The title of the measure is provided, along with the most commonly used acronym.

Purpose

This section describes the intended use of the measure.

Population

This section describes the intended population and populations for which norms are available.

Background and Description

This section provides a brief overview of the rationale for developing the measure, as well as information on any prior versions of the measure. This section also provides a description of the structure, format, and content of the measure.

Administration

This section provides an estimate of the amount of time required to administer the measure. Any special training or equipment requirements (e.g., computers, video cameras, etc.) are also noted.

Scoring

This section provides an estimate of the amount of time required to score the measure. Any special training or inter-rater reliability concerns are noted.

Interpretation

This section summarizes the meaning attributed to any scores, scales, or subscales. Information on the range of scores or cut-off scores is also provided.

Psychometric Properties

This section provides a summative evaluation of information on norms, reliability, and validity.

Clinical Utility

This section provides a general assessment of the usefulness of the measure in applied settings. High clinical utility is often predicated on sound psychometric properties, as well as a subjective assessment of the amount of time required and the potential client benefit. The frequency with which the measure has been used in clinical settings is also considered.

Research Applicability

This section provides a general assessment of the usefulness of the measure in research settings.

High research applicability typically implies that the measure has been found useful in prior research on the specific construct being measured.

Original Citation

This section lists one of the first articles where the measure was developed and/or described.

Source

This section provides information on where the actual measure can be obtained. Often this is the address or contact information for the author or publisher.

Alternative Forms

This section provides information on whether versions of this measure are available in different languages or formats.

References

Acierno, R., Hernandez-Tejada, M., Muzzy, W., & Steve, K. (2009). *National elder mistreatment study* (NCJRS Publication No. 226456). Retrieved from http://www.ncjrs.gov/pdffiles1/nij/grants/226456.pdf

Amnesty International. (2004). *Making violence against women count: Facts and figures—A summary.* Retrieved from http://www.amnesty.org/en/library/asset/ACT77/034/2004/en/301b0c48-fabb-11dd-b6c4-73b1aa157d32/act770342004en.pdf

Anderson, C. A., Buckley, K. E., & Carnagey, N. L. (2008). Creating your own hostile environment: A laboratory examination of trait aggression and the violence escalation cycle. *Personality and Social Psychology Bulletin, 34,* 462–473. doi:10.1177/0146167207311282

Anderson, C. A., & Bushman, B. J. (2002). Human aggression. *Annual Review of Psychology, 53,* 27–51. doi:10.1146/annurev.psych.53.100901.135231

Arnold, K. A., Dupré, K. E., Hershcovis, M. S., & Turner, N. (2011). Interpersonal targets and types of workplace aggression as a function of perpetrator sex. *Employee Responsibilities and Rights Journal, 23,* 163–170. doi:10.1007/s10672-010-9155-x

Barling, J., Dupré, K. E., & Kelloway, E. K. (2009). Predicting workplace aggression and violence. *Annual Review of Psychology, 60,* 671–692. doi:10.1146/annurev.psych.60.110707.163629

Berkowitz, L. (1993). *Aggression: Its causes, consequences, and control.* Philadelphia, PA: Temple University Press.

Black, M. C., Basile, K. C., Breiding, M. J., Smith, S. G., Walters, M. L., Merrick, M. T., et al. (2011). *The National Intimate Partner and Sexual Violence Survey (NISVS): 2010 summary report.* Atlanta, GA: National Center for Injury Prevention and Control, Centers for Disease Control and Prevention.

Breiding, M. J., Black, C., & Ryan, G. W. (2008). Prevalence and risk factors for intimate partner violence in eighteen U.S. states/territories. *American Journal of Preventative Medicine, 34,* 112–118.

Brierley, F. (1934). Present tendencies in psychoanalysis. *The British Journal of Medical Psychology, 14,* 211–229. doi:10.1111/j.2044-8341.1934.tb01121.x

Bushman, B. J., & Anderson, C. A. (2001). Is it time to pull the plug on the hostile versus instrumental aggression dichotomy? *Psychological Review, 108,* 273–279. doi:10.1037/0033-295X.108.1.273

Centers for Disease Control. (2012). *Injury center: Violence prevention.* Retrieved from http://www.cdc.gov/ViolencePrevention/index.html

Chang, C. H., & Lyons, B. J. (2012). Not all aggressions are created equal: A multifocal approach to workplace aggression. *Journal of Occupational Health Psychology, 17,* 79–92. doi:10.1037/a0026073

DiGiuseppe, R., & Tafrate, C. (2007). *Understanding anger and anger disorders.* New York: Oxford University Press.

Federal Bureau of Investigation. (2009). *Uniform Crime Reports: Crime in the United States, crime clock.* Retrieved from http://www2.fbi.gov/ucr/cius2009/about/crime_clock.html

Federal Bureau of Investigation. (2010). *Uniform Crime Reports: Violent crime.* Retrieved from http://www.fbi.gov/about-us/cjis/ucr/crime-in-the-u.s/2010/crime-in-the-u.s.-2010/violent-crime

Glomb, T. M., & Cortina, L. M. (2006). The experience of victims: Using theories of traumatic and chronic stress to understand individual outcomes of workplace abuse. In E. K. Kelloway, J. Barling, & J. Hurrell (Eds.), *Handbook of workplace Violence* (pp. 517–534). Thousand Oaks, CA: Sage.

Haberstick, B. C., Schmitz, S., Young, S. E., & Hewitt, J. K. (2006). Genes and developmental stability of aggressive behavior problems at home and school in a community sample of twins aged 7-12. *Behavior Genetics, 36,* 809–819. doi:10.1007/s10519-006-9092-5

Hart, T. C., & Rennison, C. M. (2003). Reporting crime to the police, 1992–2000 (NCJRS Publication No. 195710). Washington, DC: USGPO.

Hubbard, J., McAuliffe, M., Morrow, M., & Romano, L. (2010). Reactive and proactive aggression in childhood and adolescents: precursors, outcomes, processes, experiences, and measurement. *Journal of Personality, 78,* 95–118. doi:10.1111/j.1467-6494.2009.00610.x

Kassinove, H., & Sukhodolsky, D. G. (1995). Anger disorders: Basic science and practice issues. In H. Kassive (Ed.), *Anger disorders: Definition, diagnosis, and treatment* (pp. 1–26). Washington, DC: Taylor & Francis.

Krug, E. G., Dahlber, L. L., Mercy, J. A., Zwi, A. B., & Lozano, R. (2002). *World report on violence and health*. Geneva: World Health Organization.

Mueller, S., & Tschan, F. (2011). Consequences of client-initiated workplace violence: The role of fear and perceived prevention. *Journal of Occupational Health Psychology, 16*, 217–229. doi:10.1037/a0021723

Natarajan, D., & Caramaschi, D. (2010). Animal violence demystified. *Frontiers in Behavioral Neuroscience, 4*, 9–25.

National Center on Elder Abuse. (2005). *Fact sheet: Elder abuse prevalence and incidence*. Retrieved from http://www.ncea.aoa.gov/main_site/pdf/publication/FinalStatistics050331.pdf

Sell, A. (2010). Applying adaptationism to human anger: The recalibration theory. In P. R. Saver & M. Mikulincer (Eds.), *Human aggression and violence: Causes, manifestations, and consequences*. Washington, DC: American Psychological Association.

Siever, L. L. (2008). Neurobiology of aggression and violence. *The American Journal of Psychiatry, 165*, 429–442. doi:10.1176/appi.ajp.2008.07111774

Truman, J. L. (2011). *National crime victimization survey: Criminal victimization, 2010*. (NCJRS Publication No. 235508). Retrieved from http://www.bjs.gov/content/pub/pdf/cv10.pdf

U.S. Department of Health and Human Services, Administration for Children and Families, Administration on Children, Youth and Families, Children's Bureau. (2011). *Child Maltreatment 2010*. Retrieved from http://www.acf.hhs.gov/programs/cb/stats_research/index.htm#can

Verona, E., Sadeh, N., Case, S., Reed, A., & Bhattacharjee, A. (2008). Self-reported use of different forms of aggression in late adolescence and emerging adulthood. *Assessment, 15*, 493–510. doi:10.1177/1073191108318250

Vickerman, K., & Margolin, M. (2008). Trajectories for physical and emotional aggression in midlife couples. *Violence and Victims, 23*, 18–34. doi:10.1891/0886-6708.23.1.18

Vitaro, F., & Brendgen, M. (2005). Proactive and reactive aggression: A developmental perspective. In R. E. Tremblay, W. W. Hartup, & J. Archer (Eds.), *Developmental origins of aggression* (pp. 178–201). New York: Guilford Press.

West, H. C., Sabol, W. J., & Greenman, S. J. (2010, December). Prisoners in 2009. *Bureau of Justice Statistics Bulletin*. Retrieved from http://www.bjs.gov/index.cfm?ty=pbdetail&iid=2232

World Health Organization. (2002). *World report on violence and health: Summary*. Geneva: World Health Organization. Retrieved from http://www.who.int/violence_injury_prevention/violence/world_report/en/summary_en.pdf

Assessing Anger, Aggression, and Violence

Anger, aggression, and violence are commonly observed in clinical settings. Although these responses may be the primary reason for referral in forensic assessment and anger management treatment, these responses may also occur secondary to other referral problems including psychiatric disorders, marital distress, occupational problems, or physical ailments. Given the ubiquity of anger, aggression, and violence across clinical settings, both forensic and general practitioners should be prepared to assess the risk and severity of these behaviors. Thankfully, a plethora of empirically-based instruments are available to quantify levels of anger, aggression, and violence. The instruments have been developed for use with children and adults across a variety of settings (e.g., school, work, or home) and interpersonal contexts (e.g., parent–child interaction, intimate relationship, etc.).

If the assessment goal is to quantify current level of anger, aggression, or violence, then we encourage you use the Quick View Tables that organize measures alphabetically and according to whether they can be used to assess anger, aggression, or violence. Information is provided on the purpose for which each measure was developed, the target population, the method of assessment, the amount of time required to administer the measure, and the page number where a review of the measure can be found.

Modeling Anger, Aggression, and Violence

Oftentimes the goal of the assessment is to predict the likelihood of future episodes of pathological anger, aggression, or violence. A typical referral for the assessment of pathological anger, aggression, or violence may be made by a school system, an attorney, or a court system following an episode of verbal or physical assault. In other instances an employer or significant other may initiate the referral. The overall goal is typically to determine the potential for violence, whether clinical intervention is warranted, and whether intervention is likely to decrease the probability of future acts of verbal or physical aggression. Because these aggressive behaviors tend to be context-dependent and multiply determined (Ollendick, 1996), completing such evaluations and estimating risk can be challenging.

Although conducting a thorough assessment is essential for predicting risk and developing a sound formulation of a case, many clinicians might be intimidated by the task demands. For instance, legal documents may be difficult to obtain, or collateral contacts may be unavailable. Moreover, aggression and violence are often low frequency, high amplitude behaviors such that a single instance of aggression may be difficult to predict, but can result in substantial property damage and physical harm. The challenge of risk assessment is further complicated by the fact that some individuals who engage in verbal or physical aggression do not repeat the behavior even when treatment is not provided, some individuals appear to decrease these behaviors following treatment, and other individuals repeat the behaviors even when treatment is successfully completed (e.g., Campbell, French, & Gendreau, 2009).

Miller (2000) suggested assessment be conducted using a two-step process. The first step, a general screening process, seeks to identify factors in the individual's history and current functioning that indicate increased risk of harmful behavior. Depending on the referral question, this first stage might include screening legal documents for prior violent behavior and other types of involvement with the legal system. The second step of assessment consists of obtaining information specific to the areas of identified risk. This often entails structured or semistructured interviews with the individual, in-depth document reviews to establish the developmental history of violent behavior, and discussion with collateral contacts such as parole officers, family, teachers, or employers. The findings are subsequently integrated into a theory-driven case formulation.

Historically, risk assessment has relied on two competing approaches: actuarial assessment and clinical judgment. An actuarial approach bases predictions on the presence of empirically weighted risk factors. The actuarial or formula-based approach to predicting bouts of pathological anger, aggression, and violence can be compromised when normative data relevant for populations and contexts are unavailable, and risk factors are improperly weighted in the prediction formula. The alternative of predicting risk solely on clinical judgment is fraught with other problems related to biases in clinical judgment such as availability heuristics and confirmatory search strategies (see Kahneman, Slovic, & Tversky, 1982).

Although research suggests that actuarial methods significantly outperform clinical judgment when predicting violent recidivism (Grove, Zald,

Lebow, Snitz, & Nelson, 2000), a solution that integrates both approaches involves the use of actuarial models embedded within theory-driven case formulation and clinical judgment (Hilton, Harris, & Rice, 2010). That is, a degree of interpretation is needed when assessing anger, aggression, and violence because different assessment protocols may produce disparate results and relationships between risk factors and violence may vary across samples (Coid et al., 2009; Hanson & Morton-Bourgon, 2009). In addition, statistical models may be difficult to translate into case conceptualization and treatment planning when they are not anchored in sound psychological theory (Quinsey, 2009).

We argue for an assessment approach in which actuarial data are interpreted in light of developmental psychopathology theory (Hankin, Abela, Auerbach, McWhinnie, & Skitch, 2005) and contemporary theories of anger, aggression, and violence (Anderson & Bushman, 2002). This approach is consistent with contemporary models of psychopathology that call for an integration of empirical findings with clinically relevant and theory-driven case conceptualization (Luyten & Blatt, 2011). The benefit of a theory-driven case formulation is that statistical risk factors weighted utilizing an empirically established formula can then be integrated into an organized understanding of the individual, and the structure and function of the individual's aggressive behavior. This understanding is crucial when practitioners must go beyond estimating risk and develop a treatment plan to reduce the likelihood of harmful behavior.

To assist practitioners less familiar with risk assessment, we have taken the liberty of sketching out a model for assessing and formulating a case conceptualization of pathological anger, aggression, and violence. The model is informed by theoretical and empirical models of anger, aggression, and violence and is consistent with cognitive behavioral models of case formulation. Interested readers are encouraged to review Berkowitz's (1989) Reformulated Frustration-Aggression model, Bushman and Anderson's (2002) General Aggression Model, and Gardner and Moore's (2008) Anger Avoidance Model. The model we propose relies on the use of both distant and current factors, and the measures reviewed in this text can target one or several of these factors. Because assessment requires an idiographic analysis, we will not suggest the specific measure to be employed. We will, however, suggest important empirically supported dimensions to consider when conducting such an assessment. The overall model is presented in Fig. 2.1.

This model implies that past behaviors and events (distal factors) that are non-changeable (static) are relevant for predicting pathological anger, aggression, and violence. Some static factors that positively predict future episodes of pathological anger, aggression, and violence include early modeling of aggression and violence, age at first episode of violence, number of past episodes of violence, amount of damage caused by past violence, and noncompliance with prior court-ordered conditions. Proximal factors include current personal and contextual factors. Personal factors are characteristics of the individual such as behavioral/emotional instability, disordered personality traits, poor coping skills, unrealistic plans, and treatment noncompliance. Contextual factors are aspects of the individual's external environment such as living arrangements, unemployment, and poor social supports that can foster stress and frustration. Current personal and contextual factors may mediate the relationship between static factors and current aggression. For instance, some individuals raised in abusive and violent environments (static factor) may also learn ineffective problem-solving skills (personal factor) and select relationships that are stressful and undermining (contextual factor). It is also possible that personal and contextual factors influence later aggression independently of static factors. For example, recent unemployment (contextual factor) or limited interpersonal skills (personal factor) could be unrelated to static factors but increase frustration and the probability of aggressive behavior. The following case example explicates how this case formulation model can be applied.

Jack is a 27-year-old blue collar worker who was referred by a probation officer after he was convicted of assault and battery following an incident that took place in a local bar. When asked to describe what led up to the event he reported that he was "hanging out" at a local bar when he noticed a male patron being disrespectful to a woman. He decided to intervene on her behalf and the altercation developed after he was asked to "mind his own business."

When asked, he described his childhood as "difficult." He described his father as a physically abusive alcoholic. His first fist-fight took place in the seventh grade when he came to the aid of a friend who was being picked on by a group of eighth grade students. He noted a history of several additional fist-fights, with the worst resulting in the person being treated for a broken nose and having stitches over his right eye. Jack reported being currently unemployed which he attributed to difficulty getting along with authority figures; he described himself as generally preferring to be a loner. When asked about his current living arrangements he stated, "I had no money so I was evicted from my flat. I just live with different friends."

Using the model represented above we would identify a number of distal factors that could be used to predict future aggressive behaviors. For instance, aggression as a problem-solving strategy was likely modeled by his father from an early age, and in turn Jack developed a personal learning history of using physical aggression to resolve concerns. His past aggressive behavior has resulted in significant harm to the victim, which is also relevant in understanding his increased risk for further aggressive behaviors. These are considered "static" factors because these events have previously occurred in his learning history, and as such are not directly amenable to change.

With regard to proximal factors, Jack's personal factors might include a deficit in conflict management skills, a skewed understanding of interpersonal relationships, and a worrisome level of alcohol use. It is likely that these factors were acquired through his learning history. As such we would expect that these personal factors mediate the impact of these distal experiences on his current behavior. Reduced alcohol use, enhanced conflict management skills, and a better understanding of interpersonal relationships would have a positive impact on current contextual concerns, reduce the impact of distal factors, and directly reduce the likelihood of his engaging in future episodes of pathological anger, aggression, and violence.

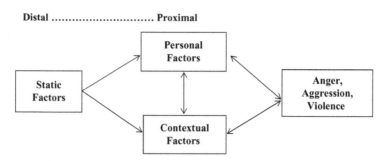

Fig. 2.1 Working model for predicting pathological anger, aggression, and violence

Other current factors for Jack might include aspects of his current context such as financial concerns, hanging out in bars, and his current living arrangement. Obtaining employment, obtaining more suitable living arrangements, and changing social settings would have a positive impact on current personal concerns, reduce the impact of distant factors, and directly reduce the likelihood of his engaging in future episodes of pathological anger, aggression, and violence.

The model presented in Fig. 2.1 is designed as a general heuristic and various components would certainly change based on the case analysis. Various procedures reviewed in this text can provide an empirically anchored assessment of most relevant factors. It is also notable that although many personal and contextual factors are potentially amenable to change in treatment, the influence of distal events and their overall predictive validity remain following treatment. A complete discussion of this possibility is beyond the scope of this chapter, but to summarize, anger, aggression, and violence once learned through distal processes are very likely to remain in the behavioral repertoire. More effective and socially desirable responses may be added to the behavioral repertoire to compete with the elicitation of aggressive behaviors, but aggression is not unlearned and may re-emerge under certain conditions.

Methods for Assessing Anger, Aggression, and Violence

Various methods exist for assessing anger, aggression, and violence. These methods include self-reports, reports from others, and behavioral

and analogue measures. Self-report information may be collected using paper-and-pencil measures or clinical interviews. This text reviews many different paper-and-pencil measures for assessing anger, aggression, and violence, as well as several structured and semistructured interview formats. These measures are used to collect demographic information, relevant historical information, and present functioning. An advantage to using interviews over paper-and-pencil measures is that interviews allow the examiner to probe ambiguous answers and to follow-up on areas eliciting concern.

Because episodes of pathological anger, aggression, and violence can result in significant social and legal consequences, people may be motivated to minimize their role and the impact of an episode. Therefore, we suggest that self-report measures routinely be combined with information collected using collateral contacts. Information obtained from other knowledgeable people can be used to corroborate an understanding of the relevant factors. In the case example provided above, copies of the police report or information collected from the probation officer might prove useful. In other cases, information could be collected from a spouse or a parent. When information provided by collateral contacts conflicts with information reported by the client, obvious motivations for the discrepancies should be highlighted and integrated into the evaluation of risk potential.

In addition to collateral information, behavioral and analogue measures can help to better gauge a client's skill level and likely behavior in a given situation. The use of behavioral rehearsals, role-play scenarios, and verbal responses to videotaped vignettes can help to provide a sample of behavior that can then be coded and quantified. An important feature of these measures is that they are less likely to succumb to bias induced by socially desirable responding, and different contexts can be used during data collection. For instance, distressed couples can be placed in high conflict situations and their communication skills can be observed (Ronan, Dreer, Dollard, & Ronan, 2004). Similarly, parent–child conflict can be recreated in the clinic and conflict management skills can be coded. Several of the measures reviewed allow for the coding of behavior samples. The following case might help to explicate how the assessment model presented in Fig. 2.1 can be used while including a variety of assessment methods.

> Trent is a 42-year-old associate professor who was referred by his probation officer after a recent arrest for domestic violence. When asked to describe the event, he stated that his wife has changed and does not listen to him anymore. They had an argument over remodeling their kitchen that "Got out of hand." He described her as having become "unreasonable." He noted that the neighbors called the police and that his wife did not want to call the police or have charges filed; the police filed the charge of domestic violence.
>
> When asked, he described his childhood as "Wonderful." He described his father as strict and definitely "the man of the house," but he denied any history of alcohol or physical abuse in his family of origin. Trent reported a past history of angry outbursts, but he denied a history of physical aggression or violence. He described the probation officer as not really wanting him to have the evaluation but as simply "Going through the procedures." He reported struggling to meet the publication and grant requirements needed to progress to the rank of full professor, which he attributed to the chairperson who routinely assigns him difficult courses. He described himself as having few friends. Trent has been living in university housing since his arrest and noted that the evaluation needs to be completed prior to his being allowed to move back home.

Using the model represented above, we would identify a number of distant, static factors that could be used to predict future aggressive behaviors. For instance, it appears as though his father modeled "male dominance" as a means for resolving marital concerns and a history of externalizing blame might be operative. He denied a history of past violence which would need to be corroborated with the spouse and perhaps the neighbors who phoned in the incident, as it is plausible that Trent intentionally denied engagement in past aggressive behavior or failed to recognize his past behavior as constituting aggression or violence. His description of the recent event is inconsistent with behavior warranting arrest, and a copy of the police report might prove useful. The text reviews measures that could be used for these purposes.

Personal factors might include a deficit in emotional regulation or self-control skills, as well as a lack of knowledge related to conflict resolution or marital problem solving skills. Having Trent complete self-report measures and his spouse rate his skills in these areas might prove useful. Because Trent is likely to be fairly bright (associate professor), he might be able to identify the appropriate responses to most paper-and-pencil measures; therefore, the use of role-play scenarios and vignettes that require him to demonstrate his responses might prove useful.

Contextual factors might include stress at work and overall problems within the marriage. Obtaining more information regarding marital stressors might prove useful in making recommendations regarding the timing of his move back home. Various measures reviewed in this text can provide an empirically anchored assessment of most relevant factors.

Summary

This text reviews many different measures that can be used to quantify levels of anger, aggression, and violence. The Quick View Tables are an efficient means of identifying measures, methods, or procedures that can be useful in completing an assessment of pathological anger, aggression, or violence. Research has identified a number of static, personal, and contextual factors to consider when assessing risk for future episodes of pathological anger, aggression, and violence. We argue for a two-step process involving screening questions followed by the collection of more detailed information in areas of identified risk. This text reviews both paper-and-pencil and structured interview formats that can be used to complete initial screenings. The text reviews a variety of self-report, other report, and direct behavioral measures that can be used to conduct a more detailed, empirically anchored assessment of areas of potential risk. Integration of the information collected is essential and raises the difficulty of determining the optimal means of weighting and combining the information. Two general methods for collecting the information are available: the clinical and the actuarial methods. Use of either method alone has drawbacks, and there is current support for supplementing clinical decision making with actuarial methods to develop a theory-based case formulation.

References

Anderson, C. A., & Bushman, B. J. (2002). Human aggression. *Annual Review of Psychology, 53*(1), 27–51.

Berkowitz, L. (1989). Frustration-aggression hypothesis: Examination and reformulation. *Psychological Bulletin, 106*(1), 59.

Campbell, M. A., French, S., & Gendreau, P. (2009). The prediction of violence in adult offenders: A meta-analytic comparison of instruments and methods of assessments. *Criminal Justice and Behavior, 36*(6), 567–590.

Coid, J., Yang, M., Ullrich, S., Zhang, T., Sizmur, S., Roberts, C., et al. (2009). Gender differences in structured risk assessment: Comparing the accuracy of fiveinstruments. *Journal of Consulting and Clinical Psychology, 77*(2), 337.

Gardner, F. L., & Moore, Z. E. (2008). Understanding clinical anger and violence: The anger avoidance model. *Behavior Modification, 32*(6), 897–912.

Grove, W. M., Zald, D. H., Lebow, B. S., Snitz, B. E., & Nelson, C. (2000). Clinical versus mechanical prediction: A meta-analysis. *Psychological Assessment, 12,* 19–30.

Hankin, B. L., Abela, J. R., Auerbach, R. P., McWhinnie, C. M., & Skitch, S. A. (2005). Development of behavioral problems over the life course: A vulnerability and stress perspective. In B. Hankin & J. Abela (Eds.), *Development of psychopathology: A vulnerability-stress perspective* (pp. 385–416). Thousand Oaks, CA: Sage.

Hanson, R. K., & Morton-Bourgon, K. E. (2009). The accuracy of recidivism risk assessments for sexual offenders: A meta-analysis of 118 prediction studies. *Psychological Assessment, 21*(1), 1.

Hilton, N. Z., Harris, G. T., & Rice, M. E. (2010). *Risk assessment for criminal justice, offender intervention, and victim services.* Washington, DC: American Psychological Association.

Kahneman, D., Slovic, P., & Tversky, A. (1982). *Judgment under uncertainty: Heuristics and biases.* New York: Cambridge University Press.

Luyten, P., & Blatt, S. J. (2011). Integrating theory-driven and empirically-derived models of personality development and psychopathology: A proposal for DSM V. *Clinical Psychology Review, 31*(1), 52–68.

Miller, M. C. (2000). A model for the assessment of violence. *Harvard Review of Psychiatry, 7*, 299–304.

Ollendick, T. (1996). Violence in youth: Where do we go from here? Behavior therapy's response. *Behavior Therapy, 27,* 485–514. doi:10.1016/S0005-7894 (96)80040-2

Quinsey, V. L. (2009). Are we there yet? Stasis and progress in forensic psychology. *Canadian Psychology, 50*(1), 15.

Ronan, G. F., Dreer, L. E., Dollard, K. M., & Ronan, D. W. (2004). Violent couples: Coping and communication skills. *Journal of Family Violence, 19*(2), 131–137. Retrieved from http://www.scopus.com

Part II

Assessment Instruments

Quick View Table for Measures of Anger

The quick-view table in this chapter provides easy access to basic descriptive information on each of the measures reviewed. The goal is to provide enough information to allow for an estimate of the likelihood that reading additional information about a particular measure would prove fruitful. Table entries are organized alphabetically and provide the name of the measure, the purpose for which the measure was developed, and the target population. The tables also provide information on the method of assessment, the amount of time involved, and the page number where additional information is available.

Quick View Table for Measures of Anger

Name	Purpose	Population	Method	Time	Page #
Anger and Hostility Scale	To assess the degree to which respondents perceive their problems as resulting from their anger	Adults	Self-report questionnaire	2–3 min	22
Anger Attacks Questionnaire	To assess the presence of anger and anger attacks	Adults	Self-report questionnaire	5 min	23
Anger Control Inventory	To assess situational and multiple response factors related to cognitive–behavioral person–situation interaction model of anger control	Adults	Self-report questionnaire	20 min	25
Anger Discomfort Scale	To assess the degree of discomfort one experiences with one's own anger	Adults	Self-report questionnaire	5 min	27
Anger Expression Scale	To assess the tendency to express, suppress, or control both the experience and expression of anger	Adults	Self-report questionnaire	5 min	28
Anger Provoking Situations	To describe situations that commonly precede anger	Children ages 12–18	Self-report questionnaire	Unknown	30

(continued)

G.F. Ronan et al., *Practitioner's Guide to Empirically Supported Measures of Anger, Aggression, and Violence*, ABCT Clinical Assessment Series, DOI 10.1007/978-3-319-00245-3_3,
© Springer International Publishing Switzerland 2014

(continued)

Name	Purpose	Population	Method	Time	Page #
Anger Response Inventories	To measure the range of constructive and destructive responses children, adolescents or adults might select when angered	Children, adolescents, and adults	Self-report questionnaire	20–30 min	32
Anger Self-Report	To measure anger awareness, expression, and amounts of personal mistrust and guilt	Ages 13 and older	Self-report questionnaire	20 min	33
Anger Situation Questionnaire	To assess anger proneness in women	Adult women	Self-report questionnaire	15–20 min	35
Articulated Thoughts in Simulated Situations	To assess anger-related cognitive processes	Adults	Think-aloud paradigm	Time varies depending on the construct being measured and the length of the stimulus tape	37
Audiotaped Anger-Provoking Situations	To examine cognitive and behavioral responses to anger-inducing stimuli	Adults	Verbal response to six audiotaped situations	Time varies depending on the length of the responses given by the participant	38
Autonomic Nervous System Response Inventory	To assess patterns of autonomic nervous system responses that occur during emotional distress	Adults	Self-report questionnaire	8–12 min	40
Brief Anger–Aggression Questionnaire	To assess anger and aggression in violence-prone men	Adult males	Self-report questionnaire	5 min	101
Burks Behavior Rating Scales	To assess psychopathology in grammar school children	Grammar school children	Questionnaire completed by child's teacher, parent, or qualified observer	15 min	104
Children's Anger Response Checklist	To assess physiological, cognitive, emotional, and behavioral aspects of anger	Children ages 7–12	Self-report checklist	15–30 min	42
Children's Inventory of Anger	To assess the subjective experience of anger in children	Children ages 7–14	Self-report questionnaire	20–25 min	44
Clinical Anger Scale	To measure clinical anger	Adults	Self-report questionnaire	20–30 min	46
Competitive Aggressiveness and Anger Scale	To measure anger and aggressiveness	Competitive athletes	Self-report questionnaire	5–10 min	118

(continued)

(continued)

Name	Purpose	Population	Method	Time	Page #
Cook and Medley Hostility Scale	To identify levels of hostility	Adults	Self-report questionnaire	10–15 min	48
Differential Emotions Scale-IV	To measure the experience of fundamental emotions	Children ages 8 and older	Self-report questionnaire	15–20 min	50
Driving Anger Expression Inventory	To assess commonly used expressions of anger while driving	Individuals old enough to legally drive an automobile	Self-report questionnaire	15–20 min	51
Driving Anger Scale	To measure the propensity to experience anger while driving	Individuals old enough to legally drive an automobile	Self-report questionnaire	10–15 min	53
Driving Vengeance Questionnaire	To assess levels of anger aroused by common, though potentially stressful, driving situations	Individuals old enough to legally drive an automobile	Self-report questionnaire	15–20 min	55
Dundee Provocation Inventory	To measure anger provocation in individuals with intellectual disabilities	Adults with intellectual disabilities	Self-report questionnaire	10–15 min	56
Framingham Anger Scales	To assess anger expression and the ability to cope with anger	Adults	Interview	2–3 min	58
Hostile Interpretations Questionnaire	To assess overall hostility and hostility in certain situations	Adult offenders	Self-report questionnaire	10 min	59
Interpersonal Process Code	To provide an observational code of childhood interactions	Children	Behavioral observation	Varies depending on the purpose for the assessment	61
Lack of Frustration Tolerance Scale	To assess levels of impatience and irritability	Adolescents and adults	Self-report questionnaire	1–2 min	63
Low Self-Control Scale	To assess levels of self-control	Adults	Self-report questionnaire	5–10 min	64
Multidimensional Anger Inventory	To measure multidimensional aspects of anger	Adults	Self-report questionnaire	10–15 min	65
Novaco Anger Scale	To assess the experience of anger	Ages 9 and older	Self-report questionnaire	30 min	67
Pediatric Anger Expression Scale—Third Edition	To measure styles of anger expression in children	Children and adolescents	Self-report questionnaire	3–7 min	69
Picture Frustration Study	To assess thought content in response to frustration	Adults	Projective technique	20–30 min	71
Reaction Inventory	To assess the degree of arousal associated with anger provoking situations	Adults	Self-report questionnaire	15–20 min	72

(continued)

(continued)

Name	Purpose	Population	Method	Time	Page #
Situations–Reactions Hostility Inventory	To assess types of situations that are typically emotion provoking and the types and intensity of responses to these situations	Adults	Self-report questionnaire	10–15 min	151
State–Trait Anger Expression Inventory	To measure the experience and expression of anger	Ages 13 and older	Self-report questionnaire	10–12 min	74
State–Trait Anger Scale	To measure anger as an emotional state and as a personality trait	Ages 16 and older	Self-report questionnaire	5–10 min	77
Subjective Anger Scale	To assess the propensity of an individual to respond with anger to frustrating situations	Ages 16 and older	Self-report questionnaire	5–10 min	80
Test of Negative Social Exchange	To measure the frequency of negative social exchanges experienced by individuals	Adults	Self-report questionnaire	10–15 min	81
Ward Atmosphere Scale	Designed to measure the social atmosphere of psychiatric wards, from the perspective of both patients and staff	Staff and patients of psychiatric wards	Self-report questionnaire	20 min	83

Anger and Hostility Scale (AHS)

Purpose

To assess the degree to which respondents perceive their problems as resulting from their anger.

Population

Adults.

Background and Description

The Anger and Hostility Scale (AHS) is a self-report measure consisting of 13 items that describe personal means for dealing with anger. Respondents rate the frequency with which the experience occurs on a 5-point rating scale, ranging from 1 ("almost never") to 5 ("almost always").

Administration

The Anger and Hostility Scale is estimated to take 2–3 min to complete.

Scoring

Responses to items are summed to produce a total score.

Interpretation

Higher scores indicate that the respondent is more likely to attribute anger as the cause of his/her problems.

Psychometric Properties

Reliability. Pilot data produced item–total correlations ranging from .59 to .82, with the exception of items on the "Acting Out" scale. These items had item–total correlations in the .20 s. Test–retest reliability over a 3-month period was .75.

Validity. Using pilot data, spouse abusers, compared with patients without anger problems, scored significantly higher on the AHS. These data provide some evidence of construct validity.

Clinical Utility

Limited. Although there are limited data on the scale's psychometric properties, the AHS allows the assessor to examine whether the respondent connects angry responses to problem situations, which may provide relevant information for treatment planning.

Research Applicability

Limited. The AHS may be valuable in investigating how lack of insight into the connection between angry responses and life problems may hinder problem-solving skills, but the scale needs further validation and replication of reliability statistics.

Original Citation

Sappington, A. A., & Kelly, P. (1995). Purpose in life and self-perceived anger problems among college students. *The International Forum for Logotherapy, 18,* 74–82.

Source

Sappington, A. A., & Kelly, P. (1995). Purpose in life and self-perceived anger problems among college students. *The International Forum for Logotherapy, 18,* 74–82.

Cost

Unknown.

Anger Attacks Questionnaire (AAQ)

Purpose

To assess the presence of anger, specifically anger attacks.

Population

Adults.

Background and Description

Anger attacks have been associated with feelings of loss of control, overt aggressive behaviors, and interpersonal problems. Anger attacks are conceptualized as rapid onset spells of anger, which are typically ego dystonic, uncharacteristic of the self, and cause subjective distress. These spells are out of proportion to the situation; they result from provocations described as trivial by the individual. Physical features consist of autonomic arousal and behaviors resembling panic attacks without the accompanying emotions of anxiety and fear. Anger attacks are accompanied by irritability and are often followed by feelings of guilt and/or regret. The Anger Attacks Questionnaire (AAQ) is a 7-item self-report measure that assesses the frequency of anger attacks during the previous 6 months. Sample items follow.

- Over the past 6 months, have you felt irritable or easily angered?
  Always Often Sometimes Never
- Over the past 6 months, have you had "anger attacks," episodes where you would become angry and enraged with other people in a way that you thought was excessive or inappropriate to the situation?
  Yes   No

Administration

The AAQ is estimated to take 5 min to complete.

Scoring and Interpretation

An individual is considered to have experienced an anger attack if the following criteria are met: presence of irritability, overreacting with anger to minor annoyances, becoming angry and enraged with others in inappropriate ways, experience 4 of 13 autonomic and behavioral symptoms (as listed in the original citation), and the recurrence of at least one of these episodes each month.

Psychometric Properties

Reliability. Unknown.

Validity. The author and colleagues reported identifying a subtype of depression characterized, in part, by anger attacks. Additionally, anger attacks occurred more frequently in depressed outpatients than in healthy individuals without a psychiatric history. Depressed outpatients with anger attacks were more likely to have greater anxiety, somatic symptoms, and hostility. Anger attacks in depressed patients were also associated with borderline, histrionic, narcissistic, and antisocial personality disorders.

Clinical Utility

Limited. Additional information on the psychometric properties of the AAQ needs to be obtained before it can be used for clinical purposes.

Research Applicability

Moderate. The AAQ can be used to assess anger, a risk factor for aggression. It takes minimal time to complete and is easily scored to assess the presence and frequency of anger, as well as concomitant autonomic and behavioral symptoms.

Original Citation

Fava, M., Rosenbaum, J. F., McCarthy, M., Pava, J., Steingard, R., & Bless, E. (1991). Anger attacks in depressed outpatients and their response to fluoxetine. *Psychopharmacology Bulletin, 27*, 275–279.

Source

Maurizio Fava, Massachusetts General Hospital, 55 Fruit Street, Boston, MA 02114, (617) 724-2513, Fax: (617) 726-2688, mfava@partners.org

Cost

Contact the source (above) for permission to use the AAQ.

Alternative Forms

A French version is available.

A shortened form of the AAQ was created. The AAQ—Simplified Definition contains 3 items that were taken from the original 7-item AAQ. The overreaction to minor annoyances item (Item 2) was found to have high agreement with the original diagnosis of anger attacks in a sample of 203 patients with major depressive disorder. This item also had high specificity. The item related to episodes of inappropriate anger or rage (Item 3) also had high agreement and specificity in the same sample. The combination of these items resulted in nearly perfect reclassification of cases ($k = .96$) and a very high specificity (.97). (Winkler, Pjrek, Kindler, Heiden, & Kasper, 2006).

Reference

Winkler, D., Pjrek, E., Kindler, J., Heiden, A., & Kasper, S. (2006). Validation of a simplified definition of anger attacks. *Psychotherapy and Psychosomatics, 75*, 103–106.

Anger Control Inventory (ACI)

Purpose

To assess situational components and multiple response factors related to a cognitive–behavioral person–situation interaction model of anger control.

Population

Adults.

Background and Description

Three clinicians familiar with the cognitive–behavioral model of anger control generated a pool of items based on a cognitive–behavioral person–situation interaction model relevant to the clinical assessment and treatment of anger control problems. The clinicians grouped items under the domains of behavior, cognition, and arousal. These items were subsequently reviewed, modified, and organized to form the current version of the Anger Control Inventory (ACI). Items are rated using a 4-point continuum reflecting the amount of anger each situation elicits. The 134 items are organized into 10 Anger Stimulus scales and 6 Anger Response scales. Anger Stimulus items were generated to represent a variety of anger-provoking situations and each of the resulting scales contains 6 items: Seeing Others Abused; Intrusion; Personal Devaluation; Betrayal of Trust; Minor Nuisance; External Control and Coercion; Verbal Abuse; Physical Abuse; Unfair Treatment; and Goal Blocking. Items for the Anger Response scales are categorized according to destructive responding (Maladaptive Behavior scale, 12 items) or passive responding (Behavioral Skill Deficit scale, 8 items), anger-provoking thoughts (Maladaptive Cognition scale, 15 items) and few adaptive cognitive alternatives (Cognitive Skill Deficit scale, 13 items), Arousal Intensity (14 items), and Arousal Duration (6 items). An additional neutral scale containing six low provocation items is included to identify random responding such as carelessness.

Administration

The ACI takes approximately 20 min to complete.

Scoring

Items for each scale are summed.

Interpretation

High scores on individual scales are interpreted as a greater tendency to be provoked by the situations represented by the scale.

Psychometric Properties

Norms. Normative data were derived from combined clinical and normal samples of equal size totaling 236 subjects. Additional evaluations of psychometric data were obtained from a sample of 190 college subjects and 118 clinical subjects (adolescents and adults).

Factor analysis. Using principal component analysis, 16 factors were extracted. Four factors were considered meaningful based on an evaluation of the resulting scree plot. All four factors together accounted for a total of 71 % of the variance in the patient sample and 71 % of the variance in the student sample. Although the specific factor pattern varied across the clinical and normative samples, the Anger Stimulus and Anger Response scales loaded on separate factors. Cross validation with additional samples has generally resulted in the Anger Stimulus scales and the Anger Response scales forming separate factors.

Reliability. Internal consistency of the scales was moderate to high and ranged from α = .54 (Minor Nuisance scale) to α = .81 (Betrayal of Trust scale). Test–retest reliability over a 1-month interval was estimated using a randomly selected sample of 49 subjects. Estimates for the Anger Stimulus scales ranged from .72 to .83. Estimates for the Anger Response scales ranged from .73 to .83.

Validity. Anger Stimulus scales were found to have moderate to high item–total correlations (range = .55–.81). The Anger Response scales also demonstrated moderate to high item–total correlations (range = .57–.71). Criterion validity of the ACI was evaluated by correlating the anger problem criterion with each of the scales. The anger problem criterion was a checklist that rated ten signs of anger problems. These signs included "expressed personal dissatisfaction with own ways of dealing with anger" and "verbal behavior disruptive of interpersonal relationships" (Hoshmand & Austin, 1987, p. 422). For the patient sample, low significant correlations of the therapist-rated criterion with nine of the Anger Stimulus scales ranged from .21 to .31. Low to moderately significant correlations were found for the Anger Response scales (.19–.47), with the two Maladaptive scales showing the strongest relationship to difficulty with anger control. Similar results were found in a student sample (Stimulus Scales = .15–.25 and Anger Response scales = .25–.56).

Overall, the Anger Stimulus scales showed low correlations with the criterion, suggesting that differential sensitivity to provoking stimuli was only marginally related to more overt forms of anger. In contrast, the Anger Response scales, particularly the behavioral and cognitive maladaptive scales, showed stronger relationships with signs of anger control problems.

Construct validity was evaluated by contrasting the results derived from 100 spouse batterers seeking voluntary or court-ordered treatment with a group of 96 community residents who did not report anger problems. Responses on four of the Anger Stimulus scales and five of the Anger

Response scales revealed significant differences, with the batterers scoring in the direction of more anger problems on many subscales.

The clinical utility of the ACI was demonstrated by its sensitivity to change with cognitive behavioral treatment in a sample of spouse batterers. Pretreatment and posttreatment scores of the 65 batterers were compared. For the Anger Stimulus scales, significant differences were found on the Betrayal of Trust, Physical Abuse, Unfair Treatment, and Goal Blocking scales, as well as for the Total Anger Stimulus score. For the Anger Response scales, significant differences were found on the Maladaptive Behavior, Behavioral Skill Deficit, Maladaptive Cognition, and Cognitive Skill Deficit scales, as well as for the Total Anger Response score. The two Arousal subscales did not show significant pretreatment to post-treatment differences.

Clinical Utility

High. Preliminary data provide evidence for acceptable psychometric properties for the ACI. The ACI also discriminated between clinical and nonclinical samples. The ACI is easy to administer and sensitive to treatment-related changes within clinical subjects who participated in anger control treatment based on a cognitive–behavioral approach. Although additional cross validation is needed, the potential for clinical use is promising.

Research Applicability

High. Most of the research being conducted on problematic anger is consonant with a cognitive–behavioral perspective. The ACI was explicitly derived from a well-researched cognitive–behavioral model of anger control problems. The measure provides useful information for testing hypothesized relationships between situations and skills related to anger control problems.

Original Citation

Hoshmand, L. T., & Austin, G. W. (1987). Validation studies of a multifactor cognitive-behavioral Anger Control Inventory. *Journal of Personality Assessment, 51*(3), 417–432.

Source

Lisa T. Hoshmand, Ph.D., Division of Counseling and Psychology, Lesley University, 29 Everett St., Cambridge, MA 02138, (617) 349-8157, lhoshman@mail.lesley.edu

Cost

Contact the source (above) for permission to use.

Anger Discomfort Scale (ADS)

Purpose

To assess the degree of discomfort an individual experiences with his/her own anger.

Population

Adults.

Background and Description

The Anger Discomfort Scale (ADS) was developed to directly assess discomfort with anger. Previous measures indirectly assessed anger discomfort by evaluating suppressed anger and guilt in individuals. However, direct measures of anger discomfort were lacking. Anger discomfort was defined as an "inner, subjective experience" linked to both intrapsychic and interpersonal factors. Assessment of anger discomfort was hypothesized to yield important information about the etiology and treatment of anger-related concerns. Individuals experiencing high levels of anger discomfort are threatened by the experience of anger and concerned about the reactions of others to their anger. The ADS was formatted similarly to the Anger Expression Scale (pp. 28–30).

The ADS is a 15-item, self-report measure designed to measure the construct of anger discomfort. Items are rated on a 4-point Likert-type scale, ranging from 1 ("almost never") to 4 ("almost always"). Sample items are listed below.
- I fear that my anger will hurt other people
- My anger scares me

Administration

The ADS is estimated to take 5 min to complete.

Scoring

Three items are reverse scored. Items are then summed for a total score.

Interpretation

Higher scores on the ADS are indicative of greater levels of discomfort with one's own anger.

Psychometric Properties

Factor analysis. Four factors were extracted using factor analysis with varimax rotation. These factors were intrapersonal discomfort related to one's own anger, positive views of and comfort with anger, interpersonal discomfort with one's own anger, and concomitants of anger (e.g., emotions or outcomes related to experiencing anger).

Reliability. Cronbach's alpha using the scores of 150 respondents revealed an internal consistency estimate of .81. One week test–retest reliability using the scores from 68 students was estimated at .87. Corrected item–total correlations on the ADS ranged from .26 to .58, although only 2 items had correlations less than .40.

Validity. Correlations were calculated between ADS scores and related constructs. Scores on the ADS correlated positively with anger-out scores ($r=.20$), anger-in scores ($r=.32$), and general anger expression scores ($r=.34$) of the Anger Expression Scale. ADS scores correlated negatively with anger control scores of the Anger Expression Scale ($r=-.16$). Additionally, a positive correlation was found between scores on the ADS and trait anxiety levels ($r=.51$). ADS scores were not related to SAT combined scores or social desirability, providing evidence for discriminate validity.

Clinical Utility

Moderate. The ADS provides information concerning how people feel about their own anger and this may be useful in treatment planning and assessing treatment outcomes. The ability to generalize to clinical samples is limited because the research on the ADS has used college students.

Research Applicability

Moderate. Although replications of the current findings are needed to establish the psychometric properties of the ADS, research using the ADS may help to clarify the relationships between discomfort with anger and other dimensions of anger, familial emotional patterns, and reactions to other's anger. Such investigations may add clarity to the understanding and conceptualization of anger-related clinical concerns.

Original Citation

Sharkin, B. S., & Gelso, C. J. (1991). The Anger Discomfort Scale: Beginning reliability and validity data. *Measurement and Evaluation in Counseling and Development, 24,* 61–68.

Source

Bruce S. Sharkin, Kutztown University of Pennsylvania, PO Box 730, Kutztown, PA 19530, (610) 683-4072, sharkin@kutztown.edu

Cost

Contact the source (above) for permission to use the ADS.

Anger Expression Scale (AX)

Purpose

To assess the tendency to express, suppress, or control both the experience and expression of anger.

Population

Adults.

Background and Description

A preliminary version of the Anger Expression Scale (AX) was administered to high school students. Responses were factor analyzed and two factors were identified: Anger-In and Anger-Out. From these items, a 20-item version of the AX was constructed with eight items representing Anger-In, eight items representing Anger-Out, and three of the four remaining items representing anger control. This version of the AX was later expanded to 24 items by adding additional items to the anger control subscale.

The current 24-item scale consists of three subscales: Anger-Out (AX/Out; 8 items), Anger-In (AX/In; 8 items), and Anger Control (AX/Con; 8 items). The Anger-Out subscale assesses the frequency one expresses feelings of anger. The Anger-In subscale measures the tendency to suppress anger. The Anger Control subscale assesses the disposition to control both the experience and the expression of anger. A total score can be calculated to gauge the tendency to respond to angry feelings, either covertly or overtly. Instructions of the AX ask respondents to indicate how often, when feeling "angry or furious," they behaved in the manner dictated by the item. Items are rated on a Likert-type scale, ranging from 1 ("almost never") to 4 ("almost always").

Administration

The AX takes about 5 min to complete.

Scoring

Total scores for the Anger-In, Anger-Out, and Anger Control subscales are obtained by summing responses to each of the 8 items on their respective scales. A total score is obtained by summing scores on the three subscales.

Interpretation

Higher total scores indicate a greater tendency to express angry feelings, either overtly or covertly. Higher scores on the Anger-In, Anger-Out, and Anger Control subscales are indicative of greater tendencies to suppress anger, to express anger, and to control the expression and experience of anger, respectively.

Psychometric Properties

Factor analysis. Factor analyses on various populations ($n = 1,023$ men and women from New Zealand, $n = 137$ inmates, high school, and undergraduate samples) revealed the same three-factor structure across gender and population, labeled anger control, anger-in, and anger-out.

Reliability. For the Anger-Out subscale, Cronbach's alpha ranged from .73 to .84. For the Anger-In subscale, alpha values ranged from .70 to .81. For the Anger Control subscale alpha value was .87. Two week test–retest reliability estimates range from .64 to .81 (.64–.70 for males and .73–.81 for females).

Validity. In a New Zealand sample of 1,023 participants, a significant, but small correlation ($r = .13$ for men and $r = .17$ for women) was found between the Anger-In and Anger-Out subscales. To examine criterion validity, correlations between the AX total scores and the State–Trait Personality Inventory (STPI, Spielberger et al., 1979) subscales were examined. The correlations between the AX and the STPI anger and anxiety-related subscales were higher than the correlation between the AX and the curiosity subscale. Additionally, the STPI trait anger temperament subscale was more highly correlated with the Anger-Out subscale than other STPI subscales, with the exception of the trait anger subscale. A negative relationship has been found between Anger Control scores and the other AX subscale scores, as well as between Anger Control scores and scores on the State–Trait Anger Scale (STAS, pp. 77–79). Trait anger on the STAS was correlated with Anger-Out, and scores on the STAS had moderate correlations with Anger-In.

Clinical Utility

High. The AX provides an efficient means of evaluating an individual's typical expression of anger, as well as the degree to which an individual is able to control his/her anger.

Research Applicability

High. The AX takes little time to administer and is useful in examining correlates related to the expression and control of anger.

Original Citation

Spielberger, C. D., Johnson, E. H., & Jacobs, C. A. (1982). *Anger Expression Scale Manual*. Tampa, FL: Human Resources Institute, University of South Florida.

Source

The manual and the Anger Expression Inventory are available from Human Resource Institute, 5959 Central Avenue Suite 200A, St. Petersburg, FL 33710, Phone: 727-345-2226, Fax: 727-345-1254.

Cost

Please contact the source (above) for additional information.

Reference

Spielberger, C. D., Jacobs, G., Crane, R., Russell, S., Westberry, L., Barker, L., Johnson, E., Knight, J., & Marks, E. (1979). *Preliminary manual for the State-Trait Personality Inventory (STPI)*. Tampa, FL: University of South Florida, Human Resources Institute.

Anger-Provoking Situations (APS)

Purpose

To describe situations that commonly precede anger.

Population

Ages 12–18.

Background and Description

A sample of 12-, 15-, and 19-year-old Swedish children were asked to describe three situations that made them angry and to explain why they became angry in the given situation. This resulted in a pool of approximately 900 situations, 60 of which were randomly selected for additional analysis. Four situations had to be replaced due to improper completion. Raters then assessed the degree of similarity between causes of anger in the descriptions on a 5-point scale, ranging from 0 ("not at all similar") to 4 ("identical"). All ratings were pairwise and completed by four independent raters. Scores were transformed to a scale, ranging from 0 to 1, by dividing all scores by 4. Resulting scores were treated as a correlation matrix. The authors developed a ten-factor classification scheme to organize situations Swedish children found to be anger provoking. Samples of anger-provoking situations were translated verbatim from Swedish to English.

Administration

The APS remains experimental and no standardized method of administration has been developed.

Scoring

The APS remains experimental and no standardized method of scoring has been developed.

Psychometric Properties

Factor analysis. Scores in the correlation matrix were factor analyzed using a principle component method. The authors interpreted ten factors, which accounted for 77 % of the variance. Factors were comprised of situations with loadings >.50. Situations with loadings .50 or greater on more than one factor were placed on the factor with the highest loading. The ten factors are described below:

- Factor 1 (13 situations): Self-opinionated. These situations described individuals who appeared to know best, who were contradicting, and who did not listen to arguments or take others' views seriously.
- Factor 2 (8 situations): People blaming. These situations described people who were blaming, slandering, bullying, or telling tales.

- Factor 3 (6 situations): Insulting. These situations described people who exhibited disparaging and depreciatory behaviors.
- Factor 4 (7 situations): Thoughtless behaviors. These situations described individuals who did foolish or thoughtless things. Positive item loadings indicated others initiated these behaviors, whereas negative loadings indicated that the respondent initiated the behaviors.
- Factor 5 (4 situations): Teasing.
- Factor 6 (5 situations): Plans thwarted. These situations reflected frustration resulting from plans being disrupted by others that were in control.
- Factor 7 (4 situations): Nagging. These situations involved yelling or quarreling.
- Factor 8 (4 situations): Physical harassment.
- Factor 9 (3 situations): Frustration environmental. These situations were vague and no persons were identified as provokers.
- Factor 10 (3 situations): People's belongings. These situations described objects that were "pinched," destroyed, or moved around.

Reliability. Data regarding the ability of raters to reliably code the similarity of situations was not provided. Additionally, internal consistency information is also unavailable.

Validity. Validity data are not available.

Clinical Utility

Limited. The procedure does not provide a means for assessing anger-provoking situations in individuals, although the given situations may provide clinicians with insight into what situations may be anger-provoking in children. Information on the psychometric properties of the APS is needed prior to clinical use of this measure.

Research Applicability

Moderate. Identification of common groups of anger-provoking situations may be useful for studying anger-provoking situations within and across a variety of ages and contexts.

Original Citation

Törestad, B. (1990). What is anger provoking? A psychophysical study of perceived causes of anger. *Aggressive Behavior, 16,* 9–26.

Source

Bertil Törestad, Department of Psychology, University of Stockholm, S-106 91 Stockholm, Sweden.

Cost

Contact the source (above) for permission to use the APS.

Alternative Forms

Participants were instructed to list and describe situations that they found anger provoking. Situations were rated by participants in another sample on such categories as anger intensity, anxiety, vividness, and typicality. Ratings were made on a 9-point scale, ranging from 1 ("not at all") to 9 ("very much").

In a separate study, 12 anger-provoking situations were derived from the theoretical literature. Undergraduate students were asked to name the emotional feeling in each situation. Two situations elicited mostly anger and two elicited only anxiety.

References

Sterling, S., & Edelmann, R. J. (1988). Reactions to anger and anxiety-provoking events: Psychopathic and non-psychopathic groups compared. *Journal of Clinical Psychology, 44,* 96–100.

Tescher, B., Conger, J. C., Edmondson, C. B., & Conger, A. J. (1999). Behavior, attitudes, and cognitions of anger-prone individuals. *Journal of Psychopathology and Behavioral Assessment, 21,* 117–139.

Anger Response Inventories (ARIs)

Purpose

To measure the range of constructive and destructive responses children, adolescents, or adults might select when angered.

Population

Children, adolescents, and adults.

Background and Description

The Anger Response Inventories (ARIs) were developed to consider a broad range of possible responses to managing anger. The ARIs assess individual differences in constructive versus destructive responses to anger from middle childhood through adulthood. The conceptual structure of the ARIs was guided by Averill's (1983) work on everyday experiences of anger. A multitiered analysis of anger-related outcomes was used with each measure considering arousal, intentions, behavioral and cognitive responses, and perceived consequences. The ARIs were developed to target the relationship between adaptive or constructive and maladaptive or destructive components of anger. The ARIs consist of three self-report inventories that consist of a series of age appropriate situations likely to elicit anger. Respondents are asked to imagine themselves in each situation and then rate their reactions using a 5-point scale: (1) how angry they would be in such a situation (anger arousal); (2) their intentions, specifically, what they would feel like doing, not what they would actually do (constructive, malicious, fractious intentions are assessed); (3) their likely behaviors including a variety of aggressive and nonaggressive responses and use of cognitive reappraisals; and finally, (4) their assessment of the long-term consequences for self, target, and the relationship. The ARI (used for adults) consists of 23 scenarios, the ARI-C (used for children) consists of 20 scenarios, and finally, the ARI-A (used for adoles-

cents) consists of 20 scenarios drawing from the child and adult scenarios. The ARI contains approximately 25 scales which include the following: Anger Arousal, Constructive Intentions, Malevolent Intentions, Fractious Intentions, Direct Physical Aggression, Direct Verbal Aggression, Direct Symbolic Aggression, Malediction, Indirect Harm, Displaced Physical Aggression, Displaced Verbal Aggression, Displaced Aggression to Object, Self-Aggression, Anger Held In, Discussion With Target, Corrective Action, Diffusion, Minimization, Removal, Doing Nothing, Cognitive Reappraisals of Target's Role, Cognitive Reappraisals of Self's Role, Long-Term Consequences for Self, Long-Term Consequences for Target, and Long-Term Consequences for Relationship.

Administration

Each of the ARIs can be completed in approximately 20–30 min.

Scoring

Total and subscale scores are derived from summing responses to items.

Interpretation

Higher scores indicate greater tendencies to engage in the particular behavior assessed. For example, high scores on the Direct Physical Aggression scale indicate greater tendencies toward engaging in such behavior, whereas high scores on the Discussion with Target or Corrective Action scale indicate greater tendencies to resolve the problem or less of a tendency to engage in high amplitude anger responses.

Psychometric Properties

Norms. Final versions of the ARIs were administered to samples of 307 children (ARI-C; Grades 4–6),

434 adolescents (ARI-A; Grades 7–11), 214 college students (ARI), and 195 adults (ARI). A subgroup of the college sample completed the ARI a second time, 3–6 weeks later. Additional normative data can be found in Tangney et al. (1996).

Reliability. With regard to internal consistency, coefficient alpha estimates of the scales were generally high, with the anger arousal, intentions, and consequences scales showing the highest internal consistency (ARI-adult .97, ARI-college .96, ARI-A .94, and ARI-C .91). Test–retest reliability based on 214 college students who completed the ARI a second time, 3–6 weeks later, was estimated at .76.

Validity. Validity of the scales has been supported by theoretically consistent patterns of correlations with global self-report indices of hostility, aggression, and anger management strategies (Buss–Durkee Hostility Inventory, pp. 109–111, and the Anger Control Inventory, pp. 25–27). Teacher reports of broad aspects of social and emotional adjustment, including aggression, delinquency, social problems, and anxiety–depression, have also revealed hypothesized correlations with the ARI-C and the ARI-A. Self and family members' reports of respondents' behaviors in specific anger episodes are also consistent with scores on the Adult ARI and ARI-A. These findings lend support for the construct validity of the ARIs.

Clinical Utility

Moderate. Preliminary data on the psychometric properties of the ARIs indicate good potential for clinical use. The ARI scales provide detailed and useful information regarding how individuals from a variety of age ranges characteristically experience and manage their anger.

Research Applicability

Moderate to high. The multitiered format for the ARIs provides descriptive information across a variety of dimensions that are typically of interest to researchers. The measures also provide the

opportunity for researchers to assess anger responses longitudinally.

Original Citation(s)

Tangney, J. P., Wagner, P. E., Hansbarger, A., & Gramzow, R. (1991). The *Anger Response Inventory for Children (ARI-C)*. Fairfax, VA: George Mason University.

Tangney, J. P., Wagner, P. E., Gavlas, J., & Gramzow, R. (1991). The *Anger Response Inventory for Adolescents (ARI-A)*. Fairfax, VA: George Mason University.

Tangney, J. P., Wagner, P. E., Marschall, D., & Gramzow, R. (1991). The *Anger Response Inventory (ARI)*. Fairfax, VA: George Mason University.

Source

June Price Tangney, Department of Psychology, George Mason University, 2007. A David J. King Hall, Fairfax, VA 22030, (703) 993–1365, email available through George Mason University Web site.

Cost

Please contact the source (above) for permission to use the ARIs.

References

Averill, J. R. (1983). Studies on anger and aggression: Implications for theories of emotions. *American Psychologist, 38*, 1145–1160.

Tangney, J. P., Hill-Barlow, D., Wagner, P. E., Marschall, D. E., Borenstein, J. K., Sanftner, J., et al. (1996). Assessing individual differences in constructive versus destructive responses to anger across the lifespan. *Journal of Personality and Social Psychology, 70*, 780–796.

Anger Self-Report (ASR)

Purpose

To measure anger awareness, anger expression, and personal mistrust and guilt.

Population

Ages 13 and older.

Background and Description

The Anger Self-Report (ASR) was designed to measure anger awareness and anger expression as two separate constructs. Eighty-nine items were reduced down to 64 after an item analysis. The ASR is a likert-type questionnaire that contains five scales and three subscales: awareness of anger; expression of anger which contains three subscales general, physical, and verbal expression; guilt; condemnation of anger; and mistrust.

Administration

The ASR requires approximately 20 min to complete.

Scoring

Scores are calculated for the five scales and three subscales.

Interpretation

Higher scores indicate a greater degree of the construct measured by the particular scale or subscale.

Psychometric Properties

Reliability. Test–retest reliability coefficients over a 2-week period ranged from .28 (guilt) to .76 (condemnation of anger) for the ASR scales and subscales. The ASR total score had a test–retest reliability .54. Split-half reliability for the scales ranged from .64 to .82.

Validity. Correlations between scores on the ASR and psychiatrists' ratings on 16 of the Problem Appraisal Scales (PAS; Endicott & Spitzer, 1972) provided evidence of convergent and discriminant validity. The ASR verbal expression scale was positively correlated ($r=.31$) with ratings of anger, belligerence, and negativism, whereas it was negatively correlated ($r=-.36$) with dependency. The ASR awareness of anger scale was positively related to antisocial attitudes and acts ($r=.24$), whereas it was unrelated to PAS expression of anger (Biaggio, 1980). In a sample of undergraduate students, scores on the ASR scales were related to criterion measures including self-reported verbal antagonism and physical antagonism (Biaggio, Supplee, & Curtis, 1981). The ASR awareness, expression, verbal expression, and mistrust/suspicion scales were all significantly related to the MMPI-2 anger scale in men, and the ASR awareness, expression, and physical expression scales were significantly related to the MMPI-2 anger scale in women (Schill & Wang, 1990).

Clinical Utility

Moderate. The ASR can aid clinicians in quantifying client's awareness and experience of anger.

Research Applicability

Limited. ASR scores may fluctuate over short periods of time, thus attenuating the relationship between ASR scores and criterion variables.

Original Citation

Zelin, M. L., Adler, G., & Myerson, P. G. (1972). Anger Self-Report: An objective questionnaire for the measurement of aggression. *Journal of Consulting and Clinical Psychology, 39*, 340.

Source

Martin L. Zelin, 419 Boston Ave, Tufts University, Medford, MA, 02155, (415) 889–5560, martin.zelin@tufts.edu

Cost

Contact source (above) for permission to use the ASR.

Alternative Forms

A 30-item short form of the ASR was created that measures a single anger factor. Items were selected from the original 89-item scale by examining item-to-test correlations and removing items that had the poorest correlations. Internal consistency, as measured by KR20, was .89. Norms were obtained for a sample of 101 men and 100 women. A full listing of the items in the 30-item ASR can be found in Reynolds, Walkey, and Green (1994).

References

Biaggio, M. K. (1980). Anger arousal and personality characteristics. *Journal of Personality and Social Psychology, 39*, 352–356.

Biaggio, M. K., Supplee, K., & Curtis, N. (1981). Reliability and validity of four anger scales. *Journal of Personality Assessment, 45*(6), 639–648.

Endicott, J, & Spitzer, R. L. (1972). What? Another rating scale? The Psychiatric Evaluation Form. *Journal of Nervous and Mental Disease, 154*, 88–104.

Reynolds, N. S., Walkey, F. H., & Green, D. E. (1994). The Anger Self Report: A psychometrically sound (30 item) version. *New Zealand Journal of Psychology, 23*, 64–70.

Schill, T., & Wang, S. (1990). Correlates of the MMPI-2 anger content scale. *Psychological Reports, 67*, 800–802.

Anger Situation Questionnaire (ASQ)

Purpose

To assess anger proneness in women.

Population

Adult women.

Background and Description

The Anger Situation Questionnaire (ASQ) was developed to account for several shortcomings of other anger measures and to better understand the relationship between proneness to anger and aggressive responding in women. The ASQ consists of 33 vignettes. Each vignette has three dimensions: emotional experience, intensity of emotional experience, and action readiness. The conflicts within each vignette are grouped into one of six categories: (1) personal failure or incompetence; (2) abuses or world events; (3) failure to be given serious consideration or the violation of privacy, trust, or promises; (4) provocation, impolite treatment, or damage to interests; (5) frustration or blocked action; and (6) inattentive behavior. The respondent is asked to imagine herself in each of the situations and to select which emotion she would experience, how intense this emotion would be, and what she would do if she found herself in the situation. In addition to a choice of five different emotion labels that are rated for intensity, each vignette contains five action tendencies which are specifically tailored to the situation under consideration. The general categories of action tendencies are (1) ducking out of the situation, denying that something is wrong, or transforming it into something positive; (2) doing nothing, although knowing that something is wrong; (3) distant anger, e.g., indirect or delayed angry behavior; (4) assertive behavior, e.g., blaming someone; and (5) aggressive behavior, e.g., verbal, indirect, antagonistic behavior. Respondents are required to choose one emotion, one intensity level, and one action tendency. Thus, the ASQ contains three subscales: Emotional Experience, Intensity of Emotional Experience, and Action Readiness. Two of the vignettes are unrelated to anger and included in an effort to conceal the character of the questionnaire; responses to these two vignettes can be used to assess general response styles.

Administration

The measure is estimated to take 15–20 min to complete.

Scoring

The Anger Scale, a subscale of the Emotional Experience Scale, consists of the number of vignettes in which the respondent labels the emotion as one of anger; scores range from 0 to 33. An anger score percent can be calculated from the number of items checked for anger (emotion category divided by the total number of items, multiplied by 100). The Intensity Scale consists of the total score on all intensity values with the two dummy situations excluded; therefore, scores range from 31 to 155. The Action Readiness Scale consists of the total score on all action tendencies with scores ranging from 31 to 155. An action readiness percent can be calculated from the sum of the items checked for assertive and aggressive behaviors divided by the total number of items, multiplied by 100.

Interpretation

Higher scores are indicative of experiencing greater anger and suggest a greater susceptibility to experiencing anger or to engage in anger-related behaviors.

Psychometric Properties

Norms. Means from 146 female psychology students are available. They are organized by each of the subscales for a low anger disposition group and a high anger disposition group.

Reliability. The internal consistency for the Intensity Scale was high (Cronbach's alpha = .90), whereas the internal consistency estimate for the Action Readiness scale was lower (Cronbach's alpha = .63). Interpreting the internal consistency estimate for the Action Readiness scale is difficult because the action tendencies for each vignette are phrased differently and this counteracts specific response consistencies that typically inflate internal consistency estimates. Correlations between the three subscales are low, with the exception of the correlation between Intensity and Action Readiness ($r = .43$).

Validity. Out of the original 146 female psychology students, 30 subjects who scored low on anger and anger readiness and 30 subjects who scored high on anger and anger readiness were identified. An anger-induction paradigm was developed consisting of a physically aversive situation, the performance of some frustrating tasks, and an unpleasant female experimenter. Subjects scoring high on the ASQ, as opposed to low scoring subjects, demonstrated greater anger reactions.

Clinical Utility

Limited. The ASQ has not yet been widely used in clinical settings or with violent populations. Research on clinical samples is needed.

Research Applicability

Moderate. This measure has not been widely studied but appears to demonstrate potential for assessing different dimensions of anger (emotional experience, intensity of emotional experience, and action readiness).

Original Citation

van Goozen, S. H. M., Frijda, N. H., Kindt, M, & van de Poll, N. E. (1994). Anger proneness in women: Development and validation of the Anger Situation Questionnaire. *Aggressive Behavior, 20*, 79–100.

Source

Stephanie van Goozen, School of Psychology, Cardiff University, Tower Building, Park Place, Cardiff, CF10 3AT, Phone: +44(0)29 208 74630, Fax: +44(0)29 208 74858, VanGoozenS@Cardiff.ac.uk

Cost

Contact the source (above) for permission to use the ASQ.

Articulated Thoughts in Simulated Situations (ATSS)

Purpose

The Articulated Thoughts in Simulated Situations (ATSS) is a think-aloud paradigm that assesses cognitive processes as they occur in structured, experimenter-controlled situations. The ATSS has been adapted to assess anger-relevant cognitive processes.

Population

Adults.

Background and Description

The ATSS was originally developed to serve as a think-aloud paradigm for exploring cognition during complex events that would allow for open-ended verbal responding which would reflect, as much as possible, ongoing thought processes in contrast to retrospective self-reporting. A second goal was to allow for the experimenter to be able to specify and manipulate the situations to which the subjects were responding.

The ATSS method requires participants to listen to a tape recording of an event and imagine that they are an active part of the interaction. The ATSS method has participants articulate their thoughts and feelings at specified intervals throughout the imagined interaction. Following the interactions, articulations are transcribed into written forms and are then rated along relevant dimensions by trained coders. The ATSS method has been used with nonclinical and clinical populations.

Administration

Respondents are asked to listen to recorded vignettes while imagining themselves in the situation. A tone sounds at the end of each segment, and respondents are asked to report what they are thinking about. Respondents usually complete a practice tape first in order to become familiar with the task. The practice session also serves to allow the experimenter to coach or teach participants how to verbalize their thoughts in detail. Upon completion of the practice tape, the stimulus tape runs for about 2–3 min. The procedure has been adapted to assess situations relevant to domestic violence (e.g., assessing jealousy; Eckhardt & Kassinove, 1998).

Scoring

Participants' articulated thoughts are tape recorded and later transcribed for content analysis by coders. The original coding system utilized a reliable method for separating the flow of verbalizations into units or categories. Examples of categories included the desire to harm the speaker, empathy with speaker, problem solving, and a critical evaluation of the speaker. High agreement has been demonstrated between raters and a majority of the verbalizations were able to be coded.

Interpretation

Variable interpretations can be inferred depending upon the coding system that is utilized.

Psychometric Properties

Reliability. A coding strategy was employed in which raters coded the number of "idea-units" in responses and then classified these responses into meaningful categories. Idea-units are discrete ideas that are contained in the response segments. Most responses were composed of one or two idea-units. Reliability was assessed by calculating the percent of agreement between two raters on the number of idea-units per segment using the Pearson product–moment correlation. The reliability was found to be good with $r = .88$. The reliability of the coding of idea-units into categories was also assessed. There was partial agreement on the coding of idea-units for 82 % of the units and total agreement for 76 % of units.

Validity. Various coding strategies have been studied and demonstrated face, concurrent, predictive, and construct validity. Some coding schemes have been related to the Spielberger State–Trait Anger Scale (pp. 77–79). The ATSS has also been examined with partner violent men and nonviolent men in a discordant marriage and nonviolent men in a satisfying marriage (Barbour, Eckhardt, Davison, & Kassinove, 1998; Eckhardt, Barbour, & Davison, 1998). Partner violent men articulated significantly more irrational thoughts and cognitive biases than did the men involved in a discordant marriage and the nonviolent men during the anger-arousing ATSS. In general, ATSS measures were better at discriminating among the three groups than were self-report measures.

Clinical Utility

Limited. Although a number of studies have examined the use of the ATSS with a variety of cognitive factors including anger, hostility and aggression, anxiety and depression, smoking cessation, and psychotherapy process, the measure requires equipment and raters, both of which are typically unavailable in a clinical setting.

Research Applicability

High. The ATSS has been used for evaluating a variety of cognitive constructs. The adaptability of the measure allows for the use of specific situations and provides critical information related to issues fundamental to cognitive behavior therapy, other cognitively oriented approaches, and cognitive theories of psychopathology. Additionally, the ATSS appears useful for examining thought processes under a wide range of conditions of interest.

Original Citations

Davison, G. C., Robins, C., & Johnson, M. K. (1983). Articulated thoughts during simulated situations: A paradigm for studying cognition in emotion and behavior. *Cognitive Therapy and Research, 7,* 17–40.

Source

Gerald C. Davison, Department of Gerontoloy, University of Southern California, Los Angeles, CA 90089-1061, (213) 740-1354, Fax: (213) 740-0792, gdaviso@usc.edu

Cost

Contact the source (above) for permission to use the ATSS.

References

Barbour, K. A., Eckhardt, C. I., Davison, G. C., & Kassinove, H. (1998). The experience and expression of anger in maritally violent and maritally discordant-, nonviolent men. *Behavior Therapy, 29,* 173–191.

Eckhardt, C. I., Barbour, K. A., & Davison, G. C. (1998). Articulated thoughts of maritally violent and nonviolent men during anger arousal. *Journal of Consulting and Clinical Psychology, 66,* 259–269.

Eckhardt, C. I., & Kassinove, H. (1998). Articulated cognitive distortions and cognitive deficiencies in maritally violent men. *Journal of Cognitive Psychotherapy, 12,* 231–250.

Audiotaped Anger-Provoking Situations (AAPS)

Purpose

To examine cognitive and behavioral responses to anger-inducing stimuli.

Population

Adults.

Background and Description

The audiotaped anger-provoking situations (AAPS) involves presenting individuals with six audiotaped anger-inducing situations. The situations were initially developed to range in intensity from low to high and to investigate responses to anger-eliciting stimuli amongst anger-prone individuals. A male and a female version are available that differ only in language content; the same female voice is used for every tape. Respondents are asked to imagine themselves in the situation and to respond to the question, "What is your reaction?" Responses are recorded and later transcribed. Responses are subsequently played back to the participants who judge their responses in terms of effectiveness (producing the desired result), appropriateness (suitable or fitting, correct), and the likely consequences (positive and negative consequences for them and the other individual in the situation). Ratings are given on a 9-point Likert scale.

Transcripts of the responses are given to peer judges, who rate them on a 9-point scale for effectiveness, appropriateness, and complexity (e.g., number alternative actions, sequence of actions, forethought, and consideration of circumstances involved in response), and response style (confrontational versus non-confrontational).

Administration

Administration time varies as a function of length of responses by the participant and the background of the peer evaluators.

Scoring

Participant ratings for each dimension (response appropriateness, response effectiveness, and potential positive and negative consequences for them and the other individual in the situation) are summed and averaged across situations. Peer ratings for each dimension (response effectiveness, response appropriateness, and response complexity) are summed and averaged across situations.

Interpretation

Higher scores for each self-rated dimension are indicative of greater response appropriateness, response effectiveness, positive consequences, and negative consequences. Higher scores for

each peer-rated dimension indicate greater response effectiveness, response appropriateness, and response complexity.

Psychometric Properties

Reliability. Internal consistency reliability of the peer ratings was assessed using the intraclass reliability coefficient based on 12 judges. Coefficient ranges were .84–.92 (appropriateness), .75–.90 (effectiveness), and .90–.94 (complexity) with the exception of one situation, which had coefficients of .69 for effectiveness and .68 for appropriateness.

Validity. When asked to rate the vividness and amount of anger evoked by each situation, responses confirmed the expected anger-arousing ability of the situations. Variation in the anger reactions was present across situations. Individuals described as high anger-prone produced ratings for high, moderate, and low-anger situations similar to those originally obtained. Additionally, individuals described as low anger-prone produced identical rank orders, but gave lower ratings.

Concerning the validity of the self-evaluations, anger-prone individuals perceived a greater number of negative consequences for the self and others than low anger-prone individuals, while the latter saw more positive consequences than the former. Using the transcriptions, peer raters were unable to differentiate between individuals described as high and low anger prone.

Construct validity was supported by evidence that high anger-prone individuals rated themselves as feeling greater anger than low anger-prone individuals when responding to the situations. Strong correlations were found between effectiveness and appropriateness ratings, indicating that self-raters were unable to discriminate between the two dimensions.

Clinical Utility

Moderate. The procedure provides a means with which to identify cognitions and emotions involved in responses to anger-inducing situations, which may subsequently be targeted by interventions. Reliability information of the self-ratings is needed.

Research Applicability

Moderate. The procedure is lengthy to complete but provides a means of accurately assessing perceptions and emotions of individuals when evaluating their responses to anger-inducing situations.

Original Citation

Tescher, B., Conger, J. C., Edmondson, C. B., & Conger, A. J. (1999). Behavior, attitudes, and cognitions of anger-prone individuals. *Journal of Psychopathology and Behavioral Assessment, 21*, 117–139.

Source

Judith C. Conger, 703 Third St, West Lafayette, IN 47907, (765) 494-6977, Fax: (765) 496-2670, jcc@psych.purdue.edu

Cost

Contact the source (above) to obtain permission to use the instrument.

Autonomic Nervous System Response Inventory (ANSRI)

Purpose

To assess patterns of autonomic nervous system responses that occur during emotional distress, pleasure, or physical activity.

Population

Adults.

Background and Description

There are numerous ways to measure psychophysiological arousal (e.g., skin conductance, heart rate, and electroencephalography). The Autonomic Nervous System Response Inventory (ANSRI) was developed as a self-report measure of autonomic nervous system responses to aid in assessing psychophysiological arousal. Items were derived from prior research on psychophysiology of emotion and from discussion with colleagues. The ANSRI consists of 51 items that assess patterns of autonomic nervous system responses across five situations (fear, anger, sadness, joy, and physical activity). Each situation is treated as a separate inventory wherein respondents are asked to choose a prototypical emotional reaction that is representative of the given situation and to reconstruct this situation from memory and imagine themselves in the situation. The examiner chooses which situations to administer. For each situation participants rate the presence or intensity of 51 self-report items using a 5-point scale.

The items are organized into 12 Physiological Scales (P Scales: cardiac, cardiovascular, skin, pseudomotor, piloerection, muscle tension, respiration, gastrointestinal, excretory, energy activation, eyes, and thermoregulation) and 7 Factor Scales (F Scales: fear, anger, sadness, joy, activity, all situations, emotional situations). F and P Scales overlap so that combining scales across situations results in 84 P Scales and 54 F Scales. Sample items follow.

• Forehead and/or upper lip perspired
• Neck muscles became tense

Administration

Each situation (51 items) is estimated to take 8–12 min to complete.

Scoring

Responses to items are summed to produce scale scores. Scores can be listed for each scale under each situation, summed across scale scores for each situation, averaged across the situation, or averaged across the four emotional situations. T-score conversions are available.

Interpretation

Patterns of responses for each situation and across situations may be examined qualitatively or scores may be compared to the available norms.

Psychometric Properties

Norms. Norms for each scale are available.

Factor analysis. A principal components method, conducted separately for each situation, revealed nine factors for fear (Gastrointestinal, Muscle Tension, Headache 1, Pseudomotor, Energy Activation, Pattern 1, Respiration, Vasoconstriction), 8 for anger (Vasoconstriction, Muscle Tension, Headache 2, Cardiac Respiration, Pattern 2, Gastrointestinal), 8 for sadness, 8 for joy, 7 for activity, 7 for all situations, and 7 for all emotional situations. Pattern 1 refers to responses involving cardiac, respiration, and piloerection. Pattern 2 refers to responses involving respiration and gastrointestinal items. Headache 1 involves mixed vascular and muscle-contraction headache symptoms. Headache 2 involves a pounding and steady, dull headache pain emphasizing vasodilation and pseudomotor responses.

Reliability. Test–retest coefficients for a 4-week period for males and females, respectively, were .69 and .79 (all situations), .70 and .73 (all emotional situations), .62 and .64 (fear), .67 and .68 (anger), .73 and .71 (sadness), .69 and .79 (joy), and .58 and .85 (activity). The 4-week test–retest coefficients for a cross-validation sample ranged from .79 (anger) to .87 (sadness) for males and .83 (anger) to .92 (activity) for females.

Cronbach's alpha for males and females, respectively, were .97 and .97 (all situations), .97

and .96 (all emotional situations), .90 and .87 (fear), .92 and .90 (anger), .92 and .91 (sadness), .92 and .92 (joy), and .92 and .93 (activity). In a cross-validation sample, alpha values ranged from .91 (fear) to .98 (all situations) for males and .91 (fear and joy) to .98 (all situations) for females.

Validity. Combinations of the P and F scales have been found to predict psychophysiological responses, as measured by electrophysiological measures during emotional imagery. In such situations, the P scales were more predictive of psychophysiological response than the F scales. The ANSRI has some support for experimental discriminant validity. P scale scores were successful in differentiating among headache groups and a control group.

Clinical Utility

Moderate. The ANSRI has potential as a self-report measure of physiological correlates of anger during anger-provoking situations. More research is needed on the clinical validity and clinical utility of the ANSRI.

Research Applicability

Moderate. The ANSRI might provide an efficient adjunctive measure of perceived physiological responses to anger-provoking situations and such information might prove useful for research targeting processes related to contextual and individual difference variables related to anger arousal levels.

Original Citation

Waters, W. F., Cohen, R. A., Bernard, B. A., Buco, S. M., & Dreger, R. M. (1984). An Autonomic Nervous System Response Inventory (ANSRI): Scaling, reliability, and cross-validation. *Journal of Behavioral Medicine, 7*(3), 315–341.

Source

William F. Waters, Louisiana State University, Department of Psychology, Baton Rouge, Louisiana 70803, wwaters@ochsner.org

Cost

Contact the source (above) for additional information on the ANSRI.

Children's Anger Response Checklist (CARC)

Purpose

To assess physiological, cognitive, emotional, and behavioral aspects of anger.

Population

Ages 7–12.

Background and Description

The Children's Anger Response Checklist (CARC) assesses the behavioral, cognitive, physiological, and affective components of anger experienced by children. Dimensions of the CARC are based on Novaco's (1975) conceptualization of anger. The overall rating incorporates components of the Children's Inventory of Anger (pp. 44–46). The current version of the CARC was developed from a series of initial investigations.

The CARC is a multidimensional self-report measure of anger. Respondents report their expected physiological, cognitive, emotional, and behavioral responses to ten hypothetical problem situations. Respondents mark expected ways of responding to each vignette; space is also provided for respondents to list novel ways of responding. Respondents then use a Likert-type scale, ranging from 1 ("I'm not angry, that situation doesn't even bother me at all") to 5 ("I can't stand it! I'm very, very angry and I feel like…

really hurting that person or destroying that thing"), to indicate the level of anger they would likely experience. The rating scale includes faces depicting increasing levels of anger in lieu of numbers. For each hypothetical situation, respondents are instructed to imagine how they might feel or behave if confronted by the scenario. The CARC consists of four domains (behavioral, cognitive, emotional, and physiological) and eight subdomains (behavioral aggressive, behavioral assertive, behavioral submissive, cognitive aggressive, cognitive assertive, cognitive submissive, cognitive perceived injustice, and cognitive self-blame). Possible responses are balanced across domains and approximately balanced across subdomains.

Administration

The CARC may be administered verbally or completed independently. The authors recommend completing the first hypothetical situation with the child to gauge his or her comprehension of directions and to monitor the completion of the response checklist and the overall anger level rating. The CARC is estimated to take 15–30 min to complete.

Scoring

For each hypothetical situation, five possible responses are listed for each domain (behavioral, cognitive, emotional, and physiological). For each situation, scores are computed for each domain and subdomain by counting the number of items endorsed within each domain. Anger ratings (scores from 1 to 5) are also recorded for each situation. Total domain, subdomain, and overall anger rating scores are obtained by summing totals from each vignette. An overall responsivity score is obtained by adding the total number of items checked for each situation (scores range from 1 to 20). Total aggressive, assertive, and submissive scores can be obtained by summing aggressive, assertive, and submissive subdomain scores in the behavioral and cognitive domains.

Interpretation

Domain and subdomain scores represent the frequency with which those types of responses are utilized. Anger ratings for each situation indicate the level of anger provoked by the situation. Overall anger ratings indicate level of anger experienced across situations. The overall responsivity score may be used as means of monitoring compliance to the task and to identify impulsive checking-off styles. The authors of the CARC stated that the responses in the assertiveness domains are representative of the most appropriate behavioral and cognitive responses. "Other" responses provide supplemental information. The scoring summary sheet, which allows the scorer to record information from each situation, allows the scorer to examine response patterns of the individual.

Psychometric Properties

Factor analysis. Principal component analyses with varimax rotation of the CARC subscales, but not the Overall Anger ratings, did not produce the expected four-component structure (behavioral, cognitive, physiological, and emotional components). The authors concluded that the CARC might be suited to facilitate children's awareness of their responses when angry. Items on the CARC were factor analyzed with items on the Children's Inventory of Anger (ChIA; pp. 44–46) and the Children's Action Tendency Scale (CATS; pp. 111–113). Items on the ChIA and the CATS loaded on a single factor with CARC Overall Anger ratings and Aggressive subscales. Items on the CARC Assertive and Submissive subscales loaded on their own separate factors. Additional analyses support the use of the CARC as a means of obtaining information over and above what can be obtained from the ChIA or the CATS.

Reliability. Internal consistency was measured using Cronbach's alpha. For the response checklist across the ten situations $\alpha = .96$. For the anger ratings across the ten situations $\alpha = .87$.

Validity. Data have supported the construct validity of the CARC. The Overall Anger rating score was not related to the domain and subdomain scales, with the exception of physiological and aggression domain scores. Overall Anger rating scores were positively related to ChIA scores and CATS Aggressiveness scores, but negatively related to CATS submissiveness scores. The CARC total assertion and submission scores, however, were not significantly correlated with the CATS assertiveness and submission scores, respectively, bringing to question the validity of the CARC as a measure of assertive and submissive behaviors.

Clinical Utility

Moderate. The CARC has potential to aid in the clinical interpretation of how a child perceives and responds to anger-provoking situations. Thus, it may be useful for treatment planning and pre/post-intervention assessment. Available data can guide the use of the CARC for the identification of response styles. More substantial normative data are needed prior to suggesting widespread clinical applications.

Research Applicability

Moderate. The CARC is useful in assessing multiple dimensions of anger. There is some question concerning the ability of the CARC to differentiate between assertive and aggressive responses. Further tests of reliability (e.g., test–retest) and validity are warranted.

Original Citation

Feindler, E. L., Adler, N., Brooks, D., & Bhumitra, E. (1993). The Children's Anger Response Checklist. In L. VandeCreek, S. Knapp, & T. L. Jackson (Eds.), *Innovations in clinical practice: A source book* (Vol. 12, pp. 337–362). Sarasota, FL: Professional Resource Press/Professional Resource Exchange.

Source

Eva L. Feindler, Long Island University, C. W. Post Campus, Brookville, NY 11548, eva.feindler @liu.edu

Cost

Please contact the source (above) for permission to use.

Children's Inventory of Anger (ChIA)

Purpose

To assess the subjective experience of anger in children.

Population

Children between the ages of 7 and 14.

Background and Description

The Children's Inventory of Anger (ChIA) was developed from the cognitive–behavioral conceptualization of anger which suggests that anger results from an interaction between anger provoking situations and the thinking errors made when provoked. Items were derived by recoding interviews with normal and emotionally disturbed children wherein they were asked to describe what made them angry. The resulting inventory requires children to indicate the amount of anger they would experience in 39 different situations. Children respond to each situation using a 4-point scale that ranges from 1 (I don't care. That situation doesn't even bother me. I don't know why that would make anyone mad) to 4 (I can't stand that; I'm furious! I feel like really hurting or killing that person or destroying that thing!). Visual aids are also used to anchor these numbers: four faces depict

increasing degrees of feeling angry. The ChIA was written at a fourth grade reading level, but is reportedly understood by children as young as 7 years old when administered verbally. Sample items follow.

- Your friends are playing a game and they won't let you play.
- You bump into a stranger on the bus. He says he will beat you up if you get near him again.

Administration

The ChIA is estimated to take 20–25 min to complete.

Scoring

Responses to each item are summed, with scores on the ChIA ranging from 39 to 156.

Interpretation

The ChIA measures anger, as opposed to aggression. Higher scores indicate that more anger was expected within the situations. A list of specific situations respondents rate as anger provoking is generated. The ratings can also provide qualitative information regarding the coping style of the child.

Psychometric Properties

Norms. Normative data for children in grades four through seven are available in Finch, Saylor, & Nelson (1987). Norms for children ages 9–14 years are available upon request.

Factor analysis. Using a sample of normal children, six factors were extracted and described as: at the mercy of authority figures; at the mercy of uncontrollable events; injustice; embarrassment or threat to self-esteem; frustration of desires;

and sibling conflict. Using a sample of emotionally disturbed children, four factors were extracted: loss of possessions; imposed events with a loss of control or helplessness; perceived injustices; and loss through accidental destruction of an object.

Reliability. Split-half reliabilities for a sample of normal children ranged from .83 to .95 and from .93 to .96 for a sample of psychiatrically hospitalized children. Kuder–Richardson reliability in a sample of normal children was .96. Overall test–retest reliability was .82, and ranged from .63 to .90 in samples of psychiatric inpatient children and normal children, respectively.

Validity. In a sample of third and fourth grade boys, a multitrait–multimethod model was employed, using the ChIA, the Child Depression Inventory (Kovacs, 1980/1981), the Peer Nomination Inventory for Depression (Lefkowitz & Tesiny, 1980), and the Peer Nomination of Anger Control Problems (Finch, Moss, & Nelson, 1993). Data from these analyses supported the convergent validity, but not the discriminate validity, of the ChIA. In a different study with a sample of emotionally disturbed children, the multitrait–multimethod procedure demonstrated poor convergent validity of the ChIA with the Quay Behavior Problem Check List (teacher rated; Quay, 1977) and the Child Behavior Checklist (unit staff reported).

To explore criterion-related validity, scores on the ChIA were correlated with scores of various other methods and populations. The ChIA was not capable of distinguishing between emotionally disturbed and normal children or between conduct-disordered children, affective/anxiety-disordered children, and dual-diagnosed children. Using a sample of emotionally disturbed children, the ChIA correlated with peer nominations of anger and individual treatment plans, but did not covary with teacher ratings. In samples of normal children, the ChIA correlated with the acting out factor on the teacher completed Walker Problem Behavior Checklist (Walker, 1970), the Children's Depression Inventory, and the depression and anxiety subscales of the Teacher-Rated

Child Behavior Checklist. The ChIA was not related to the Peer Nomination Inventory of Depression or the Peer Nomination of Anger Control Problems (Saylor, Finch, Baskin, Furey, & Kelly, 1984; Shoemaker, Erickson, & Finch, 1986). The ChIA was sensitive to treatment changes in a cognitive–behavioral treatment program for temper tantrums (Williams, Waymouth, Lipman, Mills, & Evans, 2004).

Clinical Utility

Moderate. Due to the inconsistency of the psychometric properties, especially the validity studies, it is not recommended to use the ChIA for clinical decision making wherein the classification of children is a main goal. The ChIA might be useful for conducting an idiographic analysis of the types of situations that are likely to elicit anger.

Research Applicability

Moderate. The ChIA has been used in several research studies to examine children's self-reports of anger. Validity studies have yielded inconclusive results, which makes interpretation of the ChIA's relationship with other constructs difficult. Further validation studies would be useful to clarify the construct validity of the ChIA.

Original Citation

Nelson, W. M., III & Finch, A. J., Jr. (1978). *Nelson-Finch Children's Inventory of Anger manual.* Unpublished manuscript, Xavier University (Ohio).

Source

W. M. Nelson, III, Ph.D., Psychology Department, Xavier University, 3800 Victory Parkway, Cincinnati, OH 45207, (513) 745-3298, Fax: (513) 745-3327, nelson@xavier.edu

Cost

Contact the source (above) for permission to use the ChIA.

Alternative Forms

A short version of the ChIA, consisting of 21 items, is also available.

References

Finch, A. J., Jr., Moss, J. H., & Nelson, W. M., III. (1993). Stress inoculation for anger management in children. In A. J. Finch, Jr., W. M. Nelson III & E. S. Ott (Eds.), *Cognitive behavioral procedures with children.* New York: Spectrum.

Finch, A. J., Saylor, C. F., & Nelson, W. M. III. (1987). Assessment of anger in children. In R. J. Prinz (Ed.), *Advances in behavior assessment of children and families* (Vol. 2, pp. 235–265). Greenwich, CT: JAI Press.

Kovacs, M. (1980/1981). Rating scales to assess depression in school-aged children. *Acta Paedopsychiatry, 46,* 305–315.

Lefkowitz, M. M., & Tesiny, E. P. (1980). Assessment of childhood depression. *Journal of Consulting and Clinical Psychology, 48,* 43–50. 773–782.

Quay, H. C. (1977). Measuring dimensions of deviant behavior: The Behavior Problem Checklist. *Journal of Abnormal Child Psychology, 5,* 277–287.

Saylor, C. F., Finch, A. J., Baskin, C. H., Furey, W., & Kelly, M. M. (1984). Construct validity for measures of childhood depression: Application of multitrait-multimethod methodology. *Journal of Consulting and Clinical Psychology, 52,* 977–985.

Shoemaker, O. S., Erickson, M. T., & Finch, A. J. (1986). Depression and anger in third and fourth-grade boys: A multimethod assessment approach. *Journal of Clinical Child Psychology, 15,* 290–296.

Walker, H. M. (1970). *Walker Problem Behavior Identification Checklist.* Los Angeles, CA: Western Psychological Services.

Williams, S., Waymouth, M., Lipman, E., Mills, B., & Evans, P. (2004). Evaluation of a children's temper-taming program. *Canadian Journal of Psychiatry, 49,* 607–612.

Clinical Anger Scale (CAS)

Purpose

To measure clinical anger.

Population

Adults.

Background and Description

The Clinical Anger Scale (CAS) was designed to account for a gap in the anger literature regarding measures designed to specifically assess clinical anger. Clinical anger is conceptualized as a multisymptom syndrome consisting of affective, cognitive, physiological, social, and behavioral manifestations. The items for the CAS were created by consulting previous research regarding clinical-related instruments and discussing items with professional psychologists, undergraduate psychology majors, and graduate counseling students. The CAS contains 21 groups of statements, with four statements per group. Each group of statements reflects possible symptoms of clinical anger: anger now, anger about the future, anger about failure, anger about things, angry–hostile feelings, annoying others, angry about self, angry misery, wanting to hurt others, shouting at people, irritated now, social interference, decision interference, alienating others, work interference, sleep interference, fatigue, appetite interference, health interference, thinking interference, and sexual interference. Respondents select the single statement out of the group of four that best describes how they feel.

Administration

The CAS is estimated to require 20–30 min to complete.

Scoring

Each group of statements is scored using a 4-point Likert type scale. The scores are summed to produce a total score.

Interpretation

The intensity of the statements in each group increases so that more clinical anger is associated with the later statements in a group. Total scores can range from 0 to 63. Scores from 0 to 13 are considered to be minimal clinical anger, 14–19 mild clinical anger, 20–28 moderate clinical anger, and 29–63 severe clinical anger.

Psychometric Properties

Factor analysis. Factor analyses were conducted on a sample of 405 college students (104 males, 301 females). Using varimax rotation, the factor analysis revealed a single factor that accounted for 45.4 % of the variance, suggesting that the CAS is a unidimensional measure.

Reliability. Internal consistency reliability was assessed using Cronbach's alpha on a sample of 405 college students. Internal consistency was good for males (α=.95), females (α=.92), and the total sample (α=.94). Three-week test–retest reliability was assessed on a sample of 39 college students (31 females, 8 males). Test–retest reliability was good for males (r=.85), females (r=.77), and the total sample (r=.78).

Validity. The CAS did not correlate significantly with social desirability or the EPI Lie Scale (Eysenck & Eysenck, 1968), suggesting answers on the CAS were not distorted by social desirability or lying tendencies. Scores on the CAS were significantly related to the two subscales of the State–Trait Anger Scale (pp. 77–79) and the subscales of the Anger Expression Scale (pp. 28–30). Scores on the CAS were related to symptoms endorsed on a psychopathology symptom checklist (SCL-90-R, Derogatis, 1983), wherein individuals with greater clinical anger reported more psychological symptoms related to hostility. The CAS was found to be positively related to neuroticism and negatively related to extraversion, pleasantness–agreeableness, and emotional stability. The CAS was significantly related to unhealthy, anger-related behaviors including acting-out behaviors, neurotic behaviors, and interpersonal defensiveness. The CAS was also significantly related to an early family history of conflict and exaggerated family control.

Clinical Utility

Moderate. The CAS may be a useful tool for investigating the nature of clinical anger. It may be used to examine the extent to which clients are influenced by various symptoms of clinical anger. It could be used in treatment planning and assessing treatment outcome. However, the lack of normative data for clinical and non-clinical populations limits the clinical utility of the CAS.

Research Applicability

Moderate. The CAS could be a useful tool for researching interpersonal expression of anger, the role of anger in health problems such as hypertension and coronary heart disease, and gender-related aggressiveness and anger. It could also be used to investigate the efficacy of therapeutic approaches designed to treat violent behavior or clinical anger.

Original Citation

Snell, W. E., Gum, S., Shuck, R. L., Mosley, J. A., & Hite, T. L. (1995). The Clinical Anger Scale: Preliminary reliability and validity. *Journal of Clinical Psychology, 51*, 215–226.

Source

Dr. William Snell Jr., Department of Psychology, Southeast Missouri State University, One University Plaza, Cape Girardeau, MO, 63701, (573) 651-2447, wesnell@semo.edu. The CAS can be found online at http://www4.semo.edu/snell/scales/CAS.HTM

reflect the respondent's own description of him/herself, are answered "true" or "false."

Cost

Please contact the source (above) for permission to use the CAS.

References

Derogatis, L. R. (1983). *SCL-90-R administration, scoring and procedures manual-II*. Towson, MD: Clinical Psychometric Research.
Eysenck, H. J., & Eysenck, S. B. G. (1968). *The Eysenck Personality Inventory*. San Diego, CA: Educational and Industrial Testing Service.

Cook and Medley Hostility Scale (Ho)

Purpose

To identify levels of hostility.

Population

Adults.

Background and Description

The scale was derived from the Minnesota Multiphasic Personality Inventory (MMPI), by selecting the 250 items that best discriminated between teachers scoring high and low on the Minnesota Teacher Attitude Inventory (MTAI; Cook, Leeds, & Callis, 1951). From these items, five clinical psychologists independently selected items (primarily based on item content) to comprise the Hostility scale (Ho scale), and the amount of agreement between psychologists was used to select the final 50 items.

The Cook and Medley Hostility scale is a 50-item, self-report measure assessing cynical attitudes and mistrust of others. Items, which

Administration

The scale is estimated to take 10–15 min to complete.

Scoring

Items are keyed either true or false. Respondents receive a higher score on the item when their response matches the item key.

Interpretation

A high score is most often associated with bitterness, mistrust of others, and resentment but not overt hostile actions.

Psychometric Properties

Norms. Norms were derived from the sample of the normal sample group (226 males, 315 females) used in the original clinical scales of the MMPI. Norms are listed in the original citation.

Factor analysis. In a sample of undergraduate students, researchers interpreted one factor and numerous small factors. The researchers concluded that internal consistency might be improved by deleting items (Han, Weed, Calhoun, & Butcher, 1995).

Reliability. Internal consistency, assessed using Cronbach's alpha, was .86 in the initial sample of 200 graduate students and .82 and .80 for undergraduate males and females, respectively, in later samples. Test–retest reliabilities were reported as .85 and .84 for 1-year and 4-year intervals, respectively.

Validity. The Ho scale correlated negatively with the MTAI (which predicts student–teacher rapport), and correlated positively (.65 for males, .73 for females) with the Pharisaic Virtue (Pv) scale. The Pv scale describes individuals who view themselves as preoccupied with morality and burdened with fears and tensions. These latter correlations indicate that the Pv and Ho scales are highly correlated but assess different dimensions of personality.

The Ho scale correlates with trait anger and those who score high on the scale experience anger often, are bitter and resentful, view others with distrust and resentment but may not exhibit overt aggression. The majority of items reflect cynicism or mistrust of others, but researchers have argued that it is not clear what personality dimension is being assessed by the Ho scale (Smith, Sanders, & Alexander, 1990). The scale has not been shown to correlate well with overt forms of hostility. In many studies, high Ho scores were correlated with coronary heart disease and coronary death (Pope, Smith, & Rhodewalt, 1990).

Several studies provide support for the construct validity of the scale. Scores on the Ho scale have correlated positively with trait anger, the Buss–Durkee Hostility Inventory subscales (pp. 109–111), trait anxiety, Machiavellianism, locus of control, Revised Philosophies of Human Nature Cynicism subscale (Wrightsman, 1974), and Jenkins Type A. Scores were found to correlate negatively with the Rotter Trust Scale (Rotter, 1967), the Revised Philosophies of Human Nature Trust subscale (Wrightsman, 1974), social desirability, and hardiness (Barefoot, Peterson, Dahlstrom, Siegler, Anderson, & Williams, 1991). Additionally, there were lower correlations between the scale and measures of anxiety and depression. Another study found strong correlations between the scale and measures of anger and suspicion, as well as an association with general dysphoric states.

Other researchers have found support for the construct validity in male samples, but limited support in female samples. In men, scores covaried positively with self-reported anger, anxiety, and overt hostile behavior during a high conflict discussion. Additionally, those scoring higher were more likely to blame their wives for typical disagreements and viewed more intentionality in wives' disagreement-engendering behavior. Hostility scores were not related to dominant behavior. In women, scores on the Ho scale were only weakly related to hostile behavioral responsiveness and self-reported anxiety during high conflict discussions.

Clinical Utility

Limited. The usefulness of this measure lies in its potential ability to predict health problems, but the evidence is not conclusive (Smith et al., 1990).

Research Applicability

Limited. Before this measure can be very useful for research purposes, it must be clear what is being measured. The scale is reliable but the validity is unclear.

Original Citation

Cook, W. W., & Medley, D. M. (1954). Proposed hostility and pharisaic-virtue scales for the MMPI. *Journal of Applied Psychology, 38*, 414–418.

Source

The items of the Ho scale are contained in the MMPI and the MMPI-2, and the items of the MMPI that comprise the Ho scale are listed in the original citation. The MMPI-2 may be purchased from Pearson Assessments.

Cost

Pricing information is available at http://www.pearsonassessments.com/mmpi2.aspx.

Alternative Forms

Nine items of the Ho scale were revised when the MMPI was revised in 1989. Men who scored high on the MMPI-2 Ho scale were described by their spouses as hotheaded, demanding and bossy. For women, scores on the MMPI-2 Ho scale were less strongly related to ratings of overt hostility.

References

Barefoot, J. C., Peterson, B. L., Dahlstrom, W. G., Siegler, I. C., Anderson, N. B., & Williams, R. B. (1991). Hostility patterns and health implications: Correlates of Cook-Medley Hostility Scales Scores in a National Survey. *Health Psychology, 10*, 18–24.

Cook, W. W., Leeds, C. H., & Callis, R. (1951). *Minnesota Teacher Attitude Inventory,* New York: The Psychological Corporation.

Han, K., Weed, N., Calhoun, R. F., & Butcher, J. N. (1995). Psychometric characteristics of the MMPI-2 Cook-Medley Hostility Scale. *Journal of Personality Assessment, 65*, 567–585.

Pope, M. K., Smith, T., & Rhodewalt, F. (1990). Cognitive, behavioral, and affective correlates of the Cook and Medley Hostility Scale. *Journal of Personality Assessment, 54*, 501–514.

Rotter, J. B. (1967). A new scale for the measurement of interpersonal trust. *Journal of Personality, 35,* 651–665.

Smith, T. W., Sanders, J. D., & Alexander, J. F. (1990). What does the Cook and Medley Hostility Scale Measure? Affect, behavior, and attributions in the marital context. *Journal of Personality and Social Psychology, 58*, 699–708.

Wrightsman, L. S. (1974). *Assumptions about human nature: A social-psychological approach.* Monterey, CA: Brooks-Cole.

Differential Emotions Scale-IV (DES-IV)

Purpose

To measure the experience of fundamental emotions.

Population

Children ages 8 and older.

Background and Description

The Differential Emotions Scale-IV (DES-IV) is a measure of the fundamental emotions experienced by children and adolescents. The DES-IV was adapted from an earlier form that was designed to measure emotions experienced by adults. The DES-IV expands on the DES-III and includes two additional emotional states. The 37 items of the DES-IV reflect 12 emotions: interest, enjoyment, surprise, sadness, anger, disgust, contempt, fear, shame, shyness, guilt, and self-directed hostility. Items are comprised of phrases reflecting an aspect of the experience of the emotion. Respondents rate the frequency with which they have experienced the emotion during a specified time frame (i.e., past week, past month). Alternatively, respondents can report the intensity with which they experience the emotion at the present time.

Administration

The DES-IV requires approximately 15–20 min to complete.

Scoring

Scores for each emotion are calculated by summing items comprising that emotion. This results in 12 subscale scores, one for each emotion.

Interpretation

Higher scores indicate greater intensity of a particular emotion experienced at the present time, or greater frequency of experiencing the particular emotion during the specified time frame.

Psychometric Properties

Reliability. In a sample of 145 youth, ages 10–17 years old, internal consistency ranged from .50 (guilt) to .85 (sadness). The average alpha for the

12 subscales was .69, suggesting adequate internal consistency considering 11 of the 12 subscales are comprised of three items. Four month test–retest reliability for the 12 subscales ranged from .30 (interest) to .66 (self-directed hostility).

Validity. The DES-IV subscales guilt, surprise, anger, sadness, and interest together were found to accurately discriminate between depressed and nondepressed adolescents. Sadness, anger, hostility, joy, and interest were found to predict Children's Depression Inventory scores (Kovacs & Becks, 1977). The DES-IV anger and hostility subscales were significantly related to the Pediatric Anger Expression Scale-III (PAES-III, pp. 69–70). The DES-IV anger subscale was negatively correlated with anger-in ($r=-.22$) and anger-control ($r=-.38$) and positively correlated with anger-out ($r=.42$). The hostility subscale was significantly, negatively correlated with anger-control ($r=-.26$), and positively correlated with anger-out ($r=.18$).

Clinical Utility

Moderate. The DES-IV provides clinicians with detailed information on the types of emotions experienced by an individual, which may be beneficial for treatment planning purposes.

Research Applicability

Moderate. Research with the DES-IV may clarify the pattern of emotions associated with various mental disorders in children and adolescents. The DES-IV can be used in its entirety to investigate various patterns of emotions, or individual subscales may be used to determine their individual relation to various disorders or related constructs (see Blumberg, & Izard, 1986; Carey, Finch, & Carey, 1991; Hagglund, Clay, Frank, Beck, Kashani, Hewett, et al., 1994; Kotsch, Gerbing, & Schwartz, 1982).

Original Citation

Izard, C. E., Dougherty, F. E., Bloxom, B. M., & Kotsch, W. E. (1974). *The Differential Emotions Scale: A method of measuring the subjective experience of discrete emotions.* Unpublished manuscript, Vanderbilt University, 1974.

Source

Dr. Carroll E. Izard, Department of Psychology, 108 Wolf Hall, University of Delaware, Newark, DE, 19716-2577, (302) 831-1838, Fax: (302) 831-3645, izard@psych.udel.edu

Cost

Please contact the source (above) for permission to use the DES-IV.

References

Blumberg, S. H., & Izard, C. E. (1986). Discriminating patterns of emotions in 10- and 11-year-old children's anxiety and depression. *Journal of Personality and Social Psychology, 51,* 852–857.

Carey, T. C., Finch, A. J., & Carey, M. P. (1991). Relation between differential emotions and depression in emotionally disturbed children and adolescents. *Journal of Consulting and Clinical Psychology, 59,* 594–597.

Hagglund, K. J., Clay, D. L., Frank, R. G., Beck, N. C., Kashani. J. H., Hewett, J., et al. (1994). Assessing anger expression in children and adolescents. *Journal of Pediatric Psychology, 19,* 291–304.

Kotsch, W. E., Gerbing, D. W., & Schwartz, L. E. (1982). The construct validity of the Differential Emotions Scale as adapted for children and adolescents. In C. Izard (Ed.), *Measuring emotions in infants and children* (pp. 251–278). Cambridge, UK: Cambridge University Press.

Kovacs, M., & Beck, A. (1977). An empirical clinical approach towards a definition of childhood depression. In J. G. Schulterbrandt & A. Raskin (Eds.), *Depression in children: Diagnosis, treatment and conceptual models* (pp. 1–25). New York: Raven Press.

Driving Anger Expression Inventory (DAX)

Purpose

To assess commonly used means of expressing anger while driving.

Population

Individuals that are of the appropriate age required to obtain a license to drive an automobile.

Background and Description

Sixty-two sample items relating to ways in which people express their anger while driving were created from interviews with university students, faculty members and community members. Common responses were selected for use in the Driving Anger Expression Inventory (DAX). This resulted in 49 items designed to assess the manner in which individuals express their anger while driving. The DAX contains four subscales: Verbally Aggressive Expression (12 items), Physically Aggressive Expression (11 items), Use of the Vehicle to Express Anger (11 items), and Adaptive/Constructive Expression (15 items). Respondents use a 4-point scale (1 = almost never, 4 = almost always) to indicate how often they express their anger in the specified manner while driving. Sample items follow.
- I give the other driver the finger
- I call the other driver names aloud
- I follow right behind the other driver for a long time
- I pay even closer attention to being a safe driver

Administration

The DAX requires approximately 15–20 min to complete.

Scoring

Scores are summed for the items on each of the four factors. Additionally, an aggressive expression index can be calculated by summing the scores on the items on the first three factors (all factors excluding the adaptive/constructive factor).

Interpretation

Higher scores on the factors indicate greater use of the particular expressive behavior while driving. The aggressive expression index provides information on an individual's use of various aggressive expressive behaviors while driving.

Psychometric Properties

Factor analysis. The original 62 items were used in a principal components analysis with varimax rotation. Items that loaded onto one factor .40 or greater were retained. This resulted in five factors. The factors were verbal aggressive expression, personal physical aggressive expression, use of vehicle to express anger, displaced aggression, and adaptive/constructive expression. The displaced aggression factor was dropped because it had low internal consistency and was comprised of only four items.

Reliability. The four scales of the DAX have adequate internal consistency, with Cronbach's alphas ranging from .81 (physical aggressive expression) to .90 (adaptive/constructive expression). Cronbach's alpha for the total aggressive expression index was .90.

Validity. The five scales of the DAX were submitted to correlational analyses to assess the measure's discriminant validity. The adaptive/constructive expression factor was negatively related to the other factors ($r = -.02$ to $-.22$), which was predicted given that the remaining factors were comprised of items endorsing nonadaptive forms of aggressive expression. Scores on the DAX total aggressive expression factor were significantly related to scores on other measures of driving aggression including the Driving Anger Scale ($r = .52$, DAS, pp. 53–55) and the State-Trait Anger Scale ($r = .41$, pp. 77–79) and self-reported anger experienced in ordinary traffic ($r = .19$) and heavy traffic ($r = .35$). Discriminant validity was found by correlating the aggressive expressive factors with corresponding behaviors. The verbal aggressive expression factor had the highest correlation with self-reported verbally aggressive behavior, and the use of vehicle to express aggression factor had the highest correlation with behaviors including "honked horn in anger" and "flashed lights in anger."

Clinical Utility

Moderate. The DAX can be useful for operationalizing vague complaints of "road rage"; however, the length of administration (15–20 min) may preclude repeated use with individual cases.

Research Applicability

High. The DAX is a useful measure of various types of angry and aggressive driving. It has demonstrated sound psychometric properties and is suitable for identifying risk factors for angry driving and the negative outcomes of angry driving.

Original Citation

Deffenbacher, J. L., Lynch, R. S., Oetting, E. R., & Swaim, R. C. (2002). The Driving Anger Expression Inventory: A measure of how people express their anger on the road. *Behavior Research and Therapy, 40*, 717–737.

Source

Dr. Jerry Deffenbacher, Department of Psychology, Colorado State University, 1876 Campus Delivery, Fort Collins, CO, 80523-1876, (970) 491-6871, Jerry.Deffenbacher@colostate. edu

Cost

Please contact the source (above) for permission to use the DAX.

Alternative Forms

The DAX was adapted for use in a Turkish sample of drivers (Esiyok, Yasak, & Korkusuz, 2007). This revised DAX contains 47 items and replicated the same four factors. Drivers who had a traffic offense because of running a red light, going into an oncoming lane of traffic, or exceeding the speed limit scored high on the use of physical anger expression and use of a vehicle to express anger. The revised DAX was also related to scores on the DAS (pp. 53–55), Brief Symptom Inventory (Derogatis, 1992), and Multidimensional Anger Scale (pp. 65–67).

References

Derogatis, L. R. (1992). BSI: Administration, scoring, and procedures manual-II. Towson, MD: Clinical Psychometric Research.

Esiyok, B., Yasak, Y., & Korkusuz, I. (2007). Anger expression on the road: Validity and reliability of the Driving Anger Expression Inventory. *Turkish Journal of Psychiatry, 18*, 1–12.

Driving Anger Scale (DAS)

Purpose

To measure the propensity to experience anger while driving.

Population

People who are above the legal age required to obtain a license to drive an automobile.

Background and Description

The Driving Anger Scale (DAS) was designed to measure anger that is evoked by frustrating driving conditions. Interviews with college students and faculty produced 53 driving situations that commonly evoke anger. Over 1,500 college students then rated the degree of anger provoked by each of the 53 scenarios. A cluster analysis identified six types of driving situations that lead to anger: hostile gestures, illegal driving, police presence, slow driving, discourtesy, and traffic obstructions. Item analyses identified 33 items that best measured overall driving anger and anger in response to each of the six areas of frustrating driving. The DAS asks respondents to indicate how angry they would become in response to each situation using a 5-point scale (1 = not at all, 5 = very much). Sample items are as follows.

- Someone is weaving in and out of traffic
- You are stuck in a traffic jam

Administration

The DAS is estimated to require 10–15 min to complete.

Scoring

Scores are summed for each of the six areas. A total driving anger score can also be calculated.

Interpretation

Higher scores for each of the six clusters indicate a greater amount of anger experienced in response to that specific type of driving-related problem. Higher scores on the total driving anger score indicate greater anger experienced in response to a variety of driving-related situations.

Psychometric Properties

Norms. Norms were obtained from a sample of 1,526 college freshmen (724 men, 802 women).

Cluster analysis. A cluster analysis was performed on the original 53 items and revealed six clusters: hostile gestures, illegal driving, police presence, slow driving, discourtesy, and traffic obstructions.

Reliability. Internal consistency of the six clusters was found to be adequate with Cronbach's alphas ranging from .78 (traffic obstructions) to .87 (hostile gestures).

Validity. High scores on the DAS were related to risky driving and increased numbers of accidents (Iverson & Rundmo, 2002). Scores on the DAS were significantly related ($r = .52$) to scores on the Driving Anger Expression Inventory total aggressive expression factor (pp. 51–53). Scores on the French DAS were significantly related to general anger ($r = .41$) as measured by the NEO-PI-R (Costa & McCrae, 1992).

Clinical Utility

Moderate. The DAS may be useful to assess the particular types of driving situations that are anger provoking for an individual and to evaluate the efficacy of interventions designed to reduce driving-related anger.

Research Applicability

Moderate. The DAS may be a useful tool in researching how anger relates to dangerous driving behaviors such as tailgating and speeding. The DAS may also aid in investigating other psychological correlates of driving-related anger.

Original Citation

Deffenbacher, J. L., Oetting, E. R., & Lynch, R. S. (1994). Development of a driving anger scale. *Psychological Reports, 74*, 83–91.

Source

Dr. Jerry Deffenbacher, Department of Psychology and Tri-Ethnic Center for Prevention Research, Colorado State University, Fort Collins, CO, 80523-1876, (970) 491-6871, Jerry.Deffenbacher@colostate.edu

Cost

Please contact the source (above) for permission to use the DAS.

Alternative Forms

A short form of the DAS has been created. The 14-item short DAS was developed by selecting items from each of the six previously found clusters comprising the original DAS. It has adequate internal consistency with alpha .80 and is substantially correlated with the original DAS ($r=.95$).

The DAS has been adapted for use in the UK, Norway, and France (Iverson, & Rundmo, 2002; Villieux, & Delhomme, 2007). The UK adapted DAS contains three subscales: progress impeded, reckless driving, and direct hostility. The Norway adapted DAS also contains three subscales: discourtesy, police presence and traffic obstructions, and hostile gestures. The France adaptation of the DAS has 22 items and five subscales: progress impeded, hostile gestures, illegal driving, police presence, and traffic obstructions.

References

Costa, P. T., & McCrae, R. R. (1992). *Revised NEO Personality Inventory (NEO-PI-R) and NEO Five-Factor Inventory (NEO-FFI) professional manual.* Odessa, FL: Psychological Assessment Resources.

Iverson, H., & Rundmo, T. (2002). Personality, risky driving and accident involvement among Norwegian drivers. *Personality and Individual Differences, 33,* 243–255.

Villieux, A., & Delhomme, P. (2007). Driving Anger Scale, French adaptation: Further evidence of reliability and validity. *Perceptual and Motor Skills, 104,* 947–957.

Driving Vengeance Questionnaire (DVQ)

Purpose

To assess levels of anger aroused by common, though potentially stressful, driving situations.

Population

People who drive automobiles (typically ages 16+).

Background and Description

The impetus for developing the Driving Vengeance Questionnaire (DVQ) was to measure a driver's emotional reaction in stressful, though common, driving conditions to better understand triggering incidents for aggressive responses. The DVQ consists of 37 scenarios/items that represent common driving situations in which an individual might be irritated or feel unjustly treated by another driver. Respondents are asked to indicate how they would react to each situation using a 5-point scale (1=very relaxed, 5=very angry).

Administration

The DVQ requires approximately 15–20 min to complete.

Scoring

A "Vengeance Score" is calculated from summing across the item ratings.

Interpretation

High scores indicate a greater level of anger and are interpreted as reflecting a greater potential to seek vengeance against the protagonist.

Psychometric Properties

Norms. Normative data were obtained from 266 male and female university students. The scale was subsequently administered to 271 university students (both male and female) and 74 male inmates who were classified as either violent or nonviolent offenders on the basis of the amount of force used in committing the offense that resulted in their recent incarceration.

Reliability. Cronbach's alphas for the Vengeance Scale have ranged from .81 to .83. In a separate sample of 56 drivers (28 males, 28 females), internal consistency, as measured by Cronbach's alpha, was .81.

Validity. Younger drivers (18–23 years old) have obtained higher Vengeance Scale scores than older drivers (24–66 years old). The DVQ was validated by assessing the frequency of past acts of driving aggression (Hennessy & Wiesenthal, 2001). DVQ scores correlated with self-reported driver violence, wherein vengeful drivers endorsed greater acts of past violence.

The validity of the DVQ was also evaluated in a sample of 56 drivers from Ontario, Canada. Scores on the DVQ were significantly related to the State Driver Aggression Questionnaire completed at a high congestion time ($r = .42$; Hennessy & Wiesenthal, 2001) and the Violent Driving Behavior Questionnaire ($r = .36$; Hennessy & Wiesenthal, 2001). DVQ scores were also found to be significantly predicted by history and frequency of past violent driving acts, with individuals with a history of driving-related violence receiving higher scores on the DVQ.

Clinical Utility

Moderate. The DVQ has considerable potential as a tool for screening people who may evince a propensity toward driving-related aggression.

Research Applicability

Moderate. Limited research has been conducted with this measure. However, the measure shows potential for use in research studies to examine susceptibility for driving aggression and/or vengeance.

Original Citation

Wiesenthal, D. L., Hennessy, D., & Gibson, P. M. (2000). The Driving Vengeance Questionnaire (DVQ): The development of a scale to measure deviant drivers' attitudes. *Violence and Victims, 15*(2), 115–136.

Source

David L. Wiesenthal, 288 Behavioral Science Building, York University, 4700 Keele Street, Toronto, Ontario, M3J 1P3, Canada, (416) 736-2100 ext. 30114, davidw@yorku.ca

Cost

Please contact the source (above) for permission to use the DVQ.

Reference

Hennessy, D. A., & Wiesenthal, D. L. (2001). Further validation of the Driving Vengeance Questionnaire. *Violence and Victims, 16*, 565–573.

Dundee Provocation Inventory

Purpose

To measure anger-provoking emotions in adults with intellectual disabilities.

Population

Adults with intellectual disabilities.

Background and Description

The Dundee Provocation Inventory (DPI) was developed with the assumption that anger is an emotional response to provocation and is comprised of physiological and cognitive components. As such, the 20 items on the DPI are organized into six sections that relate to emotions that may be interpreted as anger provoking: disappointment, embarrassment, jealousy, frustration, anger to self, and direct threat to self. Respondents report how they would feel in response to each situation and then report how angry they would feel using a 4-point, Likert-type scale ranging from 0 (not at all angry) to 3 (very angry). Pictures are provided that serve as scale anchors to clarify understanding for respondents.

Administration

Items can be read to respondents in order to overcome literacy deficits that are often present in individuals with intellectual disabilities.

Scoring

Scores are summed across items to calculate a total score. Scores can range from 0 to 60.

Interpretation

Higher scores indicate greater anger experienced in response to provoking situations.

Psychometric Properties

Factor analysis. An exploratory factor analysis using oblimin rotation revealed five interpretable factors that accounted for 63.8 % of the variance. The five factors were labeled: threat to self-esteem, locus of control, resentment, frustration, and rejection.

Reliability. Internal consistency, as measured by Cronbach's alpha, was .79 in the preliminary analysis sample. In a separate sample of 114 intellectually disabled individuals, Cronbach's alpha was .91 (Alder, L., & Lindsay, W. R., 2007).

Validity. The DPI was found to be significantly related to the Novaco Anger Scale ($r = .57$, pp. 67–69).

Clinical Utility

Moderate. The DPI is easy to administer and score and may be useful for assessing the effectiveness of anger treatment programs designed for individuals with intellectual disabilities. Although initial studies indicate the DPI has adequate psychometric properties, additional evidence of reliability and validity in varied samples would strengthen the clinical utility of the DPI.

Research Applicability

Moderate. The DPI may be a useful measure to investigate the types of situations that are interpreted as anger provoking for individuals with intellectual disabilities and the nature of misinterpretations that lead to anger provocation in this population. In turn, this information could aid in the development of effective treatment programs.

Original Citation

Lindsay, W. R. (2000). *The Dundee Provocation Inventory.* Unpublished manuscript, NHS Tayside

Source

Bill Lindsay, School of Health and Social Sciences, University of Abertay Dundee, Bell St, Dundee, DD1 1HG, Scotland, UK.

Cost

Please contact the source (above) for permission to use the DPI.

Reference

Alder, L., & Lindsay, W. R. (2007). Exploratory factor analysis and convergent validity of the Dundee Provocation Inventory. *Journal of Intellectual and Developmental Disability, 32*, 190–199.

Framingham Anger Scales (FAS)

Purpose

To assess anger expression and the ability to cope with anger.

Population

Adults.

Background and Description

The Framingham Psychosocial Survey is a 300-item interview measuring five areas of psychosocial stress and strain: sociodemographic situations, life events, behavior types, situational stress, and somatic strain. Items were grouped into 20 scales. The Framingham Anger Scales (FAS) were derived from the Framingham Psychosocial Survey. Items were reviewed by a panel of three outside experts, who selected items assessing a priori behavior patterns identified in the initial construction of the survey. A factor analysis was conducted and items with poor inter-item correlations, low factor loadings, and/or low item–total correlations were dropped. The Anger-In scale (FI) contains three items and assesses suppressed hostility. The Anger-Out scale (FO) contains two items and measures outward expressions of anger. The Anger-discuss scale (FD) contains two items and measures coping with anger in a socially acceptable way. An interviewer typically administers the scales with respondents asked to indicate how likely they would be to emit the specified reactions.

Administration

The FAS takes 2–3 min to complete.

Scoring

Each item is scored as either absent (0) or present (1). Scores for each scale are summed and then divided by the number of questions contained in the scale.

Interpretation

Higher scores indicate higher levels of anger-in, anger-out, and ability to effectively deal with anger.

Psychometric Properties

Reliability. Reliability estimates are not available. Internal consistency estimates are often not conducted on the FAS because of the limited number of items included in the scales (Armstead & Clark, 2002).

Validity. FI correlated positively with the anger-in subscale of the Multidimensional Anger Inventory (pp. 65–67) and was inversely related to "potential for hostility" assessed via the structured interview for Type A behavior pattern. The FI was not correlated with anger experience and hostility measured using the Multidimensional Anger Inventory, the State–Trait Anger Scale (pp. 77–80), and the Buss–Durkee Hostility Inventory (pp. 109–111). FO correlated positively with "potential for hostility" and other measures of anger experience and hostility measured by the Multidimensional Anger Inventory, the State–Trait Anger Scale, and the Buss–Durkee Hostility Inventory, but did not correlate with the FD or the Anger-out/Brooding of the Multidimensional Anger Inventory. FD correlated positively with the Anger-out subscale of the Multidimensional Anger Inventory and was inversely related to FI. FD did not correlate with measures of anger experience measured using the Multidimensional Anger Inventory and the State–Trait Anger Scale. The FI, FD, and FO scales differentiated those with coronary heart disease.

Clinical Utility

Limited. Although the FI, FO, and FD scales may be used as a quick screening device, the lack of reliability and normative data places limits on the clinical utility.

Research Applicability

Moderate. The FI, FO, and FD scales provide a quick means of assessing anger expression, but further data are needed to support the reliability and validity of these scales.

Original Citation

Haynes, S. G., Levine, S., Scotch, N., Feinleib, M., & Kannel, W. B. (1978). The relationship of psychosocial factors to coronary heart disease in the Framingham study: I. Methods and risk factors. *American Journal of Epidemiology, 107*(5), 362–383.

Source

Suzanne G. Haynes, Office on Women's Health, Department of Health and Human Services, 200 Independence Avenue, SW Room 712E, Washington, DC 20201, (202) 205-2623, Suzanne.haynes@hhs.gov

Cost

Please contact the author (above) for permission to use the FI, FO, and FD scales of the FAS.

Reference

Armstead, C. A., & Clark, R. (2002). Assessment of self-reported anger expression in pre- and early-adolescent African Americans: Psychometric considerations. *Journal of Adolescence, 25*, 365–371.

Hostile Interpretations Questionnaire (HIQ)

Purpose

To measure general levels of hostility and hostility in response to specific situations.

Population

Adult offenders.

Background and Description

Anger and hostility are variables believed to be associated with aggression that have received a lot of attention in the research community. However, most anger/hostility assessment instruments have used inconsistent definitions and have been face valid and thus prone to response bias. The Hostile Interpretations Questionnaire (HIQ) was created to address these shortcomings by providing a means of accurately assessing the concept of hostility.

The HIQ is a vignette-style questionnaire that was based on the hostile attribution bias. The hostile attribution bias is the tendency to view neutral social situations and events as threatening (as cited in Simourd & Mamuza, 2000). The HIQ contains seven vignettes that describe social situations commonly experienced by offenders. The social situations include relationships with authority figures (Authority), interpersonal relationships (Intimate/family), acquaintance relationships (Acquaintance), work relationships (Work), and stranger interactions (Anonymous)

(Simourd & Mamuza, 2000). Each vignette has five questions that are answered using a 5-point, Likert-style scale. The questions assess different components of hostility including overgeneralization, hostile attribution, personal responsibility, hostile reaction, and external blame (Simourd & Mamuza, 2000). An example for vignette and question follows.

- Fred invites a few friends to his house, and when he walks in, his common-law wife complains about how late he is.
  - How likely do you think it is that his wife always nags Fred?

Administration

The HIQ is estimated to require 10 min to complete.

Scoring

A hostility score is calculated for each type of situation, along with scores for the different components of hostility. An overall hostility score is also calculated.

Interpretation

Higher scores are associated with greater hostility.

Psychometric Properties

Reliability. The HIQ was administered to a sample of 146 male inmates at a Canadian correctional institution. Internal consistency was assessed using Cronbach's alpha for each type of situation, component of hostility, and the total score. Cronbach's alpha ranged from .42 (anonymous) to .71 (intimate/family) for the situations and .55 (overgeneralization) to .84 (external

blame) for the components of hostility. Cronbach's alpha was .86 for the total score.

Validity. The HIQ and other anger/hostility measures (Aggression Questionnaire, AQ, pp. 91–92; Novaco Anger Scale, NAS, pp. 67–69) were correlated with measures of social desirability (Paulhus Deception Scales, Paulhus 1999) to evaluate their susceptibility to response bias. All of the measures were significantly related to measures of social desirability, but the HIQ had the lowest correlations ($r = -.01$ to $-.40$).

The HIQ was correlated with other measures of anger/hostility to assess construct validity. The HIQ total score and all of the subscales, except for personal responsibility, were significantly related to the AQ anger subscale ($r = .21 - .45$) and total score ($r = .29 - .52$). The HIQ total score and the majority of the HIQ subscales were also significantly related to the AQ subscales hostility, physical aggression, and verbal aggression. These relationships remained after controlling for impression management, although at a lesser degree. The HIQ was also correlated with the NAS and similar results were found. The HIQ total score and subscales, with the exception of personal responsibility, were significantly related to the NAS cognitive ($r = .20 - .52$) and arousal ($r = .18 - .56$) subscales and the total score ($r = .18 - .59$). The HIQ total score and most of the HIQ subscales were also significantly related to the NAS behavioral subscale. These correlations remained after partialling out the effects of impression management, although to a lesser degree.

The relationship between the HIQ and external criteria were then examined to further evaluate the validity of the HIQ. The HIQ was found to be significantly related to age ($r = -.21$). The hostile reaction subscale was significantly related to number of different offenses ($r = .17$), whereas the authority subscale and intimate/family subscale were significantly correlated with misconducts ($r = .22$ and .19, respectively).

Clinical Utility

Moderate. The HIQ is brief, easy to administer, and has been shown to be less susceptible to response bias than other measures of anger and hostility. This may make the HIQ well suited for use with offender populations to identify problematic situations likely to elicit hostility or thinking errors of hostility to be targeted in treatment. It may also be useful as a measure of treatment-related changes in hostility.

Research Applicability

Moderate. The HIQ may be a useful assessment instrument for examining the relationship between anger, hostility, and aggressive behavior or criminal recidivism.

Original Citation

Mamuza, J. M., & Simourd, D. J. (1997). *The Hostile Interpretations Questionnaire.* Unpublished manual.
Simourd, D. J., & Mamuza, J. M. (2000). The Hostile Interpretations Questionnaire: Psychometric properties and construct validity. *Criminal Justice and Behavior, 27,* 645–663.

Source

Dr. David Simourd, Algonquin Correctional Evaluation Services, 86 Braemar Road, Kingston, Ontario K7M 4B6 Canada, (613) 384-6637, Fax: (613) 384-6637, dave@acesink.com

Cost

Please contact the source (above) for permission to use the HIQ.

Reference

Paulhus, D. L. (1999). *Paulhus Deception Scales.* Toronto, ON: Multi-Health Systems.

Interpersonal Process Code (IPC)

Purpose

To provide an observational code of childhood interactions.

Population

Children.

Background and Description

The Interpersonal Process Code (IPC) was developed from three decades of observational research at the Oregon Social Learning Center. The IPC was designed to assess social exchanges between two people and can be adapted to a variety of contexts. Behaviors are recorded as the interactions occur using a hand held event recorder. Each person in the interaction is assigned a number and the observer records the interactions of one individual for a 10-min interval. A five-digit entry is made for each observed behavior (initiator, content code, recipient, and emotional valence). Additionally, a toggle switch is used to record the global context of the behaviors. The interaction is coded on three dimensions: activity (i.e., the global context in which interactions occur), content (i.e., verbal, nonverbal, and physical behavior), and valence (i.e., the emotional tone accompanying the content code). Frequency is tracked each time a behavior is entered, sequence is recorded through the order in which behaviors are coded, and duration is established by the time lapse between the digit entries for each code.

Each behavior is defined, a priori, to have a positive, neutral, or negative impact on society. The following are code-able content categories: positive talk (positive verbal behaviors which do not refer directly to others involved in the interaction), talk (general conversation), negative talk (negative verbal behavior not referring directly to others involved in the interaction), positive interpersonal (verbal expression of approval of another's behavior, appearance, or state), advice (directions, instructions, or future suggestions which teach a behavior or specific skill), negative interpersonal (personalized and unqualified disapproval of a person present or a statement of unqualified negative emotion toward a person), directive (commands for behavior change which could occur within the observation), cooperative (clearly complying with another's directive), social involvement (behaviors that are interactive, but not accompanied by verbal or physical behavior), noncooperative (clearly noncompliant to another's directive), positive physical (positive and/or affectionate physical contact), physical interact (physical contact during game playing, unless this contact is unnecessarily rough or pushy), and negative physical (aversive physical contact).

Affect is coded based on facial expressions, tone of voice, and body language.

Independent affect codes are divided into the following categories: happy, caring, neutral, distress, aversive, and sad.

Activity codes for interactions on a playground include free play (unstructured play activities), participation (game with defined set of rules), parallel play (activity within 5 ft of another child, but not interacting), and alone (engaged in an activity at least 5 ft away from other children). Only one activity may be coded at a time. Activity codes for family interactions include work (household or home maintenance jobs, homework, grooming, etc.), play (activity for amusement, pleasure or diversion), read (looking at printed materials), eat (alone or with others), attend (not engaged in any activity but actively watching others in observation), and unspecified (basically inactive, involved solely in conversation, or between activities for an extended length of time).

Additionally, interactions are coded as either antisocial or neutral, providing assessment of the individual's behavior in respect to societal norms. This code should be made independent of the content codes. Activity codes for problem-solving lab tasks may also be made using the Family Process Code, which identifies the family or the group as either "on task" or "off task." The IPC manual provides detailed descriptions of all codes, as well as examples and coding numbers.

Administration

The time is dependent on the goals of the assessment.

Scoring

The computer on which codes are entered records the frequency, duration, and sequencing of the observations.

Interpretation

Interpretations are made qualitatively, based upon the research question or the clinical inquiry.

Psychometric Properties

Reliability. For two observers, the correlation of rate per minute of physical aggression was .91 for pre-intervention ratings and .88 at post-intervention ratings. In a sample of first and fifth grade children, the mean percent agreement for a laboratory task was 85 % for Content with $\kappa = .69$, and 86 % for Affect with $\kappa = .59$ (Dishion, Duncan, Eddy, Fagot, & Fetrow, 1994). In the same sample, percent agreement for playground observation was 78 % for Content with $\kappa = .67$, and 77 % for Affect with $\kappa = .48$.

Validity. Observer impressions of children's antisocial and prosocial behavior were significantly related to scores on the IPC (Dishion et al., 1994).

Clinical Utility

Moderate. The IPC provides an objective means of assessing interpersonal interactions. It is a relatively complicated system, however, that requires time to learn and normative data are not available.

Research Applicability

Moderate. The IPC requires time to learn and little information is available on its psychometric properties. It is, however, adaptable for specific research purposes, provides an objective means for scoring naturalistic observations, and is valuable in examining peer interactions.

Original Citation

Rusby, J., Estes, A., & Dishion, T. J. (1991). *The Playground Code (PGC): Observing School Children at Play.* Unpublished training manual, Oregon Social Learning Center, Eugene, OR.

Source

Oregon Social Learning Center, 160 E. 4th Street, Eugene, OR 97401-2426. The manual is also available online at: http://www.oslc.org/resources/codemanuals/interpersonalprocess-code.pdf

Cost

Please contact the Oregon Social Learning Center for additional information.

Reference

Dishion, T. J., Duncan, T. E., Eddy, J. M., Fagot, B. I., & Fetrow, R. (1994). The world of parents and peers: Coercive exchanges and children's social adaptation. *Social Development, 3*, 255–268.

Lack of Frustration Tolerance Scale (LFTS)

Purpose

To assess levels of impatience and irritability.

Population

Adolescents and adults.

Background and Description

The Lack of Frustration Tolerance Scale (LFTS) is a 3-item self-report measure designed to assess an individual's level of impatience and irritability.

Administration

The LFTS is estimated to take 1–2 min to complete.

Scoring

The score for each item is summed to create a total score.

Interpretation

A greater number of items endorsed indicate greater levels of impatience and irritability.

Psychometric Properties

Reliability. Internal consistency, measured by Cronbach's alpha is estimated at .59. In a sample of 106 college women, Cronbach's alpha was .82 (Harris, 1997). Test–retest reliability was .84 and .64 at 4 and 6 months, respectively.

Validity. Scores on the LFTS were significantly related ($r = .28$) to level of testosterone in a sample of 54 boys ages 15–17. LFTS scores in a sample of college women were found to be significantly related to various measures associated with aggression such as physical aggression ($r = .38$), hostility ($r = .50$), and anger ($r = .53$). Scores were also highly related to a measure of impatience ($r = .94$) (Harris, 1997; Olweus, 1986).

Clinical Utility

Limited. The scale provides a quick means of assessing frustration tolerance, but normative data are unavailable and additional information on the psychometric properties is needed.

Research Applicability

Moderate. The scale provides an easy means of assessing frustration tolerance in individuals. However, more data is needed on the psychometric properties of the scale.

Original Citation

Olweus, D., Mattsson, A., Schalling, D., & Low, H. (1980). Testosterone, aggression, physical, and personality dimensions in normal adolescent males. *Psychosomatic Medicine, 42*, 253–269.

Source

Dan Olweus, Research Centre for Health Promotion, (HEMIL), University of Bergen, Bergen, Norway, Phone: +47 55 58 23 27, Olweus@uni.no

Cost

Please contact the source (above) for permission to use.

References

Harris, J. A. (1997). A further evaluation of the Aggression Questionnaire: Issues of validity and reliability. *Behavior Research and Therapy, 35*, 1047–1053.
Olweus, D. (1986). Aggression and hormones: Behavioral relationships with testosterone and adrenaline. In D. Olweus, J. Block & M. Radke-Yarrow (Eds.), *Development of antisocial and prosocial behavior: Research, theories, and issues* (pp. 51–72). Orlando, FL: Academic Press.

Low Self-Control Scale (LSCS)

Purpose

To assess levels of self-control.

Population

Adults.

Background and Description

Items on the Low Self-Control Scale (LSCS) were derived from the definition of self-control proposed by Gottfredson and Hirschi (1990). The definition identifies low self-control as being related to impulse regulation, a preference for simple rather than complex tasks, risk seeking, a preference for physical rather than cognitive activity, a self-centered orientation, and a volatile temper linked to a low tolerance for frustration. These components are hypothesized to load on a single dimension of low self-control.

The LSCS contains 23 items. Some of the items were modified from the self-control subscale of the California Psychological Inventory (Gough, 1975). The scale contains the following six components: impulsivity, simple tasks, risk seeking, physical activities, self-centeredness, and temper. The physical activity component contains three items, whereas the remaining components contain four items. Respondents rate each item using a 4-point scale ranging from "strongly disagree" to "strongly agree."

Administration

The LSCS is estimated to require 5–10 min to complete.

Scoring

Responses to items are summed to calculate a component and a total score.

Interpretation

Higher scores are indicative of lower levels of self-control.

Psychometric Properties

Factor analysis. A principal components analysis of the original 24 items produced ambiguous results. Resulting six, five, and one-factor solutions were examined, with a one-factor solution representing the best fit. The authors, however, encouraged replication of the data from other samples and the development of other items to test the unidimensionality of the scale.

Reliability. The LSCS scale had a Cronbach's alpha coefficient of .81.

Validity. The factor analysis of the items provides some evidence that the six components of the scale are reflective of a single, one-dimensional trait.

Clinical Utility

Limited. The lack of validity research and normative data limit the clinical utility of the scale. Nonetheless, the content of the scale does tap components that have some support for being related to antisocial behavior, at least as defined by Gottfredson and Hirschi (1990).

Research Applicability

Moderate. There are few theoretically derived measures of self-control. More research on the scale and the construct of low self-control, as represented by the scale, would be useful.

Original Citation

Grasmick, H. G., Tittle, C. R., Bursik, R. J., Jr., & Arneklev, B. J. (1993). Testing the core empirical implications of Gottfredson and Hirschi's general theory of crime. *Journal of Research in Crime and Delinquency, 30*(1), 5–29.

Source

Harold G. Grasmick, 780 Van Vleet Oval, Kaufman Hall 331, Norman, OK 73019, hgrasmick@ou.edu

Cost

Please contact the source (above) for permission to use the LSCS.

References

Gough, H. G. (1975). *Manual for the California Psychological Inventory*. Palo Alto, CA: Consulting Psychologists Press.
Gottfredson, M. R., & Hirschi, T. (1990). *A general theory of crime*. Palo Alto, CA: Stanford University Press.

Multidimensional Anger Inventory (MAI)

Purpose

To measure multidimensional aspects of the anger construct.

Population

Adults.

Background and Description

The Multidimensional Anger Inventory (MAI) was developed to better evaluate the variety of dimensions associated with anger, particularly those relevant for cardiovascular disease. The MAI consists of 38 items selected to reflect various dimensions of anger. Some of the items were adapted from existing anger inventories and were rephrased. Other items were developed specifically for the MAI.

The 38 items contained in the MAI assess anger frequency (5 items), duration (2 items), magnitude (4 items), mode of expression (12 items), hostile outlook (6 items), and range of anger eliciting situations (9 items). Mode of expression is further divided into five related dimensions: anger-in (6 items), anger-out (5 items), guilt (2 items), brooding (4 items), and anger-discuss (1-item). Respondents rate each statement using a scale that ranges from 1 (completely undescriptive) to 5 (completely descriptive). Sample items are reprinted below.

- I try to get even when I'm angry with someone.
- I can make myself angry about something in the past just by thinking about it.
- I get so angry, I feel like I might lose control.

Administration

The MAI is estimated to require 10–15 min to complete.

Scoring

MAI scale scores are computed by summing responses to the relevant items. A total score can be computed from summing scale scores.

Interpretation

Higher scores indicate greater problems with anger.

Psychometric Properties

Norms. The MAI was initially administered to 198 male and female college students and to 288 male factory workers. The college students also completed three existing anger inventories so that comparisons could be made between the dimensions of the MAI and scores derived from existing anger inventories.

Factor analysis. All scale items, excluding the mode of expression items, were included in one-factor analysis. The mode of expression items were examined in a separate factor analysis because the authors hypothesized that mode of expression may itself include several dimensions. The factor structure for both samples resulted in a three-factor solution that was labeled anger-arousal, anger-eliciting situations, and hostile outlook. Factor analysis of the mode of expression items yielded two factors which were labeled anger-in and anger-out. Psychometric properties of the MAI were also examined in a sample of 372 male inmates (Kroner, Reddon, & Serin, 1992). Factor analysis resulted in a two-factor solution and the factors were labeled arousal/ experience and range of anger-eliciting interpersonal situations.

Reliability. A subgroup of the 60 college students completed a second MAI 3–4 weeks after the initial administration; the test–retest reliability was .75. With the exception of the alpha coefficient (.41) for the anger-out dimension in the factory sample, all of the factor-derived scales showed acceptable levels of reliability ($\alpha = .51-.83$). The overall alpha coefficient was .84 for the college sample and .89 for the factory sample. Alpha coefficients for the resulting factors and full scale scores in a sample of 372 inmates ranged from .85 to .93.

Validity. Correlations were computed among college student responses to the Harburg (Harburg et al., 1973), Novaco Anger Scale (pp. 67–69), and the Buss–Durkee Hostility Inventory (pp. 109–111), and the factor-derived MAI scales. Factor-derived MAI scales showed the expected pattern of relations with these measures.

In a sample of 52 gay couples, self-report scores on the MAI were significantly related to partner-reported psychological abuse as measured by the Psychological Maltreatment Inventory ($r = .40$, pp. 216–218). MAI scores were not significantly correlated with partner-reported physical abuse as measured by the Conflict Tactics Scale ($r = .18$, $p > .05$; pp. 177–180) (Landolt & Dutton, 1997).

Clinical Utility

High. The MAI possesses acceptable psychometric properties, provides a wealth of information related to understanding multiple dimensions of anger, and is relatively easy to administer and score. The MAI has been used with samples of depressed patients, Vietnam Veterans with PTSD, chronic pain patients, and an inmate sample.

Additional normative data would help with score interpretation.

Research Applicability

High. The MAI has been used in a number of research projects and is relatively brief and easy to score.

Original Citation

Siegel, J. M. (1986). The Multidimensional Anger Inventory. *Journal of Personality and Social Psychology, 51,* 191–200.

Source

Judith M. Siegel, Department of Community Health Sciences, UCLA School of Public Health, PO Box 951772, Los Angeles, CA 90095, jmsiegel@ucla.edu

Cost

Please contact the source (above) for permission to use the MAI.

References

Harburg, E., Erfurt, J. C., Hauenstein, L. S., Chape, C., Schull, W. J., Schork, M. A. (1973). Socio-ecological stress, suppressed hostility, skin color, and black-white male blood pressure: Detroit. *Psychosomatic Medicine, 35,* 276–296.

Kroner, D. G., Reddon, J. R., & Serin, R. C. (1992). The Multidimensional Anger Inventory: Reliability and factor structure in an inmate sample. *Educational and Psychological Measurement, 52,* 687–693.

Landolt, M. A., & Dutton, D. G. (1997). Power and personality: An analysis of gay male intimate abuse. *Sex Roles, 37,* 335–359.

Novaco Anger Scale (NAS)

Purpose

To assess the experience of anger.

Population

Ages 9 and older.

Background and Description

The Novaco Anger Scale (NAS) was based on the theory that anger is a subjective emotional state that includes physiological arousal, the cognitive labeling of that arousal, and a behavioral reaction. The measure was designed to assist with understanding the risk of violence and help with the evaluation of treatments for anger and aggression. Earlier versions of the NAS include the Novaco Anger Inventory, also known as the Provocation Inventory (Novaco, 1975). The NAS consists of two separate components. Part A, the Reaction to Provocation component, is purported to guide the understanding of anger and aggression linked to cognitive, arousal, and behavioral domains. Part B, the Index of Anger component, prompts individuals to describe anger experiences related to specific situations.

The Reactions to Provocations component of the NAS contains 48 items divided into three domains that are further divided into four subdomains. The Cognitive Domain contains subscales that assess attention, rumination, hostile attitude, and suspicion. The Arousal Domain contains subscales that assess intensity, duration, somatic tension, and irritability. Finally, the Behavioral

Domain contains subscales that assess impulsiveness, verbal aggression, physical confrontation, and indirect expression. The Index of Anger component of the NAS contains 25 items that describe situations in which individuals may become angry. These items are grouped into five subscales that summarize the nature of the provocation: disrespectful treatment, unfairness/injustice, frustration/interruptions, annoying traits, and irritations.

Administration

The NAS can typically be completed within 30 min.

Scoring

Scores assigned to each item are summed to provide total, scale, and subscale scores. Some items require reverse scoring.

Interpretation

Higher scores indicate greater problems within each of the domains sampled.

Psychometric Properties

Norms. Novaco (1994) published information on the psychometric properties of the NAS. Normative data were originally collected from a state hospital sample ($N=142$) and a student sample ($N=171$).

Reliability. Cronbach's alpha estimates of internal consistency for scale scores have ranged from .92 (Part A) to .97 (Part B). Estimates for some of the individual subscale scores have been less impressive. Two-week test–retest reliability

estimates for the scale scores have ranged from .72 to .86. A sample of 204 corrections clients obtained 1-month test–retest coefficients that ranged from .78 to .91 (Mills, Kroner, & Forth, 1998).

Validity. Using a state hospital sample, the total score on the NAS correlated .84 with the State–Trait Anger Expression Inventory (STAXI) (pp. 74–77) and .82 with the Buss–Durkee Hostility Inventory (pp. 109–111). Using an offender sample, Williams, Boyd, Cascardi, and Poythress (1996) found the Aggression Questionnaire (pp. 91–92) correlated .71, .74, and .82 with the NAS cognitive, arousal, and behavioral domains, respectively. Moderate to high correlations with other anger-related measures have been demonstrated. For instance, Mills, Kroner, and Forth (1998) used correctional offenders to further assess concurrent validity with three anger/aggression measures and clinical ratings along eight anger dimensions. Jones, Thomas-Peter, and Trout (1999) found that the NAS correctly classified 212 nonclinical sample subjects and 58 outpatient anger-management referrals with 94 % accuracy.

Clinical Utility

High. The NAS possesses acceptable psychometric characteristics and has been used frequently with violent populations. The resulting descriptive information can assist with developing interventions to target the areas of arousal, cognitions, behaviors, and situations related to anger and aggression. Some normative data are available.

Research Applicability

High. The NAS has been widely used and studied within a number of violent and nonviolent populations and taps domains likely to be of interest to researchers.

Original Citation

Novaco, R. W. (1994). Anger as a risk factor for violence among the mentally disordered. In J. Monahan & H. Steadman (Eds.), *Violence and mental disorder: Developments in risk assessment* (pp. 21–59). Chicago: University of Chicago Press.

Novaco, R. M. (1994). *Novaco Anger Scale and Provocation Inventory: Manual.* Los Angeles, CA: Western Psychological Services.

Source

Raymond W. Novaco, University of California – Irvine, School of Social Ecology, 3385 Social Ecology II, Irvine, CA 92697, (949) 824-7206, rwnovaco@uci.edu

The NAS may be purchased from Western Psychological Services, 12031 Wilshire Blvd., Los Angeles, CA 90025-1251, (800) 648-8857, Fax: (310) 478-7838, http://portal.wpspublish.com/portal/page?_pageid=53,70332&_dad=portal&_schema=PORTAL

Cost

The Novaco Anger Scale kit, which includes 25 autoscore forms and a manual, can be purchased from Western Psychological Services for $92.

References

Jones, J. P., Thomas-Peter, B. A., & Trout, A. (1999). Normative data for the Novaco Anger Scale from a non-clinical sample and implications for clinical use. *British Journal of Clinical Psychology, 38,* 417–424.

Mills, J. F., Kroner, D. G., & Forth, A. E. (1998). Novaco Anger Scale: Reliability and validity within an adult criminal sample. *Assessment, 5,* 237–248.

Novaco, R. W. (1975). *Anger control: The development and evaluation of an experimental treatment.* Lexington, MA: Lexington Books.

Williams, T. Y., Boyd, J. C., Cascardi, M. A., & Poythress, N. (1996). Factor structure and convergent validity of the Aggression Questionnaire in an offender population. *Psychological Assessment, 8,* 398–403.

Pediatric Anger Expression Scale: Third Edition (PAES-III)

Purpose

To measure styles of anger expression in children.

Population

Children and adolescents.

Background and Description

The Pediatric Anger Expression Scale—Third Edition (PAES-III) was based on the multidimensional model of anger expression used for the State–Trait Anger Expression Inventory (pp. 74–77). The PAES-III contains 15 statements that are organized into three scales: anger-in, anger-out, and anger control. A 3-point scale, ranging from 1 (hardly ever) to 3 (often) is used to rate the frequency with which children use the strategy identified in the statement when angered.

Administration

The PAES-III is estimated to take 3–7 min to complete.

Scoring

Scores for anger-in, anger-out, and anger control are obtained by summing item scores within each scale. An overall anger expression score is obtained by summing the anger-in and anger-out scores and then subtracting the anger control score.

Interpretation

Higher scores on the anger-in and anger-out scales indicate the respondent is more likely to suppress anger or overtly express it, respectively. Higher scores on the anger control scale indicate greater control of one's anger.

Psychometric Properties

Factor analysis. Studies employing principal components analyses with varimax rotation have supported a three (anger-in, anger-out, and anger control) or four factor solution (anger-in, anger-out, anger control, and anger distraction).

Reliability. Internal consistency estimates ranged from .62 to .78 for anger-in, .72–.77 for anger-out, and .54–.71 for anger control. An internal consistency estimate using a sample of Native American children revealed a coefficient of .28 for the anger control factor. Stability coefficients ranged from .45 (anger-in) to .61 (anger control) for a 1-year interval.

Validity. Scores on the PAES-III were moderately correlated with self, peer and teacher ratings of anger expression. Anger-out scores correlated with scores on the Differential Emotions Scale-IV Anger and Hostility Scales (DES-IV, pp. 50–51) and the Child Behavior Checklist Aggressive subscale (CBCL, Achenbach & Edelbrock, 1983). Anger-in correlated negatively with the DES-IV Anger Scale. Anger control correlated negatively with scores on the DES-IV Anger and Hostility Scales and the CBCL Aggressive subscale. Moderate correlations were found between the PAES-III and measures of anxiety and Type A behavior. Strong correlations were found between the subscales of the PAES-III and the corresponding subscales of the Anger Expression Scale (pp. 28–30) (Musante et al., 1999).

Clinical Utility

Moderate. The PAES-III is an efficient means of assessing the prominent style of anger expres-sion in children. Instructions and items can be administered in verbal or written formats. Additional normative data are needed prior to the widespread adoption of the PAES-III in clinical settings.

Research Applicability

Moderate. The PAES-III is time efficient in terms of administration and scoring, and instructions and items can be presented in verbal or written formats.

Original Citation

Jacobs, G. A., Phelps, M., & Rohrs, B. (1989). Assessment of anger expression in children: The Pediatric Anger Expression Scale. *Personality and Individual Differences, 10*(1), 59–65.

Source

Gerard A. Jacobs, Disaster Mental Health Institute, South Dakota Union 114, University of South Dakota, 414 E. Clark Street, Vermillion, SD 57069, gerard.jacobs@usd.edu

Cost

Please contact the source (above) for permission to use the PAES-III.

References

Achenbach, T. M., & Edelbrock, C. (1983). *Manual for the Child Behavior Checklist.* Burlington: University of Vermont.

Hagglund, K. J., et al. (1994). Assessing anger expression in children and adolescents. *Journal of Pediatric Psychology, 19*, 291–304.

Musante, L., Treiber, F. A., Davis, H. C., Waller, J. L., & Thompson, W. O. (1999). Assessment of self-reported anger expression in youth. *Assessment, 6*, 225–233.

Picture Frustration Study (PFS)

Purpose

To assess thought content in response to frustration.

Population

Adults.

Background and Description

The Picture Frustration Study (PFS) resembles the Thematic Apperception Test (Murray, 1943); the PFS uses pictures as stimuli. The assumption is that respondents identify with the frustrated individual in each situation and subsequently project their own perceptual responses. The pictorial stimuli are composed of 24 cartoon-like pictures that portray two individuals engaged in a mildly stressful, though common, situation. One figure is shown saying certain words that help to describe the frustration of the other individual. The other person, whose facial expressions are omitted, is shown with a blank caption box above. Respondents are asked to fill in the blank box. After completing each situation respondents can be asked to read their response aloud to include vocal cadence and tone in the scoring (e.g., use of sarcasm).

Situations represent either an obstacle that directly frustrates the story character or the story character dealing with accusations of misbehavior. Responses are coded into six categories: aggression directed toward the personal or impersonal environment; overt aggression directed against the self; evasion or avoidance of aggression; dealing with an obstacle; attributions of responsibility; and movement toward a solution. Scoring categories can be combined to produce a variety of different factors.

Administration

The PFS is estimated to require 20–30 min to complete.

Scoring

Scores are typically assigned within two broad dimensions representing the focus and type of aggression.

Interpretation

Scores reflect the direction and type of aggression used when dealing with two types of frustrating situations.

Psychometric Properties

Reliability. Split-half reliability was calculated by correlating the odd-numbered items with the even numbered items to assess internal consistency of the categories. After correcting correlations for attenuation using the Spearman-Brown Prophecy formula, coefficients for males ranged from .06 to .47 whereas coefficients for females ranged from .04 to .56. Cohen's Kappa was used to assess interrater agreement across two judges and revealed a median value of .40, with a range of .06–.62. Test–retest reliability for 2 and 7.5-month intervals for males ranged from .34 to .71, respectively, and for females ranged from .34 to .62, respectively. For two pictures, single item 1-month test–retest reliabilities were .54 and .57.

Validity. Coded categories correlated with comparable measures from the Thematic Apperception Test. Scores also correlated with scale scores on the Buss–Durkee Hostility Inventory (pp. 109–111). Exposure to stress led to measurable changes in scores on the PFS and physiological correlates were found for scores on direction of aggression. In a sample of normals, chronic alcoholics, and paranoid schizophrenics, PFS scores demonstrated some discriminating capacity in the form of trends but did not reveal any clear-cut differences between groups.

Clinical Utility

Limited. The PFS may provide insight into the direction and type of aggression used by individuals in frustrating situations. The lack of clear normative data in combination with the available psychometric data make interpretation difficult.

Research Applicability

Limited. Several researchers have questioned the theoretical validity of the instrument, and correlations between the PFS and other instruments are low. Nonetheless, the use of the instrument as an analog measure to assess thoughts elicited within each of the frustrating situations could prove useful.

Original Citation

Rosenzweig, S. (1945). The picture-association method and its application in a study of reactions to frustration. *Journal of Personality, 14*, 3–23.

Source

Rosenzweig, S. (1945). The picture-association method and its application in a study of reactions to frustration. *Journal of Personality, 14*, 3–23.

Cost

Unavailable.

Alternative Forms

The PFS has been adapted for use with children and adolescents.

Reference

Murray, H. A. (1943). *Thematic apperception test.* Cambridge, MA: Harvard University Press.

The Reaction Inventory (RI)

Purpose

To assess the degree of arousal associated with anger-provoking situations.

Population

Adults.

Background and Description

The Reaction Inventory (RI) was based on the proposition that the relationship between anger and aggression is an analog to the relationship between anxiety and avoidance. Similar to anxiety, anger was postulated as a stimulus-specific emotional reaction and, like avoidance, aggression was considered modifiable through the use of reciprocal inhibition. The RI was designed as a clinical instrument that could be used to identify relevant situational determinants. Respondents use a 5-point scale to rate the degree to which 76 rationally derived situations are likely to elicit anger (1 = not at all, 5 = very much).

Administration

The RI is estimated to take 15–20 min to complete.

Scoring

Ratings for each of the 76 items are summed to derive a total score.

Interpretation

Higher scores indicate higher degrees of anger.

Psychometric Properties

Norms. Norms were obtained from 275 participants from four different samples (29 females and 16 males from a summer school undergraduate course, 21 females and 10 males in a regular undergraduate course, 108 females and 30 males in a regular undergraduate course, and 33 females and 28 male non-university students). Median ages for the samples were 25, 22, 18, and 26, respectively. Median educations for the latter three samples were 15, 13, and 14 years, respectively.

Factor analyses. A principal component analysis revealed ten factors: minor chance annoyances, destructive people, unnecessary delays, inconsiderate people, self-opinionated people, frustration in business, criticism, major chance annoyances, people being personal, and authority.

Reliability. Internal consistency for the 76 items was estimated at .95. Two-week test–retest reliability for a sample of 28 male and 32 female undergraduate students was .70.

Validity. Scores on the RI correlated positively with the Assault, Indirect, Irritability, Negativism, Resentment, Verbal, and Guilt subscales of the Buss–Durkee Hostility Inventory (BDHI. pp. 109–111), the total score on the BDHI (for three independent samples), the Awareness, General, Physical, Verbal, and Mistrust scales of the Anger Self-Report (ASR, pp. 33–35), and the total score of the ASR. The RI correlated negatively with social desirability. In a different sample, the RI correlated positively with verbal antagonism and physical antagonism, and correlated negatively with constructive action.

Clinical Utility

Moderate. The RI offers clinicians a thorough and nonintrusive means of identifying anger-eliciting situations that may be targeted in treatment. The lack of normative data for clinical samples limits the ability of the RI to identify clinically significant reactions.

Research Applicability

Moderate. The RI may be valuable in identifying anger-eliciting situations and exploring how these situations relate to the use of aggression.

Original Citation

Evans, D. R., & Stangeland, M. (1971). Development of the Reaction Inventory to measure anger. *Psychological Reports, 29*, 412–414.

Source

ASIS National Auxiliary Publications Service, c/o CCM Information Corp., 909 Third Ave., 21st Floor, New York, NY 10022.

Cost

Contact the source (above) for permission to use the RI.

Reference

Biaggio, M. K., Supplee, K., & Curtis, N. (1981). Reliability and validity of four anger scales. *Journal of Personality Assessment, 45*(6), 639–648.

State–Trait Anger Expression Inventory (STAXI)

Purpose

To measure "the experience and expression of anger."

Population

Ages 13 and older.

Background and Description

The State–Trait Anger Expression Inventory (STAXI) reflects the multidimensional nature of anger as expression style, emotion, and trait. The scale is a composite of the State–Trait Anger Scale (pp. 77–79) and the Anger Expression Scale (pp. 28–30). Constructs measured by the STAXI include trait anger (comprised of anger temperament and anger reaction), state anger, and anger expression (comprised of anger-in, anger-out, and anger control).

The STAXI is a 44-item self-report measure assessing components of anger, including dimensions of control and frequency of expressed anger. Written at a fifth-grade reading level, the instrument consists of six scales: State Anger (10 items), Trait Anger (10 items), Anger-In (8 items), Anger-Out (8 items), and Anger-Control (8 items). The latter three scales make up the Anger Expression Scale. The two subscales are derived from the Trait Anger scale: Anger Temperament and Anger Reaction.

Instructions are given in three parts and ask respondents to answer questions about "How I feel right now" (10 items), "How I generally feel" (10 items), and "When angry or furious" (24 items). Respondents are asked to rate their responses on a 4-point Likert-type scale, ranging from "not at all" to "almost always."

Administration

The STAXI takes approximately 10–12 min to complete.

Scoring

Scoring may be completed by hand or machine and takes approximately 5 min or less to complete. Machine-scored tests must be sent to the publisher and are returned with percentiles and T-scores. All raw scores are transformed into T-scores and percentiles. Eight scores are obtained from the STAXI: State Anger, Trait Anger, Angry Temperament, Angry Reaction, Anger-In, Anger-Out, Anger Control, and Anger Expression.

Interpretation

Higher scores on the Trait-Anger scale of the STAXI are indicative of a higher predisposition to anger, and higher scores on the State Anger scale are indicative of higher levels of anger while completing the inventory. Higher scores on Angry Temperament reflect greater likelihood to become angry, independent of the provocation. Higher scores on Angry Reaction reflect a tendency to become angry in response to criticism or unfair treatment. Higher scores on the Anger-In scale indicate the individual is more likely to suppress anger; higher scores on the Anger-Out scale indicate greater likelihood of directing the anger towards a person or object in the environment. Higher scores on Anger Control scale reflect more attempts to control the expression of anger, whereas higher scores on the Anger Expression scale are indicative of more expressed anger, regardless of whether it is suppressed (anger-in) or directed toward an object (anger-out).

Scores should be compared with the appropriate scale norms. Percentile ranks between the 25th and 75th percentiles are considered in the normal range, with scores above the 75th percentile indicating that anger may interfere with optimal functioning.

Psychometric Properties

Norms. Norms were developed from a sample of over 9,000 individuals. Separate norms are provided in the STAXI manual for gender, and adolescents, college, and adult populations. Norms have been criticized for an overrepresentation of African-American students in the adolescent sample, little ethnicity and racial data for other norms, and an adult and college sample comprised mostly of individuals from the National Defense University and the US Military Academy.

Factor analysis. In a sample of 655 women and 606 men (mean ages of 45 and 49 years, respectively), an exploratory factor analysis revealed seven factors: state anger, feel-like-expressing-anger, trait anger reaction, trait anger temperament, anger-out, anger-in, and anger control. A confirmatory factor analysis, using structural equation modeling with cross-validation procedures to examine six and seven-factor models, revealed that the seven-factor model had the best fit across gender.

In a sample of 714 undergraduate students, male and female scores underwent separate principal-components analyses. For both genders, six factors were obtained: state anger, trait anger temperament, anger control, anger-in, anger-out, and trait anger reaction. For men, the seventh factor was difficult to interpret. For women, the seventh factor appeared to be a second state anger factor, labeled "feel like expressing anger." A principal components analysis for the ten state anger items revealed two factors: feel angry and feel like expressing anger.

In a sample of 455 undergraduate students, a principal-components analysis revealed seven factors: state anger, anger control, anger-in, anger-out, trait temperament, trait reaction, and an uninterpretable factor. In another sample of college students, seven factors were again obtained, the first six corresponding to five of the six primary scales (with trait temperament and trait reaction loading on separate factors). The seventh factor appeared to be a second state anger factor, representing the instigation to express angry feelings in aggressive behavior (see Forgays, Forgays, & Spielberger, 1997; Forgays, Spielberger, Ottaway, & Forgays, 1998; Fuqua, Leonard, Masters, Smith, Campbell, & Fischer, 1991).

Reliability. Internal consistency was measured using Cronbach's alpha. The STAXI manual reported alphas for state anger and trait anger ranging from .84 to .93, .84 to .89 for trait temperament and .73 to .85 for the anger expression scales. Reported alpha values for the scales have ranged from .69 to .94 in a sample of 1,010 adults. In this sample, for undergraduate students and navy recruits, alpha values were .90 or higher on the state anger scale, .82–.89 for the trait-anger and trait temperament scales, and .70 for trait reaction.

In a sample of 455 undergraduate students, alpha values were .91 (state anger), .82 (trait anger), .85 (trait temperament), .73 (trait reaction), .76 (anger-in), .75 (anger-out), .82 (anger control), and .58 (anger expression). In a sample of 968 participants, alpha values for males, females, Chinese, Indian, and Malay individuals ranged from .87 to .94 (state anger), .82 to .85 (trait anger), .81 to .87 (trait temperament), .72 to .76 (trait reaction), .84 to .86 (anger control), .68 to .72 (anger-in), .66 to .77 (anger-out), and .73 to .78 (anger expression). In a sample of 1,235 university students, high school students, Pilot Academy Recruits, and Police Academy Recruits, alpha values ranged from .66 (anger-in, female high school students) to .94 (state anger, female high school students).

In a sample of 968 participants, who were predominantly Chinese, test–retest values for males and females, respectively, were .05 and −.09 (state anger), .71 and .75 (trait anger), .74 and .76 (anger temperament), .48 and .55 (anger reaction), .63 and .79 (anger control), .81 and .82 (anger-in), .64 and .92 (anger-out), and .86 and .92 (anger expression). Test–retest values in a different sample for a 2-week period ranged from .64 (trait reaction) to .84 (anger-out), except for state anger (.01). For a 4-week period, values ranged from .52 (anger control) to .75 (trait anger), except for state anger (.17). Other research has indicated that test–retest values for undergraduates over a 2-week period ranged from .62 to .81.

Validity. All items have been found to have a high degree of face validity. In a sample of 137 male sex offenders, correlations between scales ranged from .27 to .62, with the exception of the trait anger, trait temperament, and trait reaction scales, whose interscale correlations were in the .80s. Scores for this group were similar to those of normal adult males, with the exception of state anger. State anger scores were higher, corresponding to scores at the 85th percentile in normal males. The authors further reported that mean scores for sex offenders were relatively low in comparison to median scores of prison inmates; authors provided T-score conversions from raw scores, defining scores of 65 or higher as significantly high (Dalton, Blain, & Bezier, 1998; Foley, Hartman, Dunn, Smith, & Goldberg, 2002).

In a study of predominantly Chinese participants, all STAXI scales for females, and all but one scale for males, correlated with the Cook & Medley Hostility Scale (pp. 48–50). State anger correlated positively with the number of diseases, and disease score on the Seriousness of Illness Rating Scale (Wyler, Masuda, & Holmes, 1968), and scores on the Pennebaker Inventory of Limbic Languidness (PILL, Pennebaker, 1982). Trait anger scores correlated positively with the number of diseases, disease scores, and the PILL, and negatively with diastolic blood pressure. Trait temperament correlated positively with number of diseases, disease scores, and the PILL, and correlated negatively with systolic blood pressure. Anger reaction scores correlated positively with number of diseases, disease scores, and scores on the PILL. Anger-out correlated with number of diseases, disease scores, diastolic blood pressure and the PILL and correlated negatively with systolic blood pressure. Anger-in scores correlated with number of diseases, disease scores, and the PILL. Anger control correlated positively with systolic blood pressure. Anger expression scores correlated positively with number of diseases, disease scores, and PILL scores and negatively with systolic blood pressure (see Spielberger, Sydeman, Owen, & Marsh, 1999).

Clinical Utility

High. The STAXI is an efficient measure used to assess various components of anger. A drawback to using the STAXI is the lack of a validity scale; the high face validity of the instrument may makes it easy to fake either bad or good.

Research Applicability

High. Critics have noted that scores are positively skewed on both the state and trait anger scores, which may prevent discrimination among those with low scores. The STAXI has been successfully used in many studies to investigate cognitive correlates of anger (e.g., behavior, attitudes, and cognitions of anger-prone individuals), and to examine the relationships among anger, anger themes, gender, and age.

Original Citation

Spielberger, C. D. (1988). *State-Trait Anger Expression Inventory: STAXI Professional Manual.* Odessa, FL: Psychological Assessment Resources.
Spielberger, C. D., Krasnor, S., & Solomon, E. (1988). The experience, expression, and control of anger (pp. 89–108). In M. P. Janisse (Ed.), *Health psychology: Individual differences and stress.* New York: Springer-Verlag.

Source

Psychological Assessment Resources, Inc., 16204 N. Florida Ave, Lutz, FL 33549, 1-800-331-8378, Fax: 1-800-727-9329, http://www3.parinc.com/products/product.aspx?Productid=STAXI-2

Cost

An introductory kit including manual, 25 reusable item booklets, 50 rating sheets, and 50 profile forms, costs $248 from PAR.

Alternative Forms

A Russian version has been found to have a similar factorial model and adequate to good internal consistencies for all scales except the Anger-In scale.

References

Dalton, J. E., Blain, G. H., & Bezier, B. (1998). State-Trait Anger Expression Inventory scores of male sexual offenders. *International Journal of Offender Therapy and Comparative Criminology, 42*(2), 140–147.

Foley, P. F., Hartman, B. W., Dunn, A. B., Smith, J. E., & Goldberg, D. M. (2002). The utility of the State-Trait Anger Expression Inventory with offenders. *International Journal of Offender Therapy and Comparative Criminology, 46*(3), 364–378.

Forgays, D. G., Forgays, D. K., & Spielberger, C. D. (1997). Factor structure of the State-Trait Anger Expression Inventory. *Journal of Personality Assessment, 69*(3), 497–507.

Forgays, D. K., Spielberger, C. D., Ottaway, S. A., & Forgays, D. G. (1998). Factor structure of the State-Trait Anger Expression Inventory for middle-aged men and women. *Assessment, 5*(2), 141–155.

Fuqua, D. R., Leonard, E., Masters, M. A., Smith, R. J., Campbell, J. L., & Fischer, P. C. (1991). A structural analysis of the State-Trait Anger Expression Inventory. *Educational and Psychological Measurement, 51,* 439–446.

Pennebaker, J.W. (1982). *The psychology of physical symptoms.* New York: Springer.

Spielberger, C. D., Sydeman, S. J., Owen, A. E., & Marsh, B. J. (1999). Measuring anxiety and anger with the State-Trait Anxiety Inventory (STAI) and the State-Trait Anger Expression Inventory (STAXI). In M. E. Maruish (Ed.), *The use of psychological testing for treatment planning and outcomes assessment* (2nd ed.,pp. 993–1021). Mahwah, NJ: Lawrence Erlbaum Associates.

Wyler, A. R., Masuda, M., & Holmes, T.H. (1968). Seriousness of illness rating scale. *Journal of Psychosomatic Research,* 11, 363–374.

State–Trait Anger Scale (STAS)

Purpose

To measure anger as an emotional state and as a personality trait.

Population

Ages 16 years and older.

Background and Description

Using the definitions for state anger (S-Anger) and trait anger (T-Anger), the authors selected 15 S-Anger items and 15 T-Anger items from an item pool to create a preliminary form of the State–Trait Anger Scale (STAS). Some items were adapted from other measures of anger and hostility, and some were new. The T-Anger scale was given to university students, and both scales (T-Anger and S-Anger) were administered to Navy recruits. Based on analyses of data collected from these samples, the T-Anger and S-Anger scales were shortened to 10 items each. Items with high item–remainder correlations and low correlations with measures of anxiety were selected.

The STAS is a 20-item self-report measure assessing state and trait anger. State anger is conceptualized as an emotional condition comprised of feelings of tension, annoyance, irritation, or rage. Trait anger is conceptualized as the frequency with which a person feels state anger over time. Thus, the STAS measures anger as both an emotional state and as a relatively stable personality trait. Items on the STAS are rated on a Likert-type scale, ranging from 1 ("not at all") to 4 ("very much so"). Questions tapping state anger ask the respondent to answer how they feel in a particular moment, whereas items assessing trait anger ask the respondent to answer how they generally feel or react.

Administration

The STAS is estimated to take 5–10 min to complete.

Scoring

Scores on the STAS range from 20 (low anger) to 80 (high anger). Scores on the trait anger and state anger scales range from 10 to 40.

Interpretation

Higher scores on the STAS indicate that respondents have higher levels of anger. Higher scores on the state anger scale indicate that respondents have higher levels of emotions such as tension, annoyance, irritation, and rage. Higher scores on the trait-anger scale indicate that respondents experience state anger more frequently and tend to express anger more outwardly, negatively, and in a less controlled and constructive manner.

Psychometric Properties

Factor analysis. An initial factor analysis of the 20-item STAS on 280 undergraduate college students (95 males, 185 females), using the principal factor method with varimax rotation, revealed a single dimension for the state anger scale and a dual dimension for the trait-anger scale. Trait anger consisted of Angry Temperament (T-Anger/T) and Angry Reaction (T-Anger/R).

A Dutch version of the STAS was given to 1,085 Dutch male draftees. Scores were factor analyzed using the principal axis method and varimax rotations. Results supported the presence of state and trait factors. Further factor analyses revealed that items on the state anger scale loaded on the factors state anger feeling and expression, and items on the trait-anger scale loaded on the factors trait anger temperament and reaction. These results provided further support for a two-dimensional conceptualization of the STAS.

Using a sample of 137 male inmates, Kroner and Reddon (1992) examined the factor structure of the STAS using principal component analysis. Three factors were identified: anger/hostility (all items from the state anger subscale), anger arousal (seven items from the trait anger subscale), and situational anger when devalued (three items from the trait anger subscale). This latter factor seems to describe the factor labeled as angry reaction in other factor analyses.

Reliability. Using a sample of male inmates, Kroner and Reddon (1992) assessed test–retest reliability at 1-week ($n = 48$) and 1-month ($n = 46$) intervals. Test–retest coefficients indicated that the state anger subscale ($r = .70$, $r = .88$) had greater stability than the trait anger subscale ($r = .57$, $r = .64$) for both 1-week and 1-month intervals, respectively. Test–retest coefficients for the three identified factors (anger/hostility, anger arousal, and situational anger) were $r = .70$, $r = .60$, and $r = .64$, respectively, for the 1-week interval, and $r = .88$, $r = .78$, and $r = .77$, respectively, for the 1-month interval.

Internal consistency, using Cronbach's alpha, was examined for the 20-item STAS. In a sample of college and navy recruits, alpha coefficients for the Angry Temperament and Angry Reaction components of the T-Anger scale ranged from .84 to .89 and .70 to .75, respectively. To further evaluate internal consistency of the STAS, the 20-item scale was administered to a sample of junior and senior high school students, military recruits, college students, and working adults. Analyses were done based on group and gender. Alpha coefficients ranged from .88 to .97 for the S-Anger scale, .81 to .92 for the T-Anger scale, .81 to .95 for T-Anger/T, and .64 to .93 for T-Anger/R, suggesting that the STAS has adequate to excellent internal consistency across gender and various populations.

Validity. Concurrent validity of the 20-item STAS was assessed by correlating scores on the STAS with scores on the Buss–Durkee Hostility Inventory (BDHI, pp. 109–111) and the Cook and Medley Hostility Scale (Ho, pp. 48–50) in 280 college students and 270 Navy recruits. Results revealed moderately high correlations between the measures of hostility and trait anger for both men and women, supporting the relationship between trait anger and hostility. Additionally, moderate correlations were found between trait anger and the Neuroticism scale of the Eysenck Personality Questionnaire (Eysenck & Eysenck, 1975) and between trait anger and trait anxiety measured by the State–Trait Personality Inventory (STPI, Spielberger et al., 1979). These findings were consistent with clinical observations indicating that neurotics experience anger they cannot easily express.

Discriminant validity was assessed by examining the relationship between anger and hostility. Responses to trait anger items on the BDHI total and subscale scores, the Ho scores, the STPI trait anxiety scores and trait-curiosity scores were compiled and factor analyzed using promax rotation. A three-factor solution produced an anger/hostility dimension, an anxiety dimension, and a curiosity dimension. A four-factor solution produced separate anger and hostility dimensions, an anxiety dimension, and a curiosity dimension. These factors were found for both men and women. It was concluded that anger and hostility are different but related constructs.

Deffenbacher (1992) reviewed numerous studies supporting the construct validity of the STAS T-Anger scale. Respondents scoring higher on the T-Anger scale, in comparison to low scorers, reported more intense anger-related physiological arousal, higher levels of state anger in analog provocations, more verbal and physically antagonistic behaviors and less constructive behaviors in response to analog provocations, and experienced more negative, anger-related consequences.

Clinical Utility

High. The STAS is valuable for assessing two conceptualizations of anger (state anger and trait anger). Additionally, the measure allows the clinician to differentiate between anger temperament and anger reaction.

Research Applicability

High. The STAS has been used in research to assess the multiple aspects of anger and the relationship between trait anger and self-concept. Additionally, the STAS has been used repeatedly to examine the nature of trait anger and its relationship to other variables (e.g., irrational beliefs). The STAS has adequate to excellent internal consistency across gender and

various populations and requires little time to complete.

Original Citation

Spielberger, C. D., Jacobs, G., Russell, S., & Crane, R. S. (1983). Assessment of anger: The State-Trait Anger Scale. In J. N. Butcher and C. D. Spielberger (Eds.), *Advances in personality assessment, Vol. 2* (pp. 161–189). Hillsdale, NJ: Lawrence Erlbaum Associates.

Source

Charles D. Spielberger, University of South Florida, Psychology Department, PCD 4118G, 4202 Fowler Avenue, Tampa, FL 33620-7200

Cost

Please contact the source (above) for permission to use the STAS.

Alternative Forms

A Dutch version of the STAS has been created.

References

Deffenbacher, J. L. (1992). Trait anger: Theory, findings, and implications. In C. D. Spielberger and J. N. Butcher (Eds.), *Advances in personality assessment, Vol. 9* (pp. 177–201). Hillsdale, NJ: Lawrence Erlbaum Associates.

Eysenck, H. J., & Eysenck, S. B. G. (1975). *Manual of the Eysenck Personality Questionnaire*. London: Hodder and Stoughton.

Kroner, D. G., & Reddon, J. R. (1992). The Anger Expression Scale and State–Trait Anger Scale: Stability, reliability, and factor structure in an inmate sample. *Criminal Justice and Behavior, 19*(4), 397–408.

Spielberger, C. D., Jacobs, G., Crane, R., Russell, S., Westberry, L., Barker, L., Johnson, E., Knight, J., & Marks, E. (1979). *Preliminary manual for the State-Trait Personality Inventory (STPI)*. Tampa, FL: University of South Florida, Human Resources Institute.

Spielberger, C. D., Sydeman, S. J., Owen, A. E., & Marsh,
    B. J. (1999). Measuring anxiety and anger with the
    State-Trait Anxiety Inventory (STAI) and the State-
    Trait Anger Expression Inventory (STAXI). In M. E.
    Maruish (Ed.), *The use of psychological testing for
    treatment planning and outcomes assessment* (2nd
    ed.,pp. 993–1021). Mahwah, NJ: Lawrence Erlbaum
    Associates.

Subjective Anger Scale (SAS)

Purpose

To assess the propensity of an individual to
respond with anger to frustrating situations.

Population

Ages 16 and older.

Background and Description

Items on the Subjective Anger Scale (SAS) were
taken from previous measures of anger. It was
developed as an attempt to assess more general
facets of anger. The SAS is based on an interac-
tionist perspective on personality measurement,
and is partially focused on responses to specific
situations in an attempt to remain congruent with
anger-management interventions. The measure
consists of 36 items, divided into two subscales:
Situations and Modes of Response. Nine situations are presented with four possible modes of
response. Respondents report how much they
endorse each mode of response using a 5-point
scale ranging from 1 (very much) to 5 (not at all).
An example situation and modes of response are
listed below.
- Situation: someone persistently contradicts
  you when you know you are right
  - Feel irritated
  - Feel tense
  - Feel like shouting
  - Feel angry

Administration

The SAS is estimated to take 5–10 min to
complete.

Scoring

A total score is obtained by summing ratings on
each of the items. Scores range from 36 to 180.

Interpretation

Higher scores are indicative of a higher degree of
anger responsiveness.

Psychometric Properties

Norms. Normative data were obtained for 492
males and females ages 16 to 71+. Normative
information is organized into seven categories
based on age.

Factor analysis. Principal components factor
analysis with varimax criterion revealed two factors, one for situations and the other for modes of
response. Additionally, further analyses revealed
no overlap between the anger and the anxiety
situations and no overlap among the modes of
response.

Reliability. Internal consistency was calculated
using Cronbach's alpha coefficient. Cronbach's
alpha for the total scale score was .93. Coefficients
for the "feel irritated," "feel tense," "feel like
shouting," and the "feel angry" subscales on the
Modes of Response scale were .80, .84, .84, and
.83, respectively. Additional analyses on a sample of 69 undergraduate psychology students
resulted in an alpha value of .95 for the total scale
and a test–retest coefficient of .88 for a period of
over 3 weeks. Item–remainder correlations
ranged from .48 to .69 for the Situation
subscales.

Validity. The factor analysis supports the construct validity of the SAS and supports the measure's sensitivity to anger responsiveness. Concurrent validity of the SAS was assessed by comparing the SAS to the S-R Inventory of Hostility (Endler & Hunt, 1968), using a sample of 69 (49 female, 20 male) undergraduate psychology students. The correlation between the two measures was .84. Using a sample of 54 undergraduate psychology students, the SAS was compared to the trait anger scale on the State–Trait Anger Scale (STAS; pp. 77–79), the Rathus Assertiveness Schedule (Rathus, 1973), the trait scale of the State–Trait Anxiety Inventory (Spielberger et al., 1970), the Crowne-Marlowe Social Desirability Scale (Crowne & Marlowe, 1960), and the Self-Esteem Scale (Rosenberg, 1965). Significant correlations were found between the SAS and trait anxiety on the State–Trait Anxiety Inventory ($r=.38$), trait anger on the STAS ($r=.70$), the Rathus Assertiveness Schedule ($r=-.34$), and the Crowne-Marlowe Social Desirability Scale ($r=.48$).

Clinical Utility

High. The SAS allows clinicians to gain knowledge of the types of situations that elicit angry responses in individuals and the range of responses elicited.

Research Applicability

High. The SAS contains scales to examine situations provoking anger and typical response types, allowing for more flexibility and more generalization when examining correlates of anger provoking situations and responses.

Original Citation

Knight, R. G., Ross, R. A., Collins, J. I., & Parmenter, S. A. (1985). Some norms, reliability and preliminary validity data for an S-R inventory of anger: The Subjective Anger Scale (SAS). *Personality and Individual Differences, 6*(3), 331–339.

Source

Robert G. Knight, Department of Psychology, University of Otago, P.O. Box 56, Dunedin, New Zealand, rknight@psy.otago.ac.nz

Cost

Please contact the source (above) for permission to use the SAS.

References

Crowne, D. P., & Marlowe, D. (1960). A new scale of social desirability independent of psychopathology. *Journal of Consulting Psychology, 24,* 349–354.

Endler, N. S., & Hunt, J. M. (1968). S-R inventories of hostility and comparisons of the proportions of variance from persons, responses, and situations for hostility and anxiousness. *Journal of Personality & Social Psychology, 9,* 309–315.

Rathus, S. A. (1973). A 30-item schedule for assessing assertive behavior. *Behavior Therapy, 4,* 398–406

Rosenberg, M. (1965). *Society and the Adolescent Self-Image.* Princeton, NJ.: Princeton University Press.

Spielberger, C. D., Gorsuch, R. L., & Lushene, R. E. (1970). *Manual for the State-Trait Anxiety Inventory.* Palo Alto, CA: Consulting Psychologists Press.

Test of Negative Social Exchange (TENSE)

Purpose

To measure the frequency of negative social exchanges experienced by individuals.

Population

Adults.

Background and Description

The Test of Negative Social Exchange (TENSE) was created to provide researchers with a scale that assesses multiple aspects of negative social interactions encountered across a person's entire social network (rather than just their family). Negative social interactions were defined as "affectively unpleasant, resistive, conflictual, hostile, or hurtful transactions" (Ruehlman & Karoly, 1991). The TENSE is an 18-item measure that contains four scales: Hostility/Impatience, Insensitivity, Interference, and Ridicule. Respondents report how often individuals in their lives engaged in the specified behavior during the previous month using a 5-point rating scale ranging from 0 (not at all) to 4 (about every day). The TENSE can also be adapted so respondents report how often they engaged in the specified behaviors represented by the 18 items using the same 5-point rating scale.

Administration

The TENSE is estimated to require 10–15 min to complete.

Scoring

Scoring can be done in two ways. Scores can be summed across items to obtain a total score. Alternatively, items for each of the scales can be summed and then averaged to obtain unit weightings.

Interpretation

Higher scores indicate greater frequency of negative social exchanges.

Psychometric Properties

Factor analysis. A principal components analysis with varimax rotation revealed five factors. The fifth factor only contained two items and was subsequently deleted. The remaining for four factors were: Hostility/Impatience, Insensitivity, Interference, and Ridicule. A confirmatory factor analysis using maximum likelihood estimation

procedures was conducted on data from an independent college sample. The previously specified four-factor model fit the data.

Reliability. The internal consistency of the TENSE scales, as measured by Cronbach's alpha, ranged from .70 (Ridicule) to .83 (Hostility/Impatience) in a sample of 510 undergraduate students. Test–retest reliability for the scales ranged from .65 (Interference) to .80 (Hostility/Impatience). In a sample of newlywed couples, Cronbach's alphas ranged from .89 to .92 for the total score and .62 to .89 for the subscale scores. The correlations for inter-spousal agreement were .46 and .36 for husbands' and wives' TENSE total scores, respectively. Inter-spousal agreement on the subscales ranged from .21 to .59.

Validity. TENSE scales and related constructs were correlated when social desirability was partialled out. The results indicated the TENSE scales were inversely related to social support and life satisfaction and positively related to social hindrance, anxiety, loneliness, and depressed affect. The TENSE was significantly correlated with other measures of psychological aggression including the Multidimensional Measure of Emotional Abuse ($r=.64$, pp. 206–208) and the Conflict Tactics Scale ($r=.48$, pp. 177–180).

Evidence of divergent validity for the TENSE is mixed. The TENSE was found to correlate more highly with measures of psychological aggression compared to behavioral observation measures of positive and negative affect thus supporting divergent validity. However, correlations between the TENSE and communication measures were as high as correlations between the TENSE and psychological aggression measures, suggesting that the TENSE may measure communication styles and not psychological aggression per se (see Finch, Okun, Pool, & Ruehlman, 1999; Ro & Lawrence, 2007).

Clinical Utility

Moderate. The TENSE is a brief measure that has adequate psychometric properties when the full scale is used. The TENSE subscales have not been found to have good internal consistency, so additional research is needed prior to the wide spread use of the individual subscales. The TENSE may be useful to determine the specific types of negative social exchanges an individual is experiencing that may be targeted for treatment. The TENSE assesses a broad range of negative social exchanges and therefore may be especially useful for assessing subtle forms of psychological aggression in couples.

Research Applicability

Moderate. The measure may be of general use for investigating how negative social exchanges affect an individual's social functioning. It can also be utilized by stress researchers to determine the relationship between negative social exchanges and stress.

Original Citation

Ruehlman, L. S., & Karoly, P. (1991). With a little flak from my friends: Development and preliminary validation of the Test of Negative Social Exchange (TENSE). *Journal of Consulting and Clinical Psychology, 3,* 97–104.

Source

Dr. Linda Ruehlman, Consultants in Behavioral Research, 8621 S Maple Ave, Tempe, AZ, 85284, ruehlman@asu.edu. The TENSE may also be purchased from Psychological Assessment and Training, LLC, 8621 South Maple Avenue, Tempe, Arizona 85284, 602-751-5433, order@ psychassessmentonline.com

Cost

The cost for 25 booklets and scoring instructions is $22.50 plus shipping and handling from Psychological Assessment and Training, LLC.

Alternative Forms

A revised, 24-item version of the TENSE exists that measures six types of negative social interactions: anger, insensitivity, manipulation, ridicule, impatience, and rejection. It contains three subscales: anger, insensitivity, and interference/hindrance. Internal consistency of the full scale was adequate, with $\alpha = .81$.

References

Finch, J. F., Okun, M. A., Pool, G. J., & Ruehlman, L. S. (1999). A comparison of the influence of conflictual and supportive social interactions on psychological distress. *Journal of Personality, 67,* 581–621.

Ro, E., & Lawrence, E. (2007). Comparing three measures of psychological aggression: Psychometric properties and differentiation from negative communication. *Journal of Family Violence, 22,* 575–586.

Ward Atmosphere Scale (WAS)

Purpose

Designed to measure the social atmosphere of psychiatric wards, from the perspective of both patients and staff.

Population

Staff and patients of psychiatric wards.

Background and Description

The Ward Atmosphere Scale (WAS) was developed in response to interest in understanding the nature of the ward atmosphere to help predict behaviors in patients and staff. The concept of a beta press underlies the measure. The beta press is the unique and private perceptions held by individuals of the events he/she is experiencing. The consensual beta press is the perceptions held by interacting individuals, the common interpretation of events that they participate in. The initial item pool of the WAS was developed through the utilization of three methods: (1) the College Characteristics Index (CCI; Stern, 1963) was used to generate ideas about the types of behavior that would discriminate between wards, (2) professional and popular books were read for ideas, and (3) two trained observers examined the behaviors of staff and patients of three wards for several weeks.

The "real ward" WAS is a 100-item, self-report measure used to characterize the social atmosphere of psychiatric wards. The measure consists of ten subscales, grouped into three categories: relationship variables (involvement, support, and spontaneity subscales), treatment program variables (autonomy, practical orientation, personal problem orientation, and anger and aggression subscales), and administrative structure variables (order and organization, program clarity, and staff control subscales). Items are answered true/false.

- Patients often gripe
- Staff sometimes argue openly with each other
- Patients here rarely become angry

(These items were reproduced with permission. Copyright 1996; Permission to reproduce these items should be obtained either from the author [Rudolf Moos; email: rmoos@stanford.edu) or from the publisher, Mindgarden (Web site: http://www.mindgarden.com)].

Administration

The WAS can be given as a paper-and-pencil questionnaire or using tape-recorded instructions. The WAS is estimated to take 20 min to complete.

Scoring

Items denoted as "true" or "false" in the scoring manual receive one point if the respondent also marks "true" or "false," in agreement with the indicated direction. For each subscale, the total score is the number of items marked in the indicated direction.

Interpretation

Sample profiles are discussed in Moos, R. H. (1974). *Evaluating treatment environments: A social ecological approach.* New York: John Wiley & Sons.

Psychometric Properties

Norms. Norms are available for both British and American samples.

Factor analysis. A principal-components factor analysis was conducted on 87 inpatient volunteers at a psychiatric institution for the criminally insane. Results revealed three factors. All but two subscales (anger and staff control) loaded on the first factor. The second two factors each consisted of one subscale, anger and staff control. In a different study, a factor analysis was conducted on a sample of 49 wards and produced three factors: general activity, anger and chaos, and control.

Reliability. Internal consistency was measured using KR20. Coefficients for patient and staff ratings, respectively, for each subscale are as follows: Involvement .78, .82; Support .65, .60; Spontaneity .55, .65; Autonomy .55, .69; Practical Orientation .59, .63; Personal Problem Orientation .76, .78; Anger and Aggression .76, .74; Order and Organization .75, .82; Program Clarity .59, .70; and Staff Control .59, .63. Test–retest reliabilities for a 1-week period are as follows: Involvement .79, Support .78, Spontaneity .69, Autonomy .76, Practical Orientation .68, Personal Problem Orientation .83, Anger and Aggression .71, Order and Organization .75, Program Clarity .76, and Staff Control .77.

Intraclass correlations were calculated to evaluate stability of overall ward profiles. Correlations for patient and staff ratings, respectively, are as follows: 1-week .92, .91; 1–2 months .76, .85; 4–7 months .77, .89; 9 months .70, .78; 14–15 months .70, .92; 2–2.5 years .76, .83; and 3 years, 4 months .73, .96.

Validity. Scores on the WAS were compared with similar scales to assess construct validity. Scores on the WAS Support subscale significantly correlated with Perception of Ward (POW, Ellsworth, Maroney, Klett, Gordon, & Gunn, 1969) subscales of Inaccessible Staff (negative) and Receptive-Involved Staff. The WAS Autonomy subscale correlated with the POW Involvement in Ward Management subscale. The WAS Autonomy subscale covaried with the POW Satisfaction with Ward and the Expectation for Patient Autonomy subscales. (Kellam, Shmelzer, & Berman, 1966).

WAS scores of 640 staff members and 424 inpatients in Norway psychiatric wards were examined. The WAS scores of inpatients were significantly related to three patient satisfaction questions; similarly staff WAS scores were significantly related to staff satisfaction questions. Patient and staff WAS scores were moderately correlated (average $r = .41$). The results suggested patients and staff members perceive the ward atmosphere differently, and ward atmosphere is more important for patient satisfaction than staff satisfaction (Rossberg & Friis, 2004). In a more recent study, the WAS subscales involvement, practical orientation, angry and aggressive behavior, and staff control were found to be strongly related to patient satisfaction (Rossberg, Melle, Opjordsmoen, & Friis, 2006).

Clinical Utility

High. The WAS provides an efficient means of assessing actual and ideal conditions and both behavioral and interpersonal interactions on a ward from the perspective of both patients and staff.

Research Applicability

High. The WAS is a useful tool for examining effects of ward atmospheres on patient and staff behaviors, as well as to assess differential effects of the ward atmosphere on individuals.

Original Citation

Moos, R. H. (1974). *Evaluating treatment environments: A social ecological approach.* New York: John Wiley & Sons.

Moos, R. H. (1974). *The Ward Atmosphere Scale manual.* Palo Alto, CA: Consulting Psychologists Press.
Moos, R. H., & Houts, P. S. (1968). Assessment of the social atmospheres of psychiatric wards. *Journal of Abnormal Psychology, 73*(6), 595–604.

Source

Dr. Rudolf Moos, Department of Psychiatry, Stanford University, Palo Alto, CA 94305, rmoos@stanford.edu Items may also be obtained from Mindgarden, http://www.mindgarden.com

Cost

Costs varying depending on the quantity requested. A sampler set, which includes the WAS manual and non-reproducible measure, may be purchased from Mindgarden for $40.

Alternative Forms

A short form of the WAS (Form S) has been created that contains 40 items, 4 items from each of the 10 subscales.

Items from the WAS have been reworded to create the Ideal (Form I) and Expectations (Form E) forms of the WAS. The WAS-I form asks patients and staff to rate what an ideal ward would be. The WAS-E form asks patients and staff to rate what they expect from the ward they are entering.

The WAS has been translated into several languages including German and French (Burti, Glick, & Tansella, 1990). A complete listing of translations is available from http://www.mindgarden.com.

References

Burti, L., Glick, I. D., & Tansella, M. (1990). Measuring the treatment environment of a psychiatric ward and a community mental health center after the Italian reform. *Community Mental Health Journal, 26*(2), 193–204.
Ellsworth, R. B., Maroney, R., Klett, W., Gordon, H., & Gunn, R. (1969). *Milieu characteristics of successful psychiatric treatment programs.* Paper presented at

14th Annual Conference of VA Cooperative Studies in Psychiatry, Houston, TX.

Kellam, S. G., Shmelzer, J. L., & Berman, A. (1966). Variation in the atmosphere of psychiatric wards. *Archives of General Psychiatry, 14*, 561–570.

Rossberg, J. I., & Friss, S. (2004). Patients' and staff's perceptions of the psychiatric ward environment. *Psychiatric Services, 55*, 798–803.

Rossberg, J. I., Melle, I., Opjordsmoen, S., & Friis, S. (2006). Patient satisfaction and treatment environment: A 20-year follow-up study from an acute psychiatric ward. *Nordic Journal of Psychiatry, 60*, 176–180.

Stern, G. G. (1963). Characteristics of the intellectual climate in college environments. *Harvard Educational Review, 33*, 5–41.

Measures of Aggression

4

Quick View Table for Measures of Aggression

The quick-view table in this chapter provides easy access to basic descriptive information on each of the measures reviewed. The goal is to provide enough information to allow for an estimate of the likelihood that reading additional information about a particular measure would prove fruitful. Table entries are organized alphabetically and provide the name of the measure, the purpose for which the measure was developed, and the target population. The tables also provide information on the method of assessment, the amount of time involved, and the page number where additional information is available.

Quick View Table for Measures of Aggression

Name	Purpose	Population	Method	Time	Page #
Aggression Questionnaire	To measure different facets of aggression	Children and adults	Self-report questionnaire	10	91
Antisocial Behavior Scale—Teacher Rating Scale	To measure reactive and proactive aggression in school settings	School-aged children	Questionnaire completed by teachers	5–10 min	93
Antisocial Personality Questionnaire	To assess antisocial characteristics in dangerous mentally disordered offenders	Adult criminal offenders	Self-report questionnaire	20 min	94
Assessing Influencing Strategies	To assess the various strategies used by partners to influence each other	Adults	Self-report questionnaire	15–20 min	96
Bergen Questionnaire on Antisocial Behavior	To assess antisocial behavior	Preadolescents and adolescents	Self-report questionnaire	45 min	98

(continued)

G.F. Ronan et al., *Practitioner's Guide to Empirically Supported Measures of Anger, Aggression, and Violence*, ABCT Clinical Assessment Series, DOI 10.1007/978-3-319-00245-3_4,
© Springer International Publishing Switzerland 2014

(continued)

Name	Purpose	Population	Method	Time	Page #
Bredemeir Athletic Aggression Inventory	To assess overall arousal and aggressive tendencies in athletes	Athletes	Self-report questionnaire	20–30 min	100
Brief Anger–Aggression Questionnaire	To assess anger and aggression in violence-prone men	Adult males	Self-report questionnaire	5 min	101
Bullying-Behavior Scale and the Peer-Victimization Scale	To assess bullying and victim problems within a school system	Children ages 8–11	Self-report questionnaire	5–10 min	103
Burks Behavior Rating Scales	To assess psychopathology in grammar school children	Grammar school children	Questionnaire completed by child's teacher, parent, or qualified observer	15 min	104
Buss Aggression Machine	To directly measure physical aggression	Adults	Experimental paradigm involving reinforcement and punishment of a confederate	30–45 min	107
Buss–Durkee Hostility Inventory	To assess factors related to the propensity to act aggressively	Children and adults	Self-report questionnaire	15–20 min	109
Children's Action Tendency Scale	To assess aggressive, assertive, and nonassertive behavior	Children ages 6–12	Self-report questionnaire	15–20 min	111
Children's Attitudes toward Aggression Scale	To measure attitudes held by preadolescents toward various types of aggression	Children ages 8–12	Self-report questionnaire	8–12 min	113
Children's Hostility Inventory	To evaluate aggression and hostility in children	Children ages 6–12	Questionnaire completed by child's parent(s)	10–15 min	115
Coding Audiotaped Aggressive Episodes	To objectively code conversations for elements of aggression	Adults	Conversation between individuals	2.5–4 h	116
Coercive Sexual Fantasies Scale	To assess fantasies of sexual aggression	Adult men	Self-report questionnaire	5–10 min	117
Competitive Aggressiveness and Anger Scale	To measure anger and aggressiveness	Competitive athletes	Self-report questionnaire	5–10 min	118
Competitive Reaction Time Task	To measure aggression emitted in a competitive situation	Adults	Reaction task against fictitious opponent	Varies depending on procedure used	120

(continued)

(continued)

Name	Purpose	Population	Method	Time	Page #
Conflict Tactics Scale	To assess the strategies partners use for resolving conflicts	Adults in marital, cohabiting, or dating relationships	Self-report questionnaire	10–15 min	177
Dissipation–Rumination Scale	To measure the level of dissipation and rumination in an individual as a means of predicting aggressive behavior and hostility	Adults	Self-report questionnaire	5–10 min	121
Expressive Representations of Aggression Scale	To determine whether a person views aggression in instrumental or expressive terms	All ages	Forced-choice questionnaire	5–10 min	123
Hypermasculinity Inventory	To assess a constellation of characteristics related to a conceptualization of the macho personality style	Adults	Forced-choice questionnaire	15–20 min	125
Multidimensional Aggression Scale for the Structured Doll Play Interview	To assess multidimensional aggressive responses in children	Children ages 4–5	Structured Doll Play Interview	45–60 min	127
Multidimensional Peer-Victimization Scale	To assess and identify peer victimization	Children and adolescents ages 11–16	Self-report questionnaire	15–20 min	128
Offense Scenario	To assess the likelihood of an individual responding aggressively in situations in which an offense occurs	Adults	Scenarios and accompanying questions	3–5 min per scenario	129
Overt Aggression Scale	To assess different forms of aggression emitted within a hospital setting	Adult and child psychiatric inpatients and brain-injured patients within rehabilitation settings	Checklist completed by nursing staff	5–10 min	131
Peer Nomination Inventory	To measure social adjustment for groups of preadolescent boys and to reflect the behavior systems of aggression, dependency, withdrawal, and depression	Preadolescent boys	Sociometric peer ratings	1 h	133
Personality Assessment Inventory	To assess personality style, psychopathology, and current functioning	Adults	Self-report questionnaire	40–50 min	134

(continued)

(continued)

Name	Purpose	Population	Method	Time	Page #
Point Subtraction Aggression Paradigm	To measure aggressive behavior	Children, adolescents, and adults	Experimental paradigm	Varies depending on the assessment needed	136
Problem-Solving Measure for Conflict	To assess the problem-solving skills of children in the contexts of peer, teacher–student, and parent–child conflict	Children	Story completion task	25–35 min	138
Propensity for Angry Driving Scale	To identify people who are likely to engage in hostile driving behaviors or acts of "road rage"	Individuals above the legal age required to drive an automobile	Scenarios and accompanying responses	20 min	140
Rating Scale for Aggressive Behavior in the Elderly	To assess aggressive behavior in geriatric inpatients	Geriatric inpatients on a psychiatric ward	Questionnaire completed by ward nursing staff	5 min	141
Revised Behavior Problem Checklist	To assess externalizing and internalizing behavior problems	Children and adolescents	Questionnaire completed by teachers, parents, or other qualified adults	20–30 min	143
Richardson Conflict Response Questionnaire	To measure direct and indirect aggression	Ages 13 and older	Self-report questionnaire	5–10 min	146
Right-Wing Authoritarianism Scale	To assess the authoritarianism attitudes of submission to authority, aggression, and conventionalism	Adults	Self-report questionnaire	5–10 min	148
Sentences	To explore attribution biases in ambiguous situations	Adults	Sentence completion task and memory recognition task	25–30 min	149
Situations–Reactions Hostility Inventory	To assess types of situations that are typically emotion provoking and the types and intensity of responses to these situations	Adults	Self-report questionnaire	10–15 min	151
Staff Observation Aggression Scale	To monitor the degree and frequency of aggressive, violent, and assaultive acts in psychiatric inpatients	Inpatients on psychiatric wards	Observational measure completed by ward staff	5 min	153

Aggression Questionnaire (AQ)

Purpose

To measure aggressive tendencies.

Population

Children and adults.

Background and Description

The Aggression Questionnaire (AQ) was created by Buss and Perry (1992) to provide a more specific measure of aggression than the widely used Buss–Durkee Hostility Inventory (BDHI; pp. 109–111). The AQ was modeled after the BDHI, and retained several of the features of the BDHI including an assessment of the various facets of aggression. Items were selected from the BDHI that related to physical aggression, verbal aggression, anger, indirect aggression, resentment, and suspicion (Buss & Perry, 1992). Several items were rewritten to improve clarity, and new items were added. The initial item pool consisted of 52 items. Item content was refined, and the 29-item Buss–Perry Aggression Questionnaire was developed.

The Aggression Questionnaire was revised, and a 34-item version was released in 2000 (Buss & Warren, 2000). The 34-item AQ contains five scales: Physical Aggression, Verbal Aggression, Anger, Hostility, and Indirect Aggression. For both versions of the AQ respondents are asked to rate the degree to which the items describe their behavior using a 5-point scale ranging from 1 (not at all like me) to 5 (completely like me).

Administration

The AQ is estimated to require 10 min to complete.

Scoring

Some items are reverse scored. Items are then summed for each subscale and the total score.

Interpretation

Higher scores indicate greater aggressive tendencies.

Psychometric Properties

Norms. Normative data are based on information from 2,138 individuals. It is given in three age groups: 9–18, 19–39, and 40–88. Normative data are available separately by sex for the Verbal Aggression and Physical Aggression scales.

Factor analysis. The initial 52-item AQ was subjected to factor analytic techniques to refine the scale content. Principal axis factoring with oblimin rotation was used on data from 406 participants. The analysis indicated a four-factor solution: Physical Aggression, Verbal Aggression, Anger, and Hostility. This factor structure was replicated in two separate samples.

Reliability. Internal consistency, assessed using Cronbach's alpha, ranged from .72 (Verbal Aggression) to .85 (Physical Aggression) for the scales of the 29-item AQ, and $\alpha = .89$ for the total score. Nine-week test–retest reliability ranged from .72 (Anger and Hostility) to .80 (Physical Aggression) in a sample of 372 participants.

Internal consistency for the 34-item AQ is acceptable, with Cronbach's alphas ranging from .71 (Indirect Aggression) to .88 (physical aggression). The total score reliability was reported as .94 (Buss & Warren, 2000, as cited in Lambert, 2001).

Validity. The 29-item AQ was correlated with measures of other personality traits to assess construct validity. The AQ Anger and Hostility scales were significantly, positively correlated with emotionality, public self-consciousness, and private self-consciousness and negatively correlated with self-esteem. All of the scales were significantly related to impulsiveness, assertiveness, and competitiveness. Physical Aggression (for men), Anger (for men), and Verbal Aggression were all significantly related to activity.

The 29-item AQ was correlated with peer nominations to further assess construct validity. The AQ scales were significantly related to peer nomination for the same facet of aggression ($r = .20$ to $.45$).

The validity of the 34-item AQ has also been well established. Children and adolescents' scores on the AQ have been shown to significantly correlate with the Attitudes Toward Guns and Violence Questionnaire (Shapiro, 2000) and the Children's Inventory of Anger (pp. 44–46). Adults' scores on the AQ have been shown to significantly correlate with the Novaco Anger Scale (pp. 67–69).

Clinical Utility

High. The Aggression Questionnaire has been widely used in a variety of clinical settings for treatment planning and program evaluation. It can also be used to help determine appropriate service allocation in correctional settings.

Research Applicability

High. Both versions of the Aggression Questionnaire (29-item or 34-item) have demonstrated acceptable psychometric properties. Both versions have also been used in many research settings to evaluate aggression and its relation to other constructs.

Original Citation

Buss, A. H., & Perry, M. (1992). The Aggression Questionnaire. *Journal of Personality and Social Psychology, 63,* 452–459.

Source

The AQ is available from Western Psychological Services, 2031 Wilshire Blvd, Los Angeles, CA 90025-1251, 1-800-648-8857, Fax: (310) 478-7838, http://portal.wpspublish.com/portal/page?_pageid=53,70488&_dad=portal&_schema=PORTAL

Cost

An introductory kit that includes the 34-item AQ manual and 25 autoscore answer forms may be purchased for $99 from Western Psychological Services.

Alternative Forms

A short form of the AQ (AQ-SF) has been created that contains 12 items and the same four scales as the 29-item AQ (Bryant and Smith, 2001). It has demonstrated acceptable internal consistency and construct validity (Diamond & Magaletta, 2006; Diamond, Wang, & Buffington-Vollum, 2005).

The AQ has been adapted for use in several other languages and cultures including Chinese, Dutch, German, Greek, Italian, Japanese, Spanish, and Swedish.

References

Bryant, F. B., & Smith, B. D. (2001). Refining the architecture of aggression: A measurement model for the Buss-Perry Aggression Questionnaire. *Journal of Research in Personality, 35,* 138–167.

Buss, A. H., & Warren, W. L. (2000). *Aggression Questionnaire: Manual.* Los Angeles, CA: Western Psychological Services.

Diamond, P. M., & Magaletta, P. R. (2006). The short-form of the Buss-Perry Aggression Questionnaire (BPAQ-SF): A validation study with federal offenders. *Assessment, 13,* 227–240.

Diamond, P. M., Wang, E. W., & Buffington-Vollum, J. (2005). Factor structure of the Buss-Perry Aggression Questionnaire (BPAQ) with mentally ill male prisoners. *Criminal Justice and Behavior, 32,* 546–564.

Lambert, S. (2001). *Test review: The Aggression Questionnaire (AQ)*. Retrieved from http://aac.ncat. edu/newsnotes/y01sum.html

Shapiro, J. P. (2000). *Attitudes Toward Guns and Violence Questionnaire (AGVQ): Manual*. Los Angeles, CA: Western Psychological Services.

Antisocial Behavior Scale: Teacher-Rating Scale

Purpose

To measure reactive and proactive aggression in school settings.

Population

School-aged children.

Background and Description

The Antisocial Behavior Scale—Teacher Rating Scale was designed to measure reactive and proactive aggression that occurs in school settings. Reactive aggression is aggression that occurs in response to frustration and hostile attributions of others' behavior. In contrast, proactive aggression is aggression that occurs without provocation. The 28 items for the Teacher Rating Scale were created after reviewing existing scales, primarily the scale created by Dodge and Coie (1987). The items were designed to assess proactive aggression, reactive aggression, covert antisocial behavior, and prosocial behavior. Teachers rate the frequency with which students engage in the specified behavior using a 3-point scale ranging from 0 (never) to 2 (very often). Sample items are listed below.

• Gets mad for no good reason
• Has hurt others to win a game or contest
• Won't admit anything is ever his/her fault

Administration

The Teacher Rating Scale requires approximately 5–10 min to complete.

Scoring

Responses are summed across items to form factor scores.

Interpretation

Higher scores indicate greater occurrence of reactive aggression or proactive aggression.

Psychometric Properties

Factor analysis. A principal components analysis with oblique rotation was conducted on the antisocial items of the Teacher Rating Scale for a sample of third and fifth grade boys. The analysis revealed two interpretable factors, proactive aggression and reactive aggression. The proactive aggression factor contained items related to proactive aggression and covert antisocial behavior. The reactive aggression factor contained items related only to reactive aggression.

Reliability. Internal consistency, as measured by Cronbach's alpha, was high for the two scales with $\alpha = .94$ for proactive aggression and $\alpha = .92$ for reactive aggression.

Validity. Six independent raters classified the 21 antisocial items into one of three categories: proactive aggression, reactive aggression, and covert antisocial behavior. Perfect agreement was achieved for 17 of the items, with kappa .93. The reactive aggression scale and the proactive aggression scale were both significantly related to negative peer status ($r = .26$ for each). Both scales were also significantly correlated with detentions ($r = .42$ for proactive aggression and .49 for reactive aggression). Reactive aggression was significantly correlated with detentions after the influence of proactive aggression was factored out (partial $r = .31$).

Clinical Utility

Moderate. The Teacher Rating Scale may aid in clarifying the type of aggression used by children in the classroom, which could be a target for treatment. Available psychometric information is promising. However, information on the psychometric properties of this instrument when used in a female sample, and with older school-aged children, is needed.

Research Applicability

Moderate. The Teacher Rating Scale may be a useful measure for investigating the relationship between reactive and proactive aggression and other aggression characteristics. It may also be useful in research regarding factors that predict disruptive behavior in the classroom. Additional research on the psychometric properties of this instrument in a sample of females is needed.

Original Citation

Brown, K., Atkins, M. S., Osborne, M. L., & Milnamow, M. (1996). A revised Teacher Rating Scale for reactive and proactive aggression. *Journal of Abnormal Child Psychology, 24*, 473–480.

Source

Dr. Marc Atkins, Institute for Juvenile Research, 1747 W. Roosevelt Rd, Chicago, IL, 60608, (312) 413-1048, atkins@uic.edu

Cost

Please contact the source (above) for permission to use the Teacher Rating Scale.

Reference

Dodge, K. A., & Coie, J. D. (1987). Social-information processing factors in reactive and proactive aggression in children's peer groups. *Journal of Personality and Social Psychology, 53*, 1146–1158.

Antisocial Personality Questionnaire (APQ)

Purpose

To assess antisocial characteristics in dangerous mentally disordered offenders.

Population

Adult criminal offenders.

Background and Description

The Antisocial Personality Questionnaire (APQ) is based on the Special Hospitals Assessment of Personality and Socialization (SHAPS; Blackburn, 1982) which was developed for use with mentally disordered offenders in English maximum security hospitals. SHAPS items were factor analyzed to identify internally consistent and homogeneous scales having minimal overlap. The resulting APQ measures antisocial personality characteristics in adult offenders and other socially deviant groups. APQ quantifies aspects of emotional dysfunction, poor impulse control, deviant beliefs about the self and others, and problematic interpersonal behaviors. The 125 items are presented in a dichotomous (yes–no) response format to facilitate the administration for patients of low intelligence or limited literacy. The measure consists of eight primary scales (self-control, self-esteem, avoidance, paranoid suspicion, resentment, aggression, deviance, and extraversion) and two higher order dimensions (impulsivity-aggression versus control, withdrawal versus sociability). The first higher-order dimension is known as the Impulsivity scale (33 items), which consists of items from the Self-Control, Paranoid, Resentment, Aggression, and Deviance scales. The scale was intended to be a general awareness factor that assesses the expression of dysfunctional impulses including hostile, rebellious, and aggressive behaviors. The second higher order dimension is the Withdrawal scale (24 items), which contains items drawn from the Avoidance and Extraversion scales. In general, the APQ provides comprehensive sampling of deviant traits implicated in antisocial personality disorder and also taps three of the Big Five personality dimensions (Neuroticisim, Extraversion, and Agreeableness). Sample items are reprinted below.

• Have you ever done anything dangerous just for the thrill of it?
• When you were a youngster did you ever indulge in petty stealing?

Administration

It is estimated that the APQ requires 15 min to complete.

Scoring

Items are scored dichotomously (yes or no) and responses in the keyed direction are summed.

Interpretation

High scores indicate greater endorsement of the undesirable attributes represented by each scale. For instance, high scores on the Self-Control scale suggest defensiveness and a socially desirable response style. Extreme high scores on the Self-Control scale are similar to the concept of overcontrol. It is recommended that the profile configuration be interpreted rather than examining individual scale elevations in order to gain a more complete understanding of the person's behavior.

Psychometric Properties

Norms. Scores for male mentally disordered offenders and non-offender volunteers are provided in Blackburn and Fawcett (1999).

Reliability. Internal consistency reliability, as measured by Cronbach's alpha, ranged from .77 to .87 for the total sample, .79 to .88 for patients, and .75 to .84 for non-offender volunteers. Average inter-item correlations ranged from .13 to .28, suggesting adequate homogeneity of scales.

Validity. Scales differentiated between samples of male mentally disordered offenders ($n=499$) and male volunteer non-offenders ($n=238$). Cluster analyses of APQ scores from the mentally disordered offender sample produced four profile patterns.

The APQ scales were also examined to determine whether they would differentiate between psychopathic offenders ($n=38$) and offenders legally classified as suffering from mental illness ($n=90$). The APQ scales differentiated between these offender groups. Moreover, scale intercorrelations were similar within patient and psychopathic samples. Significant correlations were found between APQ scales and scales from the Million Multiaxial Clinical Inventory (Millon, 1983), which provide support for using the APQ to assess deviant personality characteristics. Several of the APQ scales also demonstrated a relationship with an observer rating scale (Closed Living Environments: Blackburn & Renwick, 1996) which supports the validity of the APQ as a measure of social dispositions. Finally, several APQ scales correlated with relevant data gleaned from a review of 132 criminal records (e.g., age of first conviction, total number of convictions, violence, robbery, sex offenses, criminal damage, and arson) (Blackburn, 1999).

Clinical Utility

Moderate. The APQ is easily administered and has demonstrated acceptable psychometric properties. The APQ is useful for identifying intrapersonal and interpersonal characteristics among offenders and might serve as a useful aide when determining the classification and placement of inmates. The APQ might also help with the conceptualization and formulation or functional analysis of an individual's problems. Additional research with clinical samples would help to solidify the clinical utility of APQ.

Research Applicability

High. The APQ is easily administered and demonstrates acceptable psychometric characteristics. The APQ can be used to assess deviant personality characteristics among offenders and some data suggest utility for identifying psychopathic inmates.

Original Citations

Blackburn, R., & Fawcett, D. J. (1996). *Manual for the Antisocial Personality Questionnaire (APQ)*. Unpublished manuscript.

Source

Ronald Blackburn, University of Liverpool, Department of Clinical Psychology, The Whelan Building, Quadrangle, Brownlow Hill, Liverpool, L69 3GB, UK, ronb@liverpool.ac.uk

Cost

Contact the source (above) for permission to use the APQ.

References

Blackburn, R. (1982). *The Special Hospital Assessment of Personality and Socialization (SHAPS)*. Unpublished manuscript.
Blackburn, R. (1999). Personality assessment in violent offenders: The development of the Antisocial Personality Questionnaire. *Psychologica Belgica, 39*, 87–111.
Blackburn, R., & Fawcett, D. (1999). The Antisocial Personality Questionnaire: An inventory for assessing personality deviation in offender populations. *European Journal of Psychological Assessment, 15*, 14–24.

Blackburn, R., & Renwick, S. J. (1996). Rating scales for measuring the interpersonal circle in forensic psychiatric patients. *Psychological Assessment, 8*, 76–84.
Millon, T. (1983). *Millon Clinical Multiaxial Inventory* (3rd ed.). Minneapolis, MN: Interpretive Scoring Systems.

Assessing Influencing Strategies (AIS)

Purpose

To assess the various strategies used by partners to influence each other.

Population

Adults.

Background and Description

The Assessing Influencing Strategies (AIS) measure was derived from research examining the strategies people use to influence each other in face-to-face relationships. Results from the research were adapted and combined with additional strategies to examine influencing strategies employed by married couples. Theory and factor analyses guided the grouping of items into six categories.

The AIS contains 20 items designed to assess the strategies partners use to influence each other's thoughts, emotions, and feelings. Items are grouped into six basic categories: Positive-Direct (consists of a single item, "Talk it over"), Other Direct (being an expert, using past experience as basis of power, or making reference to what others do), Coercive-Direct (consisting of two subcategories, verbal and physical coercion; verbal coercion consists of verbal fighting, getting angry, and cursing/swearing; physical coercion consists of physical fighting and physical violence toward the spouse), Positive-Indirect (being affectionate, being nice, and praising spouse), Ignore-Indirect (pretending there was no disagreement, ignoring, and not showing feeling), and Withdraw-Indirect (emotional withdrawal, stopping sex, and threatening to leave). Respondents answer each item using a 5-point scale, ranging from 1 ("never") to 5 ("always"). Wording can be altered so respondents can report strategies used by themselves or their spouse. A sample question follows.

• Do you [Does he] ever try to get what you [he] want[s] by doing any of the following to him [you]?
  Emotionally withdraws.
  Stops having sex.
  Threatens to leave.

Administration

The measure can be completed in 5–10 min.

Scoring

Items can be summed to determine the use of direct versus indirect strategies employed by either the husband or wife. A qualitative analysis can also be used wherein the use of various direct and indirect strategies are evaluated.

Interpretation

Higher scores indicate greater use of the particular strategy. The qualitative analysis provides information relating to specific strategies used by either the husband or wife.

Psychometric Properties

Reliability. Women from a sample of 272 couples completed the AIS. Their results were used to calculate internal consistency of the measure. Cronbach's alpha was calculated for five of the six basic categories: Other Direct (.39 for women, .58 for men), Coercive-Direct (verbal coercion: .55 for women, .66 for men; physical coercion: .75 for women, .90 for men), Positive-Indirect (.75 for women, .81 for men), Ignore-Indirect (.63 for women, .64 for men), and Withdraw-Indirect

(.68 women, .61 men). An alpha value for the Positive-Direct category was not calculated because this category consists of a single item.

Validity. Research has indicated that women married to violent men use more influencing strategies ($M = 19.4$), including verbal and physical aggression than women married to nonviolent men ($M = 17.6$). Data also indicate that use of positive influence strategies by either spouse is positively related to marital happiness, whereas use of physical coercion is negatively related to marital happiness.

Clinical Utility

Limited. Although the measure might be an efficient way to track changes in strategies used by couples to influence each other, the lack of normative data for the use of these strategies in maritally satisfied, maritally distressed, and maritally violent couples makes interpreting scores within a clinical context difficult.

Research Applicability

Moderate. The measure is time efficient and could be used to assess the relationship between influencing strategies and other factors related to marital satisfaction. However, additional validity and reliability data are needed.

Original Citation

Frieze, I. H., & McHugh, M. C. (1992). Power and influence strategies in violent and nonviolent marriages. *Psychology of Women Quarterly Special Issue: Women and power, 16(4)*, 449–465.

Source

Irene H. Frieze, Department of Psychology, University of Pittsburgh, Pittsburgh, PA 15260, (412) 624-4336, Fax: (412) 624-4428, frieze@pitt.edu

Cost

Contact the source (above) for permission to use the AIS.

Bergen Questionnaire on Antisocial Behavior (BQAB)

Purpose

To assess antisocial behavior amongst preadolescents and early adolescents.

Population

Preadolescents and early adolescents.

Background and Description

The Bergen Questionnaire on Antisocial Behavior (BQAB) measures antisocial acts and behaviors in preadolescents and adolescents. The antisocial acts vary in seriousness (major and minor offenses) and the BQAB permits comparisons of the same dimensions or acts while taking into account age dependent variations. The 33 core items are grouped under the headings: high prevalence, low prevalence, and sanctions. Items consist of school-related problem behaviors, nonschool-related antisocial acts, and fraud. Items include questions about "object directed" aggressive/violent behavior in the form of vandalism, aggression/opposition against teachers, use of alcohol with the intent of getting drunk, smoking, and reactions on the part of the school. A special set of 13 additional items contain five questions about antisocial behavior of an aggressive/violent nature which have been administered to ages 13–14. The additional items correspond to the domains of illegal drug use, violence, and antisocial group activity.

Detailed instructions on how to respond are written on the front page. Subjects are asked to respond "Yes" or "No" to each question to indicate whether they had ever committed the specific antisocial act. If they answer "Yes," they are asked to estimate about how many times they committed the act. Responses are coded as 2 ("in the recent past"), 1 ("in the distant past"), and 0 ("never"). The number of times (including 0) the student committed the act in the past 5 months is recorded.

Administration

The BQAB requires approximately 45 min to complete.

Scoring

Core scales consist of the Total score, High Prevalence, Low Prevalence, and Sanction Scales. Cumulative or lifetime prevalence rate measures the proportion or percentage of subjects in a specified group who have ever committed a certain antisocial act or offense. Period of prevalence rate measures the proportion or percentage of subjects who have committed the antisocial act within a certain age or time limit. The dichotomous item values (i.e., having or not having committed a particular offense or antisocial act in the past 5 months) are summed for each subject. It is assumed that each item in a scale represents a different offense act or type (narrowly defined). A subject's variety scale score, which is a sum score, indicates the range or number of offense types or antisocial acts within a scale an individual committed. Although the variety scales do not take into account the frequency with which the various antisocial acts were committed, such scales are generally regarded as good indicators of a respondent's degree of antisocial involvement. An upper limit sets 50 as the highest permissible value for the frequency of any item within the past 5 months.

Interpretation

The measure provides specific information regarding lifetime prevalence, period of prevalence, and incidence estimates and these can be compared to other individuals of the same age as the respondent.

Psychometric Properties

Norms. Normative information was collected from four relatively large cohorts of students ($n = 571$ to 689) from the city of Bergen, Norway. Subjects were in grades four to seven at the time of the first assessment and 87 % of these students participated during a second testing. Seventy-one percent participated in the third testing.

Reliability. Internal consistency estimates for ages 13 and 14 revealed better reliability estimates for boys than girls. Across all three time spans, Cronbach's alpha coefficients for the total and high prevalence scales were .73 and .86 for boys and .67 and .74 for girls. The alpha coefficients for the two younger cohorts (ages 11 and 12) for the total and the high prevalence scales were .75 and .70 for age 11 cohort and .66 and .65 for age 12 cohort. However, for the younger girls the coefficient alpha estimates for the total and the high prevalence scales were .18 and .15 for the age 11 cohort and .59 and .57 for the age 12 cohort. For the low prevalence scale, the younger girls had too many items with zero prevalence rates for a meaningful calculation. For the two groups of younger boys, the coefficients were .44 and .42, respectively.

For girls and for students in younger age groups, stability of scores was lower. The stability coefficients for the total and high prevalence scales were of moderate size and averaged approximately .54 for boys and .48 for girls for the 1-year interval. For the 2-year interval, the stabilities were .42 for both boys and girls. The stability across both intervals was somewhat higher for the older (age 14) cohort and more so for boys. Individual differences in antisocial behavior displayed substantial stability over both a 1-year interval (.80) and 2-year interval (.60) for boys belonging to the oldest cohort. The sta-

bility of the low prevalence scale and the violence scale (for the age 14 boys) was somewhat lower than for the other two scales. Several of the coefficients were based on fairly skewed distributions, with a sizeable proportion of zero scores.

Validity. The core scales revealed expected relationships with gender, age, and self-reported arrest rates. The scales were also related to a number of criterion variables such as personality characteristics including bullying, aggression and impulsivity, and negative/positive family relationships.

Clinical Utility

Moderate. The measure has potential for use in clinical settings due to its ability to provide age norm references for antisocial acts. Additional reliability and validity data collected within clinical settings are needed prior to widespread clinical application.

Research Applicability

Moderate. The measure could be useful for researchers interested in studying antisocial acts committed by preadolescents and adolescents.

Original Citation

Bendixen, M., & Olweus, D. (1999). Measurement of antisocial behaviour in early adolescence and adolescence: Psychometric properties and substantive findings. *Criminal Behaviour and Mental Health, 9,* 323–354.

Source

Mons Bendixen and Dan Olweus, Research Center for Health Promotion (HEMIL), University of Bergen, Bergen, Norway, Phone: +47 55 58 23 27, Olweus@uni.no

Cost

Contact the source (above) for permission to use the BQAB

Bredemeier Athletic Aggression Inventory (BAAGI)

Purpose

To assess overall arousal and aggressive tendencies in athletes.

Population

Athletes.

Background and Description

General arousal seems to facilitate the expression of aggressive responses to aggressive cues. Although certain forms of assertive or aggressive behavior are believed to be acceptable in some sports, other aggressive. The Bredemeier Athletic Aggression Inventory (BAAGI) was developed to identify and monitor those athletes prior to competition who would be more likely to demonstrate aggression detrimental to performance (Mintah, Huddleston, & Doody, 1999).

The BAAGI consists of 100 items that measure two aggression components identified through factor analysis: Reactive Aggression and Instrumental Aggression. Reactive Aggression was defined as an aggressive act which has as its goal the infliction of injury on another person. Instrumental Aggression was defined as the assertive or aggressive act that has as its objective the attainment of a goal. A short form of the inventory has also been developed (Wall & Gruber, 1986). The short form consists of 28 items that assess hostile, instrumental, and overall aggression. Respondents indicate their agreement with the items using a 4-point Likert-type scale (1 = strong agreement, 4 = strong disagree-

ment). The short version includes 14 items from the original BAAGI Reactive Aggression subscale and 14 items from the Instrumental Aggression subscale.

Administration

The original version of the BAAGI is estimated to take 20–30 min to complete, whereas the short form is estimated to take 10–15 min to complete.

Scoring

Scores are summed for each subscale.

Interpretation

Higher scores reflect a higher aggression level, whereas lower scores reflect a lower level of aggression. Midpoints for each subscale are considered neutral.

Psychometric Properties

Norms. Twenty-one women intercollegiate basketball players responded to the BAAGI-S questionnaire before and after baseline practice sessions and what they perceived to be easy or crucial games.

Reliability. The original BAAGI revealed high coefficients of internal consistency and has been used primarily to compare aggression of athletes across different sports.

The shorter form has been more widely used when repeated applications are called for in competitive and/or research situations. Internal consistency coefficients for instrumental aggression were lower, but quite adequate for reactive aggression. Stability coefficients were .85 and .95 for the instrumental and the hostile subscales, respectively. Coefficients of internal consistency ranged from .09 to .57 for the instrumental aggression subscale and from .29 to .86 for the hostile/reactive aggression subscale.

Validity. Some evidence for the validity of the BAAGI-S has been found. Perceived aggression in hockey players, as measured by the BAAGI-S, was greater in older players than in younger players. The authors predicted this finding, because it was hypothesized that younger players focus on developing skills whereas older players focus on winning games and are expected to by aggressive (Loughead & Leith, 2001). Additionally, players' perceived hostile aggression was correlated with their observed hostile aggression ($r = .56$).

Clinical Utility

Moderate. The BAAGI-S has been used within a variety of athletic populations and settings. It shows potential as a brief measure of aggression and arousal level that can be used prior to or after an athletic contest.

Research Applicability

Limited. More studies are needed to further explore and demonstrate the psychometric properties of the BAAGI and the BAAGI-S.

Original Citation(s)

Bredemeier, B. (1975). The assessment of reactive and instrumental athletic aggression. In D. M. Landers (Ed.), *Psychology of sport and motor behavior II* (Vol. 11, pp. 71–83). State College, PA: Pennsylvania State HPER Series.

Wall, B. R., & Gruber, J. J. (1986). Relevancy of athletic aggression inventory for use in women's intercollegiate basketball: A pilot investigation. *International Journal of Sports Psychology, 17,* 23–33.

Source

Brenda Bredemeier, University of Missouri – St. Louis, One University Blvd, St. Louis, MO 63121, (314) 516-6820.

Cost

Please contact the source (above) for permission to use the BAAGI.

Alternative Forms

A 28-item short form is available.

References

Loughead, T. M., & Leith, L. M. (2001). Hockey coaches' and players' perceptions of aggression and the aggressive behavior of players. *Journal of Sport Behavior, 24,* 394–407.

Mintah, J. K., Huddleston, S., & Doody, S. G. (1999). Justifications of aggressive behavior in contact and semicontact sports. *Journal of Applied Social Psychology, 29,* 597–605.

Brief Anger–Aggression Questionnaire (BAAQ)

Purpose

To quickly assess anger and aggression levels in violence-prone men.

Population

Adult Males.

Background and Description

The Brief Anger–Aggression Questionnaire (BAAQ) was developed as a brief screening device for identifying problems with anger and aggression in violence-prone males. The measure was conceptually developed by constructing items representative of the content of the Buss–Durkee Hostility Inventory (BDHI, pp. 109–111) subscales of Assault, Indirect Hostility, Negativism, Irritability, and Verbal Hostility. Five of the six items were written to provide a composite description of the content of the scale on which the item was based. The BAAQ assesses the relative likelihood, frequency, or magnitude of a particular act or feeling using a 5-point rating scale.

Administration

The BAAQ requires approximately 5 min to complete.

Scoring

Items are summed for a total score.

Interpretation

High scores are indicative of the potential for anger and aggression.

Psychometric Properties

Norms. Normative data were obtained from four studies that were conducted on a clinical population of male outpatients ($n=401$) and a nonviolent control sample ($n=26$). All subjects were enrolled in an anger management program.

Reliability. Internal consistency, calculated using Cronbach's alpha, was found to be adequate ($\alpha=.82$). Measurements of the BAAQ items and total scores were correlated at times one and two in order to determine test–retest reliability. The results indicated a satisfactory degree of stability for the items and a respectable level of reliability for the BAAQ ($r=.84$).

Validity. Construct validity analysis was conducted using Pearson product–moment correlations between the six BAAQ items and the six corresponding BDHI subscales to assess the degree to which the items were representative of their respective parent scales. The correlations were generally highest between each item and its respective subscale ($r=.49$ to .66). The correlation between the BAAQ total score and BDHI

total score was also significant ($r=.78$). Violent and nonviolent samples were compared to assess criterion validity. An ANOVA revealed significant differences between the three assault samples and the nonviolent control sample on the BAAQ total score. However, there were no significant differences between the three assault samples on the BAAQ total score. Subsequent t-tests also revealed that each of the 6 BAAQ items were significantly higher in the assault sample as compared to the nonviolent control group. Finally, an ANOVA with repeated measures was computed between the treatment and waiting list control samples on the BAAQ total score at pre and post time period. The interaction was highly significant, indicating there were significant differences between the two groups at the post assessment period.

Overall, preliminary results support the BAAQ as a psychometrically acceptable measure for the rapid screening and assessment of overt anger and aggression levels in men who are prone to violence.

Clinical Utility

High. The measure provides for a good general estimate of the presence and likelihood of anger dyscontrol. This measure has been utilized in a violent clinical sample. Drawbacks are the explicit face validity. However, the measure requires the respondent to rate items in terms of the degree to which an item applies instead of being forced to label himself in an absolute fashion (true/false), which may moderate bias arising from the face validity of the items.

Research Applicability

Moderate. This measure has not yet been widely studied or used with populations that differ from the validation samples. However, it does have potential as a screening tool based on the results of the preliminary findings, its sensitivity to treatment change, and its brevity in administration.

Original Citation

Maiuro, R. D., Vitaliano, P. P., & Cahn, T. S. (1987). A brief measure for the assessment of anger and aggression. *Journal of Interpersonal Violence, 2*, 166–178.

Source

Roland, D. Maiuro, Cabrini Medical Tower, 901 Boren Avenue, Suite 1010, Seattle, WA 98104, (206) 624-1856, Fax: (206) 625-9475, RMaiuro@prodigy.net

Cost

Contact the source (above) for permission to use the BAAQ.

Bullying-Behavior Scale and the Peer-Victimization Scale (BBPVS)

Purpose

To assess bullying and victim problems within a school system.

Population

Children between the ages of 8 and 11.

Background and Description

The goal was to integrate the Peer-Victimization Scale and the Bullying-Behavior Scale to develop a single instrument that could classify children as victims only, as bullies only, or as bullies and victims. Both scales were developed to address the gap in the assessment literature for a subtle measure of direct bully/victim. Both measures are immersed within a widely used measure of self-perceptions used for children ages 8 to 11, the Harter's (1985) 36-item Self-Perception Profile for Children. The Bullying-Behavior Scale consists of three items that refer to being the

perpetrator of negative physical actions (i.e., hit and push, picked on, bullied) and three that refer to being the perpetrator of negative verbal actions (i.e., tease, call names, laugh at). The Peer-Victimization Scale consists of three items which refer to being the victim of negative physical actions (i.e., hit and pushed, picked on, bullied) and three of which refer to being the victim of negative verbal actions (i.e., teased, called horrible names, laughed at).

The 12-item BBPVS uses a forced-choice response format. It requires children to select which response is most like them and then rate the degree to which the item reflects their behavior. Children are taken through a few examples to ensure they know how to correctly complete the form. An item sample from each scale follows.

Really true for me	Sort of true for me	Sort of true for me	Really true for me
——	Some children do not hit and push other children but other children do hit and push other children	——	——
——	Some children are not hit and pushed about by other children but other children are often hit and pushed about by children	——	——

Administration

The BBPVS takes between 5 and 10 min to complete.

Scoring

For each scale, the total score is computed by summing the 6 items and dividing them by 6. Some items are reverse scored so that high scores indicate greater bullying/victimization behavior.

Interpretation

Higher scores on the BBPVS suggest a greater degree of bullying behavior or victimization. Previous studies that have shown mean scores between 2.20 and 2.33 are related to peer identification of bullies/victims, whereas mean scores of 2.70–2.82 relate to self-identification as a bully/victim. As a result, cutoff scores of 2.50 on both scales were used to classify children into four groups: bully only group (high bully behavior scores and low victimization scores), victim only group (low bully behavior scores and high victimization scores), bully/victim group (high bully behavior scores and high victimization scores), and not involved group (low bully behavior scores and low victimization scores).

Psychometric Properties

Norms. Normative data were collected for 425 schoolchildren (204 boys and 221 girls) aged 8 and 11 years.

Reliability. Internal consistency was found to be satisfactory for both scales (Cronbach's alpha .83 and .82, respectively). No significant difference was found between boys and girls on the Peer-Victimization Scale. However, boys did score higher than girls on the Bullying-Behavior Scale. Forty-six percent of children were classified as bullies, victims, or both: 22 % were classified as victims only, 15 % as bully/victims, and 9 % as bullies only.

Validity. Some evidence of the validity of the BBPVS has been found, as high scores on the Peer-Victimization Scale were related to high scores on the Birleson Depression Inventory ($r = .41$ for boys, $r = .36$ for girls).

Clinical Utility

Limited to moderate. The instruments have not been widely used in clinical settings. The measures have potential for usefulness in determining or classifying children as bullies or victims of bullying.

Research Applicability

Limited to moderate. The instruments have limited empirical studies supporting their psychometric properties. The measures have potential as a quick screening tool to classify children as bullies, victims, or both. More research, however, needs to be conducted to assess the psychometric properties of the scales and to further evaluate cut-offs to classify individuals.

Original Citation

Austin, S., & Joseph, S. (1996). Assessment of bully/victim problems in 8–11 year-olds. *British Journal of Educational Psychology, 66*, 447–456.

Source

Dr. Stephen Joseph, School of Sociology and Social Policy, University of Nottingham, University Park, Nottingham NG7 2RD, Phone: 0115 951 5410, Fax: 0115 951 5232, Stephen.joseph@nottingham.ac.uk

Cost

Contact the source (above) for permission to use the BBPVS.

Reference

Harter, S. (1985). *Manual for the Self-Perception Profile for Children*. Denver, CO: University of Denver.

Burks Behavior Rating Scales (BBRS)

Purpose

To assess the nature and severity of psychopathology in grammar school children.

Population

Grammar school children.

Background and Description

The Burks Behavior Rating Scales (BBRS) was revised from an earlier checklist developed by Burks and contains 110 items that describe 19 clusters of behaviors infrequently observed in children. The BBRS clusters are Excessive Self-Blame, Excessive Anxiety, Excessive Withdrawal, Poor Ego Strength, Poor Physical Strength, Excessive Suffering, Excessive Dependency, Poor Coordination, Poor Intellectuality, Poor Academics, Poor Attention, Poor Impulse Control, Poor Reality Contact, Poor Sense of Identity, Poor Anger Control, Excessive Sense of Persecution, Excessive Aggressiveness, Excessive Resistance, and Poor Social Conformity. Respondents indicate the frequency of the behavior using a 5-point scale, ranging from 1 ("You have not noticed this behavior at all") to 5 ("You have noticed the behavior to a very large degree"). The BBRS is typically completed by a parent or a teacher, but can be completed by any qualified observer who has observed the child's behavior for more than 2 weeks.

Administration

The BBRS requires approximately 15 min to complete.

Scoring

BBRS scores are obtained by summing the scores on items within each cluster.

Interpretation

Plotting category scores on a profile sheet allows for a visual analysis, and the manual provides directions and guides to interpretation.

Psychometric Properties

Norms. The scale was standardized using teachers' ratings of 494 (50 % male, 50 % female) primary school-age children and 69 middle school children. Both Mexican American (70 %) and Anglo American (30 %) children were rated. The sample included normal, educable mentally retarded, educationally handicapped, orthopedically handicapped, speech/hearing impaired, and "disturbed" children.

Factor analysis. Scale scores for 268 children, grades 1 through 9 resulted in three factors labeled: Neurotic, Immature, and Hostile-Aggressive. There was some overlap in behavior scales represented in each of these factors.

Reliability. Internal consistency estimates and interrater reliability for teacher–teacher and between teacher–parent dyads were calculated by Wright and Piersel (1992) using a sample of 34 boys and 19 girls from grades 1 to 6. Internal consistencies of the subscales ranged from .64 (Poor Coordination) to .92 (Poor Anger Control), indicating that the subscales had reasonable internal consistency. Interrater reliability for teacher–teacher dyads ranged from .36 (Poor Reality Contact) to .84 (Excessive Aggressiveness), whereas interrater reliability between teacher–parent dyads ranged from .04 (Poor Physical Strength) to .50 (Excessive Aggressiveness). Thus, interrater reliabilities for teacher–teacher were better than those for teacher–parent, although neither set of reliabilities was adequate for all subscales. Additionally, several subscale scores contained high levels of error variance (e.g., Excessive Dependency, Poor Reality Contact, and Excessive Withdrawal). Subscale scores containing relatively high levels of true variance included Poor Impulse Control, Poor Anger Control, and Excessive Aggressiveness. Test–retest reliabilities for the 19 clusters ranged from .74 to .96.

Validity. Correlations were computed between parent and teacher ratings and between ratings by two different teachers (Wright, Edelbrock, & Reed, 1983). Parent and teachers rated one sample containing 25 boys and 13 girls, aged 6–12 years. Two teachers rated a second sample of 26 boys and 14 girls, aged 6–12 years. Multitrait multimethod matrices were used to examine convergent and discriminant validity. Using findings from both samples, convergent and discriminant validity was established for the following scales: Excessive Self-Blame, Excessive Anxiety, Excessive Withdrawal, Poor Coordination, Poor Impulse Control, Poor Anger Control, Excessive Aggressiveness, and Poor Social Conformity. The validity of nine other scales (all but Excessive Suffering and Poor Intellectuality) was supported by data from one of the two samples. Concerning the broad factors obtained from factor analyses (Neurotic, Immature, and Hostile-Aggressive), neither convergent nor divergent validity were established. That is, parent–teacher correlations failed to support convergent validity and discriminant validity was not supported by the teacher–teacher correlations.

Clinical Utility

Moderate. The BBRS has been reported to be useful for screening for emotional handicaps and behavior disorders and has been described as a useful tool for school psychologists to aid in assessing placement and need for services. The author stated that the measure is quick to administer and to score and provided additional interpretive information, diagnostic suggestions, and specific intervention strategies in a separate volume. However, the validity of making decisions based on the BBRS scores has been questioned due to the high amount of error variance found in several of the subscales (Wright & Piersel, 1992). Additionally, items have been criticized as containing sexist language and requiring the rater to interpret behavior. Classification levels have the same cutoff scores across ages, calling into question whether all ages should have the same developmental expectations.

Research Applicability

Moderate. The BBRS has been found to have factors in common with other behavior checklists (Harris, Drummond, Schultz, & King, 1978). However, the scale has been criticized for its lack of psychometric rigor, because its subscale reliabilities are not provided by the author in the manual, and no rationale is given for the score severity designations (Wright & Piersel, 1992).

Original Citation

Burks, H. F. (1969). *Manual for the Burks' Behavior Rating Scales.* Huntington Beach, CA: Arden Press.
Burks, H. F. (1977). *Burks Behavior Rating Scales: Manual.* Los Angeles, CA: Western Psychological Services.

Source

Western Psychological Services, 12031 Wilshire Boulevard, Los Angeles, CA 90025-1251, 1-800-648-8857, Fax: (310) 478-7838, custsvc@wpspublish.com, http://portal.wpspublish.com/portal/page?_pageid=53,70127&_dad=portal&_schema=PORTAL

Cost

The BBRS-2 kit, which includes 25 parent autoscore forms, 25 teacher autoscore forms, and the manual, costs $105 from Western Psychological Services.

Alternative Forms

The BBRS has been adapted for use with younger children in the Preschool and Kindergarten Edition (ages 3–6 years). The BBRS has also been updated with new norms, simpler administration and scoring, and fewer scales. The BBRS-2 contains seven scales: disruptive behavior, attention and impulse control problems, emotional problems, social withdrawal, ability deficits, physical deficits, and weak self-confidence. The BBRS-2 is designed to assess preschool to grade 12 children. Parent and teacher-rating forms are available.

References

Harris, W. J., Drummond, R. J., Schultz, E. W., & King, D. R. (1978). The factor structure of three teacher rating scales and a self-report inventory of children's source traits. *Journal of Learning Disabilities, 11*, 56–58.

Wright, D., Edelbrock, C., & Reed, M. L. (1983). Convergent and discriminant validity of the Burks Behavior Rating Scales. *Journal of Psychoeducational Assessment, 1*, 253–260.

Wright, D., & Piersel, W. C. (1992). Components of variance in behavior ratings from parents and teachers. *Journal of Psychoeducational Assessment, 10*, 310–318.

Buss Aggression Machine

Purpose

To directly measure physical aggression.

Population

Adults.

Background and Description

The impetus behind the development of the Buss Aggression Machine was to develop a way to assess direct aggression. The standard Buss paradigm involves a respondent and a confederate who are told that the task is concerned with the effects of punishment on learning. A rigged lottery procedure is used to assign the real respondent to the teacher role and the confederate to the role of learner. Respondents are informed that the teacher's task is to present the stimulus materials to the learner over an intercom system. The materials to be administered by the respondent are lists of nonsense syllables. The Buss procedure involves telling the respondent to flash a "correct" light on the confederate's portion of the apparatus each time the confederate makes a correct response (reinforcement) and that he or she is to administer an electric shock each time the confederate makes an error (punishment). When the learner makes errors, which are prearranged by the experimenter, the teacher is told to deliver a shock to the learner as punishment. Prior to the actual task beginning, respondents are sometimes angered by the confederate in order to obtain a measure of "angry" aggression. Respondents are instructed to continue the experiment until the confederate makes five correct responses in succession. The respondent is then shown the shock buttons numbered from 1 to 10 and told that he/she could vary the intensity of shock from weak (button 1) to strong (button 10). A stop clock can be employed to measure the duration of shocks administered by respondents to the learner. The respondent is told that he/she can push any button he/she wishes. The measure of aggression is the number on the button pushed. The dependent measures used are intensity and/or duration of shock. To demonstrate the differing increments of shock, an electrode is placed on the respondent's finger and buttons 1, 3, and 5 are pressed. After a practice session, the confederate is brought back into the room and the task is continued. The confederate is disconnected to the shock unbeknownst to the respondent. Each session is programmed to continue for 61 trials, 31 of which are shock trials. The first 10 trials terminate in shock, whereas the remaining 21 shock trials are distributed randomly. After the completion of the task, all respondents are debriefed by explaining the purpose of the task.

Administration

The administration time varies but is estimated to take 30–45 min to complete.

Scoring

The total amount of noxious stimulation directed against the confederate by respondents is measured in terms of the product of shock intensity by shock duration.

Interpretation

Higher scores are indicative of displaying more intense direct aggression.

Psychometric Properties

Reliability. Reliability data have not been published for the Buss Aggression Machine.

Validity. The Buss Aggression Machine has been shown to have evidence of construct validity when compared to other forms of rated aggression (Shemberg, Leventhal, & Allman, 1968). Wolfe and Baron (1971) examined 20 male college students and 20 male prisoners of comparable age using the Buss Aggression Machine paradigm. Before aggressing, half of the subjects in each of the two groups were exposed to the behavior of an aggressive model, while the remaining individuals attacked the investigator in the absence of such experience. Results indicated that the prisoners delivered significantly more intense shocks to the victim than did the students, regardless of if they had been exposed to an aggressive model or not. In another study, the Buss Aggression Machine was found to be correlated with another aggressive paradigm (the Taylor paradigm). Bernstein, Richardson, and Hammock (1987) also found support for the discriminant validity of the measure. The scores from the Buss paradigm were correlated to a significantly greater extent with the Taylor paradigm than they were with either of two helping measures administered.

Clinical Utility

Moderate. The Buss Aggression Machine provides information related to direct physical aggression against another person which can be assessed in the laboratory without harm to the participants or the learner. However, a disadvantage is that there is no opportunity for retaliation as in real-life circumstances. Also, the respondent does not expect direct retaliation. In some studies this limitation has been addressed by allowing the respondent to believe that he/she will later switch roles with the learner and become the recipient of the shock.

Research Applicability

High. The Buss Aggression Machine had been used in a number of studies and appears to be a good measure for examining direct aggression in a controlled setting.

Original Citation(s)

Buss, A. H. (1961). *The psychology of aggression.* New York: Wiley.

Source

Arnold H. Buss, (512) 475-8492, buss@psy.-utexas.edu

Cost

Please contact the source (above) for permission to use.

References

Bernstein, S., Richardson, D., & Hammock, G. (1987). Convergent and discriminant validity of the Taylor and Buss measures of physical aggression. *Aggressive Behavior, 13,* 15–24.

Shemberg, K. M., Leventhal, D. B., & Allman, L. (1968). Aggression machine performance and rate aggression. *Journal of Experimental Research in Personality, 3,* 117–119.

Wolfe, B. M., & Baron, R. A. (1971). Laboratory aggression related to aggression in naturalistic social situations: Effects of an aggressive model on the behavior of college and student prisoner observers. *Psychonomic Science, 24,* 193–194.

Buss–Durkee Hostility Inventory (BDHI)

Purpose

To assess factors related to the propensity to act aggressively.

Population

Children and adults.

Background and Description

Many of the earliest hostility inventories consolidated various aggressive behaviors into a single summary score despite the many ways in which hostility can be manifested. The Buss–Durkee Hostility Inventory (BDHI) was designed to correct for this shortcoming by creating a multidimensional scale of hostility. It contains 75 true–false items which are organized into seven theoretically derived subscales: assault or direct physical violence against persons; indirect hostility through gossip, practical jokes, slamming doors, or breaking things; irritability or explosiveness and exasperation at the slightest stimulus; negativism as either active rebellion or passive compliance to rules and authority figures; resentment, anger, jealousy, and/or hate of others due to real or imaginary mistreatment; suspiciousness and the belief that others are derogatory and harmful; and verbal hostility in style or content. Sample items follow.

- Once in awhile I cannot control my urge to harm others.
- I can remember being so angry that I picked up the nearest thing and broke it.

Administration

The inventory takes approximately 15–20 min to complete.

Scoring

Scores are summed to obtain a total hostility score based on 66 items (all items minus the guilt items). A separate guilt scale can also be scored.

Interpretation

A high total score indicates a greater tendency toward aggressiveness.

Psychometric Properties

Norms. Normative studies were conducted on a college sample.

Factor analysis. Factor analyses were conducted separately for a sample of 85 male and 88 female college students. Two factors were extracted. Factor 1 was conceptualized as an emotional component of hostility and was defined by the resentment and suspicion scales for both sexes and the guilt scale for women. Factor 2 was conceptualized as a motor component of hostility and was defined by assault, indirect hostility, irritability, and verbal hostility for both sexes and also negativism for women. Additional studies have examined the factor structure of the BDHI and have generally found two factors that are conceptually similar to emotional hostility and motor hostility (Biaggio, Supplee, & Curtis, 1981; Bushman, Cooper, & Lemke, 1991; Felsten & Leitten, 1993; Hennig, Reuter, Netter, Burk, & Landt, 2005).

Reliability. Test–retest reliability using a sample of college students ranged from .64 to .82. Subscales of the BDHI also demonstrated acceptable short-term stability and internal consistency with prisoners. However, inter-subscale correlation revealed only the indirect hostility, negativism, resentment, and suspicion subscales had a strong relationship to the total hostility score, with all subscales being relatively independent of one another except for covariation between the suspicion, resentment, negativism, and indirect hostility subscales (Gunn & Gristwood, 1975).

Validity. The two factor scores were correlated significantly with each other ($r = .53$) and with additional measures of anger experience, thereby providing evidence of convergent validity (Riley & Treiber, 1989). Initial studies revealed that the hostility scale had lower but significant correlations with other scales, ranging from .25 to .45. Buss and Perry (1992) found that participants' total scores were positively correlated with the intensity of the electric shocks they administered to peers as punishment for their mistakes on the Buss Aggression Machine learning task (pp. 107–109). A sample of violent drinkers was compared to control subjects on the BDHI, and violent drinkers were found to have significantly higher scores than control subjects on the total score and on subscales measuring assault, irritability, verbal hostility, indirect hostility, and resentment. Additionally, men imprisoned for violent crimes have reported higher scores on the total inventory compared to men incarcerated for nonviolent offenses, providing further evidence for validity.

Clinical Utility

High. The BDHI is one of the most widely used hostility inventories and has been used with a variety of clinical populations.

Research Applicability

High. The BDHI has been one of the most widely used assessment instruments of hostility in research investigations.

Original Citation

Buss, A. H., & Durkee, A. (1957). An inventory for assessing different kinds of hostility. *Journal of Consulting Psychology, 21,* 343–349.

Source

Arnold H. Buss, (512) 475-8492, buss@psy.-utexas.edu

Cost

Unavailable.

Alternative Forms

The BDHI has been translated into Dutch and Spanish.

Boone and Flint (1988) developed a brief 24-item adaptation of the BDHI to assess hostile attitudes, verbal aggression, and physical aggression toward family members as well as toward people in general, including all nonfamily members except close friends and strangers. For reliability estimates using the alpha coefficient and Guttman's split-half to compute reliability estimates for the adapted BDHI, Boone and Flint (1988) reported reliabilities ranging from .88 to .96. The items can be found in Boone and Flint (1988).

A modified version of the BDHI has also been adapted for children (Treiber et al., 1989). Preliminary findings indicated that test–retest reliabilities of the scales (mean $r = .57$) are comparable to those of other self-report measures of emotion with young children. Concurrent validity has been demonstrated with significant positive correlations between experienced and expressed hostility ($r = .28$) and children's self-reported levels of anger ($r = .44$) and a positive correlation between expressed hostility and parental ratings of negative peer interactions ($r = .28$). The full listing of the items can be found in Treiber et al. (1989).

A brief 29-item Aggression Questionnaire (AQ; pp. 91–93) has been developed from the BDHI.

References

Biaggio, M. K., Supplee, K., & Curtis, N. (1981). Reliability and validity of four anger scales. *Journal of Personality Assessment, 45*(6), 639–648.

Boone, S. L., & Flint, C. (1988). A psychometric analysis of aggression and conflict-resolution behavior in Black adolescent males. *Social Behavior and Personality, 16*(2), 215–226.

Bushman, B. J., Cooper, H. M., & Lemke, K. M. (1991). Meta-analysis of factor analyses: An illustration using the Buss–Durkee Hostility Inventory. *Personality and Social Psychology Bulletin. Special Issue: Meta-analysis in Personality and Social Psychology, 17,* 334–349.

Buss, A. H., & Perry, M. (1992). The Aggression Questionnaire. *Journal of Personality and Social Psychology, 63*(3), 452–459.

Felsten, G., & Leitten, C. L. (1993). Expressive, but not neurotic hostility is related to cardiovascular reactivity during a hostile competitive task. *Personality and Individual Differences, 14,* 805–813.

Gunn, J., & Gristwood, J. (1975). Use of the Buss–Durkee Hostility Inventory among British prisoners. *Journal of Consulting and Clinical Psychology, 43*(4), 590.

Hennig, J., Reuter, M., Netter, P., Burk, C., & Landt, O. (2005). Two types of aggression are differentially related to serotonergic activity and the A779C TPH polymorphism. *Behavioral Neuroscience, 119,* 16–25.

Riley, W. T., & Treiber, F. A. (1989). The validity of the multidimensional self-report anger and hostility measures. *Journal of Clinical Psychology, 45*(3), 397–404.

Treiber, F. A., Musante, L., Riley, W., Mabe, P. A., Carr, T., Levy, M., et al. (1989). The relationship between hostility and blood pressure in children. *Behavioral Medicine, 15*(4), 173–178.

Children's Action Tendency Scale (CATS)

Purpose

To assess aggressive, assertive, and nonassertive behavior in children.

Population

Ages 6–12 years.

Background and Description

The Children's Action Tendency Scale (CATS) was developed as an aid to identify children who may benefit from assertiveness training, as well as a means for assessing changes resulting from such training. The scale was developed in three steps. First, a survey was conducted of situations likely to elicit aggressive, assertive, and submissive responses for children ages 6–12. Second, a list of potentially discriminating responses was developed for each situation. Finally, responses were rated for aggressiveness, assertiveness, and submissiveness.

The 13 situations involve provocation, frustration, loss, or conflict. Aggressive, assertive, and submissive response alternatives are presented for each situation. A paired-comparisons format is used to ensure that all combinations of responses are paired. Respondents choose three responses for each situation, one from each pair of items. Respondents are instructed to choose the response most reflective of what they would do in the given situation. Scores are obtained for aggressiveness, assertiveness, and submissiveness.

Administration

The CATS requires 15–20 min to complete.

Scoring

Three scores are computed: aggressive, assertive, and submissive. Each score is computed by tallying the number of aggressive, assertive, and submissive responses chosen for each vignette. Scores on each subscale range from 0 to 26, and the total sum of all responses is always 39.

Interpretation

Higher scores on a subscale indicate that the child responds more frequently with that type of response (i.e., assertive, aggressive, or submissive).

Psychometric Properties

Reliability. Test–retest reliability for a period of 2 weeks in a Dutch sample was .77 for aggressiveness, .61 for assertiveness, and .77 for submissiveness. In a different sample, test–retest reliability for a 4-month period was .48 for aggressiveness, .60 for assertiveness, and .57 for submissiveness.

In a sample of fourth and fifth grade students, internal consistency coefficients were .92 for aggressiveness, .70 for assertiveness, and .81 for submissiveness. In a sample of 112 Dutch children in the fourth through sixth grades, internal consistency coefficients, as measured by Cronbach's alpha, were .76 for aggressiveness, .34 for assertiveness, and .64 for submissiveness.

Validity. In a sample of 46 parochial school children, grades three through six, CATS aggressiveness scores were positively correlated with peer-rated physical aggression, teacher-rated verbal aggression scores, and the combination of all peer and teacher ratings. The CATS assertiveness scores were positively correlated with teacher-rated assertiveness scores. The CATS submissiveness scores were positively related to total submissiveness scores, peer- and teacher-rated submissiveness scores and negatively related to self-reported self-esteem. When individual situations were correlated with the above scores, all correlated significantly, with the exception of three situations which were eliminated to create the short, 10-item version of the CATS. Finally, CATS scores were negatively related to social desirability scores, as measured by Crandall, Crandall, and Katkovsky (1965) Children's Social Desirability Questionnaire.

Similar results were found for Latino and Dutch samples enrolled in public school grades four through seven. Aggression scores correlated positively with peer- and teacher-rated physical aggression, aggression scores obtained from behavioral observations (in boys), the negative subscale of the Children's Assertiveness Inventory (Ollendick, 1984), observed overall assertiveness in negative conflict situations for boys, and Children's Assertive Behavior Scale (Michelson & Wood, 1982) aggressiveness scores. A negative correlation was found between submissiveness scores obtained from behavioral observations, as well as CATS assertiveness and

submissiveness scores. The assertiveness subscale correlated positively with peer-rated assertiveness, the positive subscale of the Children's Assertiveness Inventory, and the Children's Assertive Behavior Scale and negatively with aggression scores obtained from behavioral observations (in boys). The submissiveness subscale correlated positively with peer-rated submissiveness, peer-rated assertiveness, and submissiveness scores obtained from behavioral observations and was negatively correlated with total scores on the Children's Assertiveness Inventory. The CATS subscales also correlated with self-esteem, social anxiety, social desirability, and perceived competence, but these correlations did not clearly discriminate between assertive and passive or submissive response tendencies. High scores on the aggressiveness subscale combined with low scores on the assertiveness subscale did differentiate between hyperaggressive/highly disruptive children and public school boys.

In a Latino sample, self-esteem in boys was related to lower assertiveness and submissiveness scores and higher aggressiveness scores. Children scoring higher on assertiveness and submissiveness also indicated less perceived self-control and lower state and trait anger scores, whereas children with higher scores of aggressiveness indicated more perceived control and had higher anger scores.

Clinical Utility

Moderate. The CATS is a useful measure for identifying children with preclinical or clinical deficits in assertive behaviors and may be used to track the efficacy of assertiveness training programs. Additional normative data would be useful.

Research Applicability

High. The CATS is a useful tool in researching correlates of assertive and unassertive behavior in children. A reliable and valid short version (10 items) exists to decrease administration time.

Original Citation

Deluty, R. H. (1979). Children's Action Tendency Scale: A self-report measure of aggressiveness, assertiveness, and submissiveness in children. *Journal of Consulting and Clinical Psychology, 47*, 1061–1071.

Source

Robert H. Deluty, University of Maryland, Baltimore County, 1000 Hilltop Circle, Baltimore, MD 21250, (410) 455-2420, Fax: (410) 455-1055, deluty@umbc.edu

Cost

Please contact the source (above) for additional information.

Alternative Forms

A short form (ten situations) is available. Internal consistency coefficients, using a split-half method and Spearman–Brown correlation, were .77, .63, and .72 for the aggressiveness, assertiveness, and submissiveness subscales, respectively.

References

Crandall, V. C., Crandall, V. J., & Katkovsky, W. (1965). A Children's Social Desirability Questionnaire. *Journal of Consulting Psychology, 29,* 27–36.

Michelson, L., & Wood, R. (1982). Development and psychometric properties of the Children's Assertive Behavior Scale. *Journal of Psychopathology and Behavioral Assessment, 4,* 3–13.

Ollendick, T. H. (1984). Development and validation of the Children's Assertiveness Inventory. *Child & Family Behavior Therapy, 5,* 1–15.

Scanlon, E. M., & Ollendick, T. H. (1985). Children's assertive behavior: The reliability and validity of three self-report measures. *Child & Family Behavior Therapy, 7,* 9–21.

Children's Attitudes Toward Aggression Scale (CASS)

Purpose

To measure attitudes held by preadolescents toward various types of aggression.

Population

Ages 8–12 years.

Background and Description

The Children's Attitudes Toward Aggression Scale (CASS) was designed to explore aggressive attitudes and to provide a means of evaluating interventions with preadolescents. Item content was developed from past research of marital aggression and portray reactive, as well as proactive, aggression. Half the items are "mirror images" of the other items. Thus, 20 items reflect the approval of aggression and 20 items reflect disapproval of aggression. Respondents rate their agreement with each item on a 5-point Likert scale, ranging from 0 ("disagreed a lot") to 4 ("agreed a lot"). The scale is illustrated with "thumbs up and thumbs down," and respondents mark the box under the illustration representative of his/her level of agreement (i.e., "agreed a lot" = two thumbs up, "agreed" = one thumb up, "unsure" = question mark, "disagreed" = one thumb down, and "disagreed a lot" = two thumbs down).

Administration

The CASS is estimated to take 8–12 min to complete.

Scoring

Items worded to reflect disapproval of aggression are reverse scored, such that higher numbers are indicative of agreement with aggressive attitudes. Each item score ranges from 0 to 4. The total CASS score, ranging from 0 to 160, is obtained by summing all item scores.

Interpretation

Higher scores on individual items reflect more agreement with the attitude presented in the item. Levels of aggressive attitudes are classified according to the total CASS score. Response consistency can be evaluated by contrasting the scores obtained on "mirror image" items.

Psychometric Properties

Factor analysis. A principal components analysis with varimax rotation extracted 11 factors: "lash out" (themes of reactive aggression in retaliation, anger, or punishment), "vengeance" (themes of vengeance, violence in sports, and use of nasty names), "maintain control" (destructive expression of emotions), "hitting excused" (belief that hitting out of temper is excusable), "violence natural" (belief that it is natural for angry parents to hit and for people to fight wars), "smack kids" (physically disciplining "naughty" children), "violence inevitable" (people cannot help hurting each other), "be caring" (themes of caring, helping, and not hurting), "parents control yourselves" (disapproval of parents using physical violence), "peace possible" (the item "wars will stop 1 day"), and "learn skills" (the item "learn not to hurt others").

Reliability. Internal consistency, using Cronbach's alpha, for the entire scale and individual items was .89. Variance between items and mirror image items was low (.02). Test–retest reliability was assessed by administering the CASS to 106 children at a one-week interval, resulting in a coefficient of .74 for the entire scale. Test–retest reliabilities of individual items ranged from .79 to .86.

Validity. Content analysis suggested that 28 items reflected direct aggressive behavior (e.g.,

hitting, smacking, or bashing) and 12 items reflected verbal attacks, revenge, or fighting. Criterion validity was assessed by comparing item scores on the CASS to scores on the teacher and peer's Aggressive Behavior Rating scale. Item scores reflecting revenge and aggression correlated significantly with the teacher's scores. Seven items, labeled the "aggressive behavior index," correlated significantly with both teacher and peer ratings. These items reflected values of vengeance, hitting to solve problems, venting anger, and hitting as excusable when done out of temper.

Clinical Utility

Moderate. The CASS may be valuable in assessing the effectiveness of cognitive and behavioral interventions designed to change preadolescent attitudes toward aggression. However, the lack of normative data limit the utility of the scale.

Research Applicability

Moderate. The CASS presents an array of attitudes toward aggression, which could be useful in exploring attitudes toward aggression held by preadolescents and making comparisons between groups. Attitudes presented are mostly reactive and therefore limit the usefulness of the scale to explore proactive beliefs about aggression.

Original Citation

Maud, M. M., & De Mello, L. R. (1999). The development of the Children's Attitudes Towards Aggression Scale (CASS). *Psychological Studies, 44*, 103–111.

Source

Dr. Lesley R. Demello, Psychology Department, University of Ballarat, P.O. Box 663, Ballarat, Victoria, Australia-3350

Cost

Please contact the source (above) for permission to use the CASS.

Children's Hostility Inventory (CHI)

Purpose

To evaluate aggression and hostility in children.

Population

Parents rate the behaviors of their 6–12-year-old children.

Background and Description

The Children's Hostility Inventory (CHI) was developed to investigate alternative modes of expressing hostility and aggression among children, thus permitting an examination of the developmental continuities among antisocial children. The structure of the CHI is similar to that of the Buss–Durkee Hostility Inventory for adults (pp. 109–111); the 38 items were reworded to increase the applicability to children. Items are presented in a true–false format for seven aggression and hostility subscales. Four of the scales assess aggression (Assault, Indirect Hostility, Negativism, and Verbal Hostility) and two of the scales measure hostility (Resentment, Suspicion). The remaining scale (Irritability) is related to both aggression and hostility. A total score is also available.

Administration

It is estimated that the CHI takes 10–15 min to complete.

Scoring

Items are summed for each of the scales and for a total score.

Interpretation

Higher scores are more indicative of aggressive expressions and/or hostile thoughts and feelings.

Psychometric Properties

Norms. Normative data were collected on 255 psychiatric inpatient children (60 girls and 195 boys). Ratings were provided by the children's mother or maternal guardian.

Factor analysis. Factor analyses resulted in two factors. The first factor reflected aggression or the outward expressions of hostility and was composed of the subscales Assault, Indirect Hostility, and Verbal Hostility. The second factor reflected hostile or aggressive thoughts or feelings and was composed of the subscales Resentment, Suspicion, and Irritability.

Reliability. Preliminary results indicated acceptable levels of internal consistency, as reflected in significant item–total score correlations and a Spearman–Brown coefficient of .81.

Validity. Preliminary evidence revealed subscale scores (Assault, Indirect Hostility, Irritability, Negativism, Resentment, and Verbal Hostility) and factor analytically derived scores (Aggression and Hostility) distinguished children independently diagnosed as conduct disordered. CHI scores were also related to measures of antisocial and externalizing behavior derived from other measures. CHI scores were shown to be sensitive to treatment changes in a cognitive–behavioral temper-taming program (Farchione, Birmaher, Axelson, Kalas, Monk, Ehmann, et al., 2007; Williams, Waymouth, Lipman, Mills, & Evans, 2004).

Clinical Utility

Limited to moderate. Although the available evidence is quite promising, further examination is needed using populations other than those sampled during the development of the measure. More studies are needed to explore test–retest reliability and to gather normative data in clinical and nonclinical samples.

Research Applicability

Moderate. Preliminary evidence regarding the psychometric properties of the CHI are positive. The CHI could prove useful as a measure of parental perceptions regarding the levels of aggression and hostility in their children.

Original Citation

Kazdin, A., Rodgers, A., Colbus, D., & Siegel, T. (1987). Children's Hostility Inventory: Measurement of aggression and hostility in psychiatric inpatient children. *Journal of Clinical Child Psychology, 16,* 320–328.

Source

Alan E. Kazdin, Yale University, Box 208205, New Haven, CT 06520-8205, (203) 432-9993, Alan.Kazdin@yale.edu

Cost

Please contact the source (above) for permission to use the CHI.

Alternative Forms

A self-report form of the CHI exists wherein children complete the measure themselves. It contains 38 true/false items and three of the same subscales as the parent-rated form: Aggression, Hostility, and Irritability.

References

Farchione, T. R., Birmaher, B., Axelson, D., Kalas, C., Monk, K., Ehmann, M., et al. (2007). Aggression, hostility and irritability in children at risk for bipolar disorder. *Bipolar Disorders, 9,* 496–503.

Williams, S., Waymouth, M., Lipman, E., Mills, B., & Evans, P. (2004). Evaluation of a children's temper-taming program. *Canadian Journal of Psychiatry, 49,* 607–612.

Coding Audiotaped Aggressive Episodes

Purpose

To objectively code conversations for mode and form of aggression.

Population

Adults.

Background and Description

The procedure was designed to create a natural environment to encourage social talk among individuals. Conversations among individuals are audio recorded, transcribed, and coded in two phases. First, the number of anger episodes occurring in the course of a conversation are isolated and coded according to mode of aggression (direct, indirect, or no action), form of aggression (verbal, physical, or no action), setting (work, home, or public place), sex of antagonist (male or female), and relationship with antagonist (friend/acquaintance, lover/spouse, or stranger). The reason for the angry episode is coded according to the following criteria: integrity threat (i.e., an attack on one's competence in one's role or status as spouse, lover, professional, parent, or friend), jealousy, threat of or actual physical harm or violation of personal space, loyalty (i.e., fighting to protect the integrity or safety of another), incompetence of another person, and impotence (i.e., the inability to gain compliance from another). A single angry episode may be coded for more than one causal factor. The second phase of coding entails examining the conversation for recurrent themes: degree of experienced anger, self control, crying, aggressive action, behavioral restraint by self and by others, perception of action by self and others, experienced frustration, and behavioral management of aggression.

Administration

Sessions in the original study that utilized this methodology lasted between 2.5 and 4 h.

Scoring

The number of episodes that occurred for each of the six possible reasons is calculated.

Interpretation

A qualitative interpretation is used to assess the reasons why an individual experiences anger episodes.

Psychometric Properties

Reliability. Interrjudge reliability was reported as .76.

Validity. The reason for anger episodes and the relationship the individual had to his/her counterpart in the anger episode were the only "objective" correlates of the anger episodes that differed for men and women. This was consistent with previous literature that indicated few sex differences exist in self-reported anger and aggression.

Clinical Utility

Moderate. The procedure has use for examining communication patterns between couples and family members, but more information is needed on the reliability of the coding.

Research Applicability

Limited. The procedure has been used to create a schematic model of anger and aggression for

both men and women. However, the procedure is rather lengthy and little is known of its psychometric properties.

Original Citation

Campbell, A., & Muncer, S. (1987). Models of anger and aggression in the social talk of women and men. *Journal for the Theory of Social Behaviour Special Issue: Social Representations, 17,* 489–511.

Source

Dr. Anne Campbell and Dr. Steven Muncer, Psychology Department, Durham University Science Laboratories, South Road, DURHAM, DH1 3LE, Phone: +44(0)191 3343240, Fax: +44(0)191 3343241, a.c.campbell@durham. ac.uk

Cost

Please contact the source (above) for permission to use the Coding Audiotaped Aggressive Episodes.

Coercive Sexual Fantasies Scale (CSF)

Purpose

To assess fantasies of sexual aggression.

Population

Adult men.

Background and Description

Research has shown a link between sexual fantasies and behavior in criminal populations. The Coercive Sexual Fantasies Scale (CSF) was developed to examine the sexual fantasies of coercion, rape, violence, domination, and sadomasochism held by adult men. The goal was to develop a measure that could assess the relationship between aggressive sexual fantasies and acts in criminal and noncriminal populations. Respondents rate 36 sexually aggressive statements according to the degree to which they are congruent with their fantasies, preferences, and beliefs. Items are rated using a 7-point scale.

Administration

The CSF requires 5–10 min to complete.

Scoring

Some items are reverse scored and responses are then summed to create a total score.

Interpretation

Higher scores on the CSF indicate higher frequencies of sexually aggressive beliefs and fantasies.

Psychometric Properties

Reliability. Internal consistency as measured by Cronbach's alpha was .91.

Validity. Scores on the CSF were related to the likelihood to rape ($r = .51$) but were not correlated with rape myth acceptance or aggressive tendencies. Scores on the CSF were related to past physical and/or verbal sexually coercive behavior ($r = .26$).

Clinical Utility

Limited. The CSF provides information about sexual fantasies. However, no information is available regarding the relationship between scores on the CSF and the likelihood of the individual acting out these fantasies.

Research Applicability

Moderate. The CSF has potential for investigating the relationship between sexual fantasies and sexual aggression, but further data are needed to support its psychometric properties.

Original Citation

Greendlinger, V., & Byrne, D. (1987). Coercive sexual fantasies of college men as predictors of self-reported likelihood to rape and overt sexual aggression. *The Journal of Sex Research, 23*, 1–11.

Source

Donn Byrne, Ph.D., Department of Psychology, State University of New York at Albany, 1400 Washington Avenue, Albany, NY 12222, Vyaduckdb@aol.com

Cost

Please contact source (above) for permission to use the CSF.

Competitive Aggressiveness and Anger Scale (CAAS)

Purpose

To measure anger and aggressiveness.

Population

Competitive athletes.

Background and Description

The Competitive Aggressiveness and Anger Scale (CAAS) was designed to assess anger and aggressiveness exhibited in a variety of sport contexts. The 12 items were designed to reflect anger, acceptance of aggressive behavior, and aggressiveness. Respondents indicate how often they have engaged in each behavior using a 5-point scale ranging from 1 (almost never) to 5 (almost always).

Administration

The CAAS is estimated to require 5–10 min to complete.

Scoring

During test development, items were assigned severity level ratings. Participants' responses are multiplied by item severity and then summed to calculate subscale scores and a total score.

Interpretation

Higher scores on the aggressiveness subscale indicate greater acceptance of aggression and willingness to use aggression during sports. Higher scores on the anger subscale indicate greater frustration experienced in response to losing points or games, officials making mistakes, or greater anger reactivity in general.

Psychometric Properties

Norms. Normative data are available for men and women in contact and noncontact sports.

Factor analysis. A principal components analysis with oblimin rotation was conducted on the responses of 309 competitive athletes (192 males, 117 females). Analysis indicated the presence of two factors that accounted for 53.5 % of the variance: aggressiveness and anger. Confirmatory factor analysis was then conducted on a separate sample of 230 competitive athletes (158 males, 72 females). This analysis provided support for the previously specified two-factor model.

Reliability. Internal consistency was measured using Cronbach's alpha. Internal consistency was acceptable in two separate samples of competitive athletes, with alphas ranging from .78 to .84 for the subscales and .87 to .88 for the total score. Test–retest reliability was .86 for the anger subscale, .84 for the aggressiveness subscale, and .88 for the total score.

Validity. The CAAS was significantly related to the Aggression Questionnaire ($r=.54$, AQ, pp. 91–93). Correlations between the CAAS subscales and the AQ subscales ranged from .18 to .53. Scores on the CAAS were related to peer report of aggressive behavior, such that individuals rated by peers as aggressive scored significantly higher on the CAAS than individuals rated as neutral or calm. Scores on the CAAS aggressiveness subscale were found to significantly predict past use of unsanctioned aggression in Hong Kong rugby players (Maxwell & Visek, 2009).

Clinical Utility

Limited. The CAAS has not been used in clinical settings. The psychometric properties of the CAAS, and the relationship between aggression expressed during sports and outside of sports needs to be further clarified prior to the clinical use of this measure.

Research Applicability

Moderate. The CAAS is a brief measure that may be useful in researching cultural or gender differences in anger and aggressiveness expressed during sports. It may also aid in the investigation of how anger and aggressiveness impact performance in athletes.

Original Citation

Maxwell, J. P., & Moores, E. (2007). The development of a short scale measuring aggressiveness and anger in competitive athletes. *Psychology of Sport and Exercise, 8*, 179–193.

Source

Maxwell, J. P., Institute of Human Performance, University of Hong Kong, 111-113 Pokfulam Road, Hong Kong, SAR, 856-2589-0583, Fax: (852)-2855-1712.

Cost

Please contact the source (above) for permission to use the CAAS.

Reference

Maxwell, J. P., & Visek, A. J. (2009). Unsanctioned aggression in Rugby Union: Relationships among aggressiveness, anger, athletic identity and professionalization. *Aggressive Behavior, 35*, 237–243.

Competitive Reaction Time Task (CRT)

Purpose

To measure aggression emitted in a competitive situation.

Population

Adults.

Background and Description

The competitive reaction time task (CRT) was based on Buss' (1961) work, which used the intensity of electric shock used against another to define and score aggression. The CRT pits the participant against a fictitious opponent. The person with the slower reaction time receives a shock. Prior to each trial, the participant sets the level of intensity of the shock to be given to the opponent; the participant is told that the opponent is completing the same procedure. The frequency of wins and losses by the participant is predetermined, and shocks are randomly administered with two exceptions; participants do not receive a shock if they demonstrate an extremely fast reaction time and they are shocked if they demonstrate an extremely slow reaction time. Adhering to these exceptions increases the credibility of the procedure. To increase provocation against the participant, the intensity of the shock directed at the participant by the opponent is increased.

Administration

The procedure used determines the amount of time required to complete the task.

Scoring

Aggression is measured by the level of shock administered by the participant to the opponent.

Interpretation

Higher intensities of shock administered are indicative of higher levels of aggression.

Psychometric Properties

Reliability. Reliability data have not been reported for the CRT.

Validity. Researchers have found that individuals who demonstrate difficulty controlling their aggression respond with more increasing aggression than those who overcontrol their aggression. Additionally, opponents using more intense shocks induce more intense shock levels from the participant. The CRT has also been found to correlate with another aggression paradigm, the Buss Aggression Machine (pp. 107–108), wherein the level of shocks selected by participants in the CRT was significantly related to shock intensities used by the same participants in the Buss Aggression Machine ($r = .43$).

Clinical Utility

Limited. The procedure is difficult and lengthy, and produces an artificial environment in which participants demonstrate aggression. Responses to this task, therefore, may not generalize to real-life situations.

Research Applicability

Moderate. Although the procedure is lengthy and requires sophisticated equipment, the CRT allows researchers to obtain direct measures of aggression. A variety of individual difference and contextual factors can be manipulated.

Original Citation

Taylor, S. P. (1967). Aggressive behavior and physiological arousal as a function of provocation and the tendency to inhibit aggression. *Journal of Personality, 35,* 297–310.

Source

A complete description of the method and apparatus used for the competitive reaction time task is described in the original citation.

Cost

Unavailable.

Alternative Forms

The CRT has been modified to use noise as a form of punishment instead of shocks. In this modified version, scores are calculated based on

the mean noise level (ranging from 0 to 105 dB) and mean noise duration (0–5 s) used by participants (Coyne, Nelson, Lawton, Haslam, Rooney, Titterington, et al., 2008).

References

Bernstein, S., Richardson, D., & Hammock, G. (1987). Convergent and discriminant validity of the Taylor and Buss measures of physical aggression. *Aggressive Behavior, 13,* 15–24.

Buss, A. (1961). *The psychology of aggression.* New York: Wiley.

Coyne, S. M., Nelson, D. A., Lawton, F., Haslam, S., Rooney, L., Titterington, L., et al. (2008). The effects of viewing physical and relational aggression in the media: Evidence for a cross-over effect. *Journal of Experimental Social Psychology, 44,* 1551–1554.

Dissipation–Rumination Scale (DRS)

Purpose

To measure the levels of dissipation and rumination in an individual as a means of predicting aggressive behavior and hostility.

Population

Adults.

Background and Description

Dissipation and rumination may be conceived as opposite ends of a single behavioral dimension ranging from rapid dissipation or maximum rumination over a perceived injustice. Both dissipation and rumination are functions of the time lapse between the instigation to aggression and the moment in which the individual reacts aggressively. Individuals scoring high on dissipation tend to recover quickly from ill feelings, decreasing the desire to retaliate. Individuals high on rumination tend to harbor, and possibly enhance, ill feelings with the passing of time, thus increasing the desire to aggress. The Dissipation–Rumination Scale

(DRS) consists of 20 items, 5 of which are buffer items to control for response-set bias. Each item reflects aspects of dissipation or rumination. Items are worded in the present tense to elicit currently used strategies, and participants are encouraged to answer the items spontaneously. Items are rated using a 6-point Likert-type format. Sample items are listed below:

- It takes many years for me to get rid of a grudge.
- I won't accept excuses for certain offenses.
- When I am outraged, the more I think about it, the angrier I feel.

Administration

The DRS requires between 5 and 10 min to complete.

Scoring

Item scores range from 0 to 5 and are summed to form a total score.

Interpretation

Higher scores on the DRS indicate greater levels of rumination.

Psychometric Properties

Factor analysis. A principle components analysis was conducted with more than 800 participants to provide empirical support for the dissipation/rumination construct and to develop the DRS. The analysis allowed the developers to decrease the scale from 60 to 15 items and to identify 5 buffer items to control for response-set effects. The results of the principle components analysis confirmed the one-dimensional structure of the scale, and this structure held across groups of participants of different languages and nationality (Italian and American).

Reliability. Cronbach's alpha coefficients for the Italian and US groups were .79 and .87,

respectively. Using the Spearman–Brown method, a slightly higher reliability coefficient (.91) was obtained by contrasting the responses to the even and the odd items obtained from Italian participants. Test–retest reliability was .81 for Italian participants.

Validity. Evidence for the validity of the dissipation/rumination construct was initially demonstrated by two studies (Caprara, Coluzzi, Mazzotti, Renzi, & Zelli, 1985; Zelli, 1984). In both studies, participants received written communications (insulting versus not insulting) from a confederate and were allowed to reciprocate either immediately or after 24 h had passed. Reciprocation was in the form of selecting levels of shock to be administered to the confederate when the confederate made an error in an extrasensory perception task or evaluating the confederate for a staff position in the laboratory. Results from both studies supported the dissipation/rumination construct, indicating that dissipation/rumination is a good predictor of aggression and hostility. Similar results were found in a later study (Collins & Bell, 1997). Those obtaining high scores again displayed greater levels of aggression when provoked (Konecni, 1984).

Clinical Utility

Moderate. The DRS is brief and easily administered. Previous studies have supported its use as a measure of the dissipation/rumination construct, as well as its use as a predictor of aggression and hostility. Thus, this scale may be especially useful when combined with other measures to predict future aggressive behaviors. Scores on the DRS may also provide insight into the types of interventions needed to prevent future aggressive acts (e.g., an intervention that helps individuals to dissipate ill feelings at a quicker rate).

Research Applicability

High. The DRS can be administered in an individual or group format. It has been used in numerous studies whose results validate the dissipation/rumination construct. Particularly, the DRS appears to be most valuable in research examining cognitive processes in aggressive responding (Caprara, 1987). Results from previous research using this scale suggested the need to further assess both the cognitive and emotional components of aggression.

Original Citation

Caprara, G. V. (1986). Indicators of aggression: The Dissipation–Rumination Scale. *Personality and Individual Differences, 7,* 763–769.

Source

Gian V. Caprara, Department of Psychology, Sapienza University of Rome, Piazzale Aldo Moro 5, 00185 Roma, Italia, Phone: (064) 991-7532, gianvittorio.caprara@uniroma1.it

Cost

Please contact the source (above) for permission to use the DRS.

Alternate forms

A 29-item English version that has similar psychometric properties as the original DRS is also available (Caprara, Cinanni, & Mazzotti, 1989).

References

Caprara, G. V. (1987). The disposition-situation debate and research on aggression. *European Journal of Personality, 1,* 1–16.
Caprara, G. V., Cinanni, V., & Mazzotti, E. (1989). Measuring attitudes toward violence. *Personality and Individual Differences, 10*(4), 479–481.
Caprara, G. V., Coluzzi, M., Mazzotti, E., Renzi, P., & Zelli, A. (1985). Effect of insult and dissipation-rumination on delayed aggression and hostility. *Archivio di Psicologia, Neurologia, e Psichiatria, 46*(1), 130–139.
Collins, K., & Bell, R. (1997). Personality and aggression: The Dissipation-Rumination Scale. *Personality and Individual Differences, 22*(5), 751–755.

Konecni, V. (1984). Methodological issues in human aggression research. In K. Kaplan, V. Konecni, & K. Novaco, *Aggression in children and youth* (pp. 1–43). The Hague: Nijhoff Publishers.
Zelli, A. (1984). Ruolo delle differenze individuali nella condotta aggressiva: Variabili di personalitá, temperamentali, psicofisiologiche. *Tesi di Laurea.* Roma: Universita' degli Studi di roma "La Sapienza."

Expressive Representations of Aggression Scale (EXPAGG)

Purpose

To determine whether a person views aggression in instrumental or expressive terms.

Population

All ages.

Background and Description

The Expressive Representations of Aggression Scale (EXPAGG) was developed to test gender differences in the expression of aggression. The expectation was that women view aggression as a means of expressing themselves and those expressions can lead to feelings of guilt (Archer & Haigh, 1997b). Men were expected to view aggression as a vehicle for enhancing status and other advantages that lead to positive emotions after aggressive behavior. The EXPAGG consists of 20 forced-choice items that describe aggression related to social values, proximate causes, relevant emotions, relevant cognitions, and situational factors. Participants are asked to place themselves in the situation and to choose one of two options that most closely reflect how they would think, feel, or behave. One response constitutes an expressive reaction, whereas the other response reflects an instrumental reaction. The following are example items.

- I believe that my aggression comes from
  Being pushed too far by obnoxious people (instrumental)
  Losing my self control (expressive)

- In a heated argument, I am most afraid of
  Being out-argued by the other person
  (instrumental)
  Saying something terrible that I can never take
  back (expressive)

Administration

The EXPAGG can be administered in group or
individual settings and requires 5–10 min to
complete.

Scoring

Instrumental responses receive a score of 0 and
expressive responses receive a score of 1. Responses
to items are summed to produce a single score.

Interpretation

A high score on the scale indicates the use of
aggression for expressive purposes.

Psychometric Properties

Factor analysis. A factor analysis of 16 items
was interpreted as consistent with a one-factor
model, with all items loading positively on one
factor. This factor was labeled Instrumental-
Expressive Aggression. Two additional factors
were identified: Privacy and Guilt. A principal
component factor analysis of the 20-item scale
was interpreted as representative of one major
factor, with a second factor reflective of a preference for private rather than public aggression
(Campbell, Muncer, & Gorman, 1993).

Reliability. Internal consistency, measured by
Cronbach's alpha, ranged from .72 to .81.

Validity. The EXPAGG scores of men in the
armed forces were found to be lower than scores
of men and women in a nursing profession, and

women in the armed forces, as hypothesized by
the authors (Campbell & Muncer, 1994). The
EXPAGG was also correlated with a measure of
physical aggression ($r=.63$; Archer & Haigh,
1997a). In a sample of undergraduate students,
the EXPAGG correlated with gender (men had
lower scores) and the F scale of the Personal
Attributes Questionnaire (Spence, Helmreich, &
Stapp, 1974). Splitting the scale in half and scoring the first half in the direction of instrumental-
ity and the second half in the direction of
expressivity resulted in a correlation of $r=-.66$,
reflecting the unidimensionality of the scale.

Clinical Utility

Moderate. Ease of administration and scoring
increases clinical utility. Additional normative
work is necessary prior to wide spread clinical
use.

Research Applicability

High. Available evidence suggests acceptable
levels of reliability and correlations with other
known measures. The measure might be useful
for testing hypotheses related to expressive and
instrumental models of aggression.

Original Citation

Campbell, A., Muncer S., & Coyle, E. (1992). Social rep-
    resentation of aggression as an explanation of gender
    differences: A preliminary study. *Aggressive Behavior,*
    18, 95–108.

Source

Anne   Campbell,   Ph.D.,   Department   of
Psychology,   Durham   University   Science
Laboratories, South Road, DURHAM, DH1
3LE, Phone: +44(0)191 3343240, Fax: +44(0)191
3343241, a.c.campbell@durham.ac.uk

Cost

Please contact the source (above) for permission to use the EXPAGG.

Alternate Forms

A revised form for children was developed by Archer and Haigh (1997b). They developed a 42-item scale by separating the forced-choice responses into 20 items containing instrumental values and 20 items containing expressive values. They added two items concerning the nature of the aggressive incident and the sex and relationship of the respondent's opponent. Responses are based on a 5-point Likert scale (Archer & Parker, 1994).

A short form of the EXPAGG was developed by Campbell, Muncer, McManus, and Woodhouse (1999). Confirmatory Factor Analysis revealed that the 10-item short form of the EXPAGG fit the two-dimensional underlying structure better than the 16-item EXPAGG (Driscoll, Campbell, & Muncer, 2005).

References

Archer, J., & Haigh, A. (1997a). Beliefs about aggression among male and female prisoners. *Aggressive Behavior, 23*, 405–415.

Archer, J., & Haigh, A. (1997b). Do beliefs about aggressive feelings and actions predict reported levels of aggression? *British Journal of Social Psychology, 36*, 83–105.

Archer, J., & Parker, S. (1994). Social representations of aggression in children. *Aggressive Behavior, 20*, 101–114.

Campbell, A., & Muncer S. (1994). Sex differences in aggression: Social representation and social roles. *British Journal of Social Psychology, 33*, 233–240.

Campbell, A., Muncer S., & Gorman, B. (1993). Sex and social representations of aggression: A communal-agentic analysis. *Aggressive Behavior, 19*, 125–135.

Campbell, A., Muncer S., McManus, I., & Woodhouse, D. (1999). Instrumental and expressive representations of aggression: One scale or two? *Aggressive Behavior, 25*, 435–444.

Driscoll, H., Campbell, A., & Muncer, S. (2005). Confirming the structure of the ten-item EXPAGG scale using confirmatory factor analysis. *Current Research in Social Psychology, 10*, 222–234.

Spence, J. T., Helmreich, R., & Stapp, J. (1974). The Personal Attributes Questionnaire: A measure of sex role stereotypes and masculinity-femininity. *Catalog of Selected Documents in Psychology, 4*, 43–44.

Hypermasculinity Inventory (HMI)

Purpose

To assess a constellation of characteristics related to a conceptualization of the macho personality style.

Population

Adults.

Background and Description

The macho concept matriculated from Hispanic to American culture and was utilized in the women's movement as the defining characteristic of a hypermasculine style. That is, a masculine style containing three interrelated components: calloused sex attitudes toward women (i.e., the idea that sexual intercourse is a means of establishing masculine power and subjugation of the female), viewing violence as manly (i.e., the belief that violent expression is an accepted means to express power and dominance), and finding danger exciting (i.e., the belief that survival demonstrates power over the environment). Using this conceptualization of hypermasculinity, the authors developed a pool of 221 questions from all male peer-group discussions of fighting, sex, and dangerous exploits. This pool of items was administered to 60 college men and then subjected to internal consistency item analyses. The resulting 90 items were administered to 135 college men, and internal consistency item analyses were again conducted. The final scale consists of 30 forced-choice items that are equally divided into three subscales: calloused sex attitudes toward women, violence as manly, and danger as exciting.

Administration

The HMI requires approximately 15–20 min to complete.

Scoring

Items are summed to produce a single score for each factor, as well as an overall score.

Interpretation

Higher scores indicate endorsement of more hypermasculine beliefs.

Psychometric Properties

Factor analysis. Factor analysis resulted in a single factor labeled the macho personality pattern.

Reliability. Cronbach alpha coefficients ranged from .71 (Danger subscale) to .79 (Violence and Calloused Sex subscales). Cronbach's alpha for the 30-item scale was .89.

Validity. The HMI correlated with frequent use of alcohol, stimulants, depressants, marijuana, and hashish. The Danger subscale accounted for most of the shared variance between the HMI and drug or alcohol use. The Danger subscale also contributed most of the variance between the HMI and changes in driving and aggressive behavior following alcohol consumption. Finally, the HMI was significantly related to self-reported high school delinquency; the Violence subscale contributed the most variance to this relationship.

Construct validity was assessed by correlating the HMI with subscales from the Jackson Personality Research Form. The HMI correlated positively with the factors of play, impulsivity, exhibition, aggression, autonomy, and dominance. The HMI was inversely related to the factors of understanding, harm avoidance, cognitive structure, nurturance, order, and desirability. Mosher and Anderson (1986) found that scores on the HMI were positively related to total aggression, sexual force, the use of drugs and alcohol, verbal manipulation, angry rejection, anger expression, and threat. Scores on the HMI were also related to relevant scores on the Bem Sex Role Inventory and the Attitudes to Women Scale (Archer & Rhodes, 1989).

Clinical Utility

Moderate. The HMI has not been widely used in clinical settings. Scores on the inventory might provide insight into the possible attitudes and behaviors related to the mistreatment of women. For example, scores on the Calloused Sex subscale correlated with sexually aggressive behavior in college men (Mosher & Anderson, 1996).

Research Applicability

High. The HMI possesses acceptable psychometric properties and has frequently been used to identify correlates of the macho personality constellation. It requires minimal time to complete and is easily scored.

Original Citation

Mosher, D. L., & Sirkin, M. (1984). Measuring a macho personality constellation. *Journal of Research in Personality, 18,* 150–163.

Source

Donald L. Mosher, Department of Psychology, University of Connecticut, Unit 1020, Storrs, CT 06269-1020.

Cost

Please contact the author (above) for permission to use.

References

Archer, J., & Rhodes, C. (1989). The relationship between gender-related traits and attitudes. *British Journal of Social Psychology, 28,* 149–157.
Mosher, D. L., & Anderson, R. D. (1986). Macho personality, sexual aggression, and reactions to guided imagery of realistic rape. *Journal of Research in Personality, 20,* 77–94.

Multidimensional Aggression Scale for the Structured Doll Play Interview (MASSD)

Purpose

To assess aggressive responses in children.

Population

Children ages 4–5.

Background and Description

The Mulitdimensional Aggression Scale for the Structured Doll Play Interview (MASSD) expands on a prior scoring system that only assessed the frequency of aggressive responses. The child is presented with 12 doll play situations that often elicit aggressive responses. Two adult dolls and one child doll that represents the same sex, age, and race of the subject are used to structure the doll play. The first six situations assess dependency and the last six situations evoke aggressive responding. The MASSD codes the structured doll play using up to 34 categories of behavior. Categories include violent aggression by the self, violent aggression by the environment, violent aggression by the mother, violent aggression by the father, and violent aggression by others. In addition to scoring the categories, each scored response is rated along the dimensions of intensity, agent, and directionality.

Administration

The structured doll play is administered individually and estimated to require 45–60 min to complete depending upon the individual child.

Scoring

Each doll play response is scored. The intensity of the aggressive response to each of the 12 situations is rated from 0 (nonaggressive) to 3 (the actual killing of another human being or animal is present). In addition to intensity, each response is scored for the dimensions of agent and directionality. For agent, the responses are scored for the instigator of aggressive behavior. The instigator may be self, environment, mother, father, or other. For directionality, the responses are scored for whom they were directed at. Aggression may be directed toward self, environment, mother, father, or other. In addition to the categorization of aggressive responses along the dimensions of intensity, agent, and directionality, the total frequency of violent aggressive, aggressive, assertive, and nonaggressive responses are coded. A complete scoring manual can be found in Abramson, Abramson, Wohlford, and Berger (1972).

Interpretation

Higher scores indicate a greater tendency to use aggressive responses.

Psychometric Properties

Norms. The MASSD was examined in a group of 123 African American preschool age children.

Factor analysis. Six factors have been extracted: Violent Aggression Toward the Family; Violent Aggression by the Family; Aggression by the Self; Aggression Directed Toward the Self; Assertion Directed Toward Others; and Assertion Directed Toward the Family.

Reliability. Interrater reliability estimates range from .84 to 1.00.

Validity. Two different methods of scoring the responses resulted in a Spearman rank-order coefficient of .92.

Clinical Utility

Limited. As an analog procedure, the MASSD could provide useful insights into contextual factors associated with aggressive responding in 4- and 5-year-old children. The lack of validity and normative data limit the overall clinical utility.

Research Applicability

Moderate. The MASSD could prove useful as an analog procedure for eliciting aggressive and violent responding in different groups of children.

Original Citations

Abramson, P. R., Abramson, L. C., Wohlford, P., & Berger, S. (1972). A Multidimensional Aggression Scale for the structured doll play. In P. Wholford (Ed.), *Changing parental attitudes and behavior through participant group methods.* Washington, DC: U.S. Department of Health, Education, & Welfare, Office of Research & Evaluation, Office of Economic Opportunity.

Abramson, P. R., & Abramson, S. D. (1974). A factorial study of a multidimensional approach to aggressive behavior in black preschool age children. *The Journal of Genetic Psychology, 125,* 31–36.

Source

Paul R. Abramson, UCLA Department of Psychology, 1285 Franz Hall, Box 951563, Los Angeles, CA 90095, (310) 825-7214, Abramson@psych.ucla.edu

Cost

Please contact the source (above) for additional information.

Multidimensional Peer-Victimization Scale (MPVS)

Purpose

To assess and identify peer victimization.

Population

Children and adolescents ages 11–16.

Background and Description

The Multidimensional Peer-Victimization Scale (MPVS) was designed to increase understanding of the structure of peer victimization in an effort to produce a clear categorization system. The MPVS contains 45 items that represent a wide range of both direct and indirect victimizing experiences. The authors and teachers were involved in item development. Students are read a definition of bullying and told that the questionnaire they are about to complete is about their experiences of bullying. Students indicate whether they have been bullied during the current school year and, if so, whether this was mostly by boys, girls, or both. Students then indicate the frequency with which they have experienced one of the 45 events using a scale that ranges from 0 (not at all) to 2 (more than once). Sample items are listed below:

- Refused to talk to me
- Spat at me
- Accused me of something I didn't do

Administration

It is estimated that the questionnaire requires 15–20 min to complete.

Scoring

Scores are summed.

Interpretation

Higher scores indicate experiencing a greater degree of peer victimization.

Psychometric Properties

Norms. Eight hundred and twelve children (402 boys and 410 girls) ranging in age from 11 to 16 years who were attending a secondary school in England completed the MPVS.

Factor analysis. Principal component analysis resulted in a nine-factor solution that accounted for 55 % of the variance. The factors were labeled: physical victimization, forced truancy, social manipulation, verbal victimization, victimization with prejudiced content, attacks on property, being forced to do something and being made frightened, accusations of working too hard, and having money taken. Four factors were retained: Physical Victimization, Verbal Victimization, Social Manipulation, and Attacks on Property. Four factors were also found in a sample of Nigerian children (Balogun & Olapebga, 2007).

Reliability. Alpha coefficients for the four sub-scales ranged from .73 to .85. The MPVS was also given to a sample of 240 Nigerian children, which resulted in Cronbach's alpha .78 for the total score and split-half reliability .76.

Validity. The four scales correlated with self-reports of being bullied. The MPVS correlated significantly ($r=.54$) with the Buss-Durkee Hostility Inventory (pp. 109–111).

Clinical Utility

Moderate. This measure has not been widely used, but does demonstrate potential to provide useful information regarding different types of peer victimizations. It is relatively brief and has demonstrated acceptable psychometric properties.

Research Applicability

Moderate. This measure has not been widely studied but could prove useful for researchers interested in studying characteristics of peer victimization.

Original Citation

Mynard, H., & Joseph, S. (2000). Development of the Multidimensional Peer-Victimization Scale. *Aggressive Behavior, 26,* 169–178.

Source

Stephen Joseph, School of Sociology & Social Policy, University of Nottingham, University Park, Nottingham NG7 2RD, Phone: 0115 951 5410, Fax: 0115 951 5232, Stephen.joseph@nottingham.ac.uk

Cost

Please contact the source (above) for permission to use the MPVS.

Reference

Balogun, S. K., & Olapegba, P. O. (2007). Cultural validation of the Multidimensional Peer Victimization Scale in Nigerian children. *Journal of Cross-Cultural Psychology, 38,* 573–580.

Offense Scenario (OS)

Purpose

To assess the likelihood of an individual responding aggressively in situations in which an offense occurs.

Population

Adults.

Background and Description

The Offense Scenario (OS) was developed to evaluate the relationship between Agnew's General Strain Theory (1992) and assault behavior. A series of scenarios depict situations wherein a law has been violated (e.g., driving while inebriated, theft, and assault). Respondents are instructed to read each scenario and then estimate the likelihood that they would respond in a manner similar to the character in the scenario. A sample scenario follows:

• *It's Friday night and Mike and Lisa, who have been dating for 2 years, go to Santa Fe for a few beers with Mike's friends. During their beers, Mike excuses himself and goes to the bathroom. While he is away, another guy, Joe, starts to talk to Lisa and even sits down at her table and begins to talk to her. Mike comes back and asks the guy if he has a problem because Lisa is his girlfriend. Joe stands up and tells Mike that Lisa does not have a ring and is therefore allowed to talk to whomever she wants. Meanwhile, Mike's friends crowd behind him. Mike doesn't like this too much so he motions to Lisa for her hand so they can leave Santa Fe. Joe pushes Mike's hand down. Mike decides to hit Joe in the face and a large scale fight breaks out.*

For this scenario, respondents are asked to estimate the likelihood that they would behave as Mike did using a scale that ranges from 0 ("not likely") to 10 ("likely").

Administration

Completion of each scenario is estimated to take 3–5 min.

Scoring

Responses to each scenario are used to estimate the intent to respond in an aggressive manner when placed in a similar context.

Interpretation

Higher scores indicate a greater intent to respond aggressively.

Psychometric Properties

Reliability. No reliability data are available.

Validity. In a sample of 245 males, 98 % rated the scenario (described above) as "very believable." Exposure to strain and anger were found to be related to intentions to assault, as measured by the OS, which is consistent with GST.

Clinical Utility

Moderate. The OS provides a descriptive means of identifying situations in which an individual may respond aggressively. The lack of normative and reliability data, however, limit the clinical utility.

Research Applicability

Moderate. The methodology employed by the OS may generalize and allow for an evaluation of the differences between those who respond aggressively versus nonaggressively to various situations. More research on the psychometric properties of the OS is needed.

Original Citation

Mazerolle, P., & Piquero, A. (1997). Violent responses to strain: An examination of conditioning influences. *Violence and Victims, 12,* 323–343.

Source

Paul Mazerolle, Mt Gravatt campus, Griffith University, 176 Messines Ridge Rd, Mt Gravatt, Queensland 4122, Phone: (07) 373 55710, p.mazerolle@griffith.edu.au

Cost

Please contact the source (above) for permission to use the OS.

Reference

Agnew, R. (1992). Foundation for a general strain theory of crime and delinquency. *Criminology, 30*, 47–88.

Overt Aggression Scale (OAS)

Purpose

To assess different forms of aggression displayed within a hospital setting.

Population

Adult and child psychiatric inpatients and brain-injured patients within rehabilitation settings.

Background and Description

The Overt Aggression Scale (OAS) was developed as an objective and easy-to-complete tool to be used to quantify aggressive behavior. The checklist is typically completed by nursing staff. Aggressive behaviors are divided into four categories: verbal aggression, physical aggression against objects, physical aggression against self, and physical aggression against others. An observer codes the behavior exhibited during each aggressive episode, as well as the strategies used to decrease the aggressive behavior. Descriptive statements within each category define the scale points and serve to guide severity ratings from 1 (least severe) to 4 (most severe).

Administration

Completion of the OAS after each incident requires between 5 and 10 min.

Scoring

Scores can represent the number of episodes, the number of specific behaviors, and the num-ber of specific strategies employed. Both weekly frequencies of aggressive incidents in each of the four categories and weekly mean severity scores of aggressive incidents are often used to evaluate change in aggressive behavior. Recent versions generate total scores that weight the categories differently; physical aggression receives the highest weighting and verbal aggression receives the lowest weighting (Silver & Yudofsky, 1991).

Interpretation

The total number of behaviors checked indicates greater frequency of aggressive behaviors. Higher total scores indicate greater severity of aggressive behaviors.

Psychometric Properties

Norms. Initial normative data were obtained from 16 children involved in a total of 54 aggressive episodes and 21 adult psychiatric patients involved in 35 aggressive episodes. Eight psychiatric adults with 70 episodes were subsequently added. For each category of aggression, only the most severe behavior observed and the most extreme intervention used were recorded. Each behavior and intervention was assigned a weighted score according to relative severity. The reliability of the sum of weighted behavior and intervention scores was tested to provide a composite rating that indicated a global level of severity for an aggressive episode.

Reliability. Interrater reliability was estimated using intraclass correlations with coefficients ranging from .75 to .87. The total aggression score, representing the summed weighted scores for the most severe of each type of behavior and the most restrictive intervention, revealed a coefficient of .87. For children, the correlations between weighted scores of aggressive behaviors and strategies employed ranged from −.07 to .41 (Gothelf, Apter, & van Praag, 1997). Verbal aggression and the associated intervention used in children had the lowest reliability. For adult psychiatric samples, the correlations between weighted scores of aggressive behaviors and strategies employed ranged from .12 to 1.0.

Validity. Aggressive episodes documented within a chronic inpatient psychiatry setting were compared with data obtained from the OAS. The OAS recorded 98 % of documented aggressive incidents, whereas the hospital chart, the medication book, and the communication book noted only 27 %. In another sample of psychiatric patients, the OAS recorded 87 % of the approximately 2,300 aggressive incidents documented, whereas official hospital documents recorded 53 % of aggressive incidents. Additionally, Malone, Luebbert, Pena-Ariet, Biesecker, and Delaney. (1994) found OAS scores agreed with findings from a more general measure, the Global Clinical Consensus Rating (GCCR, Campbell et al., 1984), which was based on staff consensus regarding treatment outcomes.

Clinical Utility

High. The OAS has been used in a number of different settings and with a variety of populations. This scale assesses factors specific to each aggressive episode and episodes can be aggregated to obtain more global indices. It is easy to complete and reliable for rating aggressive events within a hospital setting. Criticism of the OAS has focused on its efforts to weight aggressive behaviors and to arrive at a composite score and difficulty defining the aggressive episode.

Research Applicability

High. The OAS has been widely used and has considerable potential for documenting individual patterns of aggression, week-to-week fluctuations in aggressive behaviors, patterns of aggression among patient groups, and the efficacy of pharmacological and psychosocial interventions designed to decrease aggressive behavior.

Original Citation

Yudofsky, S. C., Silver, J. M., Jackson, W., Endicott, J., & Williams, D. (1986). The Overt Aggression Scale for the objective rating of verbal and physical aggression. *American Journal of Psychiatry, 143,* 35–39.

Source

Stuart C. Yudofsky, One Baylor Plaza, BCM 350, Houston, TX 77030, (713) 798-4945, Fax: (713) 796-1615, stuarty@bcm.edu

Cost

Contact the source (above) for permission to use the OAS.

Alternative Forms

A modified 16-item aggressive classes or types of aggressive behavior form was adapted (Retrospective Overt Aggression Scale, Sorgi, Ratey, Knoedler, Markert, & Reichman, 1991). The modified version is cited in Sorgi et al. (1991).

The Modified Overt Aggression Scale (MOAS) was developed with upgraded psychometric properties to assess the nature and prevalence of aggression in a psychiatric population (Kay, Wolkenfeld, & Murrill, 1988). This scale added multivariate scaling which appeared to improve the measurement and the depiction of the construct. The MOAS relies upon weekly scores rather than critical incident reports. The scheduling of reports is helpful in terms of encouraging staff participation, but may create bias due to the effects of retrospective bias. Criticism has been raised because it does not allow the study of close precursors or triggers or immediate consequences for nurses and patients involved.

A third modified version of the OAS was developed in the measurement and assessment of aggressive behaviors following brain injury (Alderman, Knight, & Morgan, 1997).

References

Alderman, N., Knight, C., & Morgan, C. (1997). Use of a modified version of the Overt Aggression Scale in the measurement and assessment of aggressive behaviors following brain injury. *Brain Injury, 11*, 503–523.

Campbell, M., Small A. M., Green, W. H., Jennings S. J., Perry R., Bennett W.G., et al. (1984). Behavioral efficacy of Haloperidol and Lithium Carbonate: A comparison in hospitalized aggressive children with conduct disorder. *Archives of General Psychiatry, 41*, 650–656.

Gothelf, D., Apter, A., & van Praag, H. M. (1997). Measurement of aggression in psychiatric patients. *Psychiatry Research, 71*, 83–95

Kay, S. R., Wolkenfeld, F., & Murrill, L. M. (1988). Profiles of aggression among psychiatric patients: I. Nature and prevalence. *The Journal of Nervous and Mental Disease, 176*, 539–546.

Malone, R. P., Luebbert, J., Pena-Ariet, M., Biesecker, K., Delaney,M. A. (1994). The Overt Aggression Scale in a study of lithium in aggressive conduct disorder. *Psychopharmacology Bulletin, 30*, 215–218.

Silver, J. M., & Yudofsky, S. C. (1991). The Overt Aggression Scale: Overview and guiding principles. *Journal of Neuropsychiatry and Clinical Neurosciences, 3*, S22–S29.

Sorgi, P., Ratey, J., Knoedler, D. W., Markert, R. J., & Reichman, M. (1991). Rating aggression in the clinical setting: A retrospective adaptation of the Overt Aggression Scale: Preliminary results. *Journal of Neuropsychiatry and Clinical Neurosciences, 3*, S52–S56.

Peer Nomination Inventory (PNI)

Purpose

To measure social adjustment for groups of preadolescent boys and to reflect the behavior systems of aggression, dependency, withdrawal, and depression.

Population

Preadolescent boys.

Background and Description

The authors adapted Hartshorne and May's (1929) "guess who" technique for assessing social reputation by means of sociometric peer ratings. This method involves presenting statements in the form of "word pictures" and asking respondents to "guess," which classmate the statement describes. The Peer Nomination Inventory (PNI) contains 48 statements that are organized using an item-by-peer matrix consisting of statements assessing social maladjustment of an individual as perceived by classmates. Boys are asked to identify which of their classmates each statement describes.

Administration

The PNI can be easily completed within a 1-h class period.

Scoring

Scoring of the PNI uses a cumulative (or intensity) scoring model, tabulating the number of raters who nominated a certain boy on a given item and converting this score into a proportion or percentage for each of the total number of raters. These percentage scores are then combined to create a total score ranging from 0 to 1,200.

Interpretation

The larger the percentage, the greater the "intensity" of the behavior and the social impact of the behavior.

Psychometric Properties

Norms. The PNI was normed on 710 fourth, fifth, and sixth grade boys from lower, middle, and upper middle class backgrounds.

Factor analysis. A factor analysis revealed four primary factors: Social Isolation (withdrawal, rejection by peers, being alone), Hostility (aggression), Crying (sensitivity and low self-esteem, depression), and Attention Getting (dependency).

Reliability. One-year test–retest reliability was estimated from a group of 339 fourth and fifth grade boys and found to be in the range .34 to .57. Internal consistency was calculated by correlating the odd numbered items with the even numbered items. This resulted in estimates ranging from .76 to .89.

Validity. The PNI was related to both teacher and peer ratings. Spearman rank-order coefficients ranged from .42 to .70.

Clinical Utility

Moderate. The PNI allows for the assessment of individuals by their peers and can help to elucidate peer perceptions of a particular child. Gaining permission to administer the PNI to a group of children can be difficult.

Research Applicability

Limited. The resulting distribution of scores on the deviant behavior scales limits the usefulness for general studies, but might prove useful for identifying individual students who peers rate as deviant.

Original Citation

Wiggins, J. S., & Winder, C. L. (1961). The Peer Nomination Inventory: An empirically derived sociometric measure of adjustment in preadolescent boys. *Psychological Reports, 9*, 643–677.

Source

Wiggins, J. S., & Winder, C. L. (1961). The Peer Nomination Inventory: An empirically derived sociometric measure of adjustment in preadolescent boys. *Psychological Reports, 9*, 643–677.

Cost

Unavailable.

References

Landau, S., & Milich, R. (1985). Social status of aggressive and aggressive/withdrawn boys: A replication across age and method. *Journal of Consulting and Clinical Psychology, 53*, 141.

Milich, R., & Landau, S. (1984). A comparison of the social status and social behavior of aggressive and aggressive/withdrawn boys. *Journal of Abnormal Child Psychology, 12*, 277–288.

Personality Assessment Inventory (PAI)

Purpose

To assess personality style, psychopathology, and current functioning.

Population

Adults

Background and Description

The Personality Assessment Inventory (PAI) was designed to be a comprehensive profile of response bias, diagnostic categorization, treatment orientation, and general personality. The 344 items require a fourth grade reading level and are organized into 22 non-overlapping scales: 4 validity scales, 11 clinical scales, 5 treatment scales, and 2 interpersonal scales. The four validity scales assess response inconsistency, careless or random responding, unfavorable impression management and malingering, and favorable impression management. The clinical scales assess alcohol problems, antisocial features, anxiety, anxiety related disorders, borderline features, depression, drug problems, mania, paranoia, schizophrenia, and somatic complaints. Treatment scales assess aggression, nonsupport, stress, suicidal ideation, and treatment rejection. Interpersonal scales assess dominance and warmth. Thirty-two additional subscales cover a variety of clinical constructs. Items are rated using a scale that ranges from 0 ("totally false") to 3 ("very true").

Administration

The PAI may be administered using a paper-and-pencil or a computer-administered format and requires 40–50 min to complete.

Scoring

Responses are computer scored.

Interpretation

Interpretation of the PAI takes place at four levels: item, subscale, full scale, and configuration (e.g., mean profiles, 2-point code types, cluster analysis, actuarial analyses, or configural rules). An elevated validity scale score indicates that the profile should be interpreted with caution. Subscale and scale scores are compared with norms obtained from community and clinical samples. T-scores of 60 or higher indicate areas of concern. The manual provides descriptions of average profiles from 24 groups, each with a particular diagnosis, to aid in forming hypotheses and making diagnoses.

Psychometric Properties

Norms. Norms are provided for community ($n = 1,000$), clinical ($n = 1,246$), and student ($n = 1,051$) samples.

Factor analysis. An initial principal axis factor analysis of the 22 scales produced five factors, which were difficult to interpret. Reanalyses specifying four factors produced the following interpretable factors: general psychological distress; narcissism and tendency to exploit others; rash, impulsive behavior; and functioning in social relationships. A three-factor solution was produced for the 11 clinical scales: general psy-

chological distress, antisocial tendencies, and substance abuse.

Reliability. Mean internal consistency estimates for normative, college, and clinical samples ranged from .81 to .92. Estimates generated from a mixed clinical/normal sample revealed a median value of .84. Median estimates using alcoholic samples for the full scales and subscales ranged from .86 to .92 and .77 to .78, respectively. In a sample of psychiatric inpatients, alpha values ranged from .65 (negative impression) to .93 (anxiety). In general, median alphas have been similar across demographic characteristics such as gender and age.

The median test–retest coefficient (11 full scales) of the standardization studies over a 4-week period was .86. For a 24-day period, stability coefficients ranged from .79 to .92 for the clinical scales. Test–retest median coefficient was .73 in a normal sample for a period of 28 days. In a sample of Australian normals, alcoholics, and schizophrenics, the median stability coefficient for a 28-day period was .73 (.62 for anxiety to .86 for suicidal ideation).

Validity. Item content was initially evaluated using a panel of lay and professional individuals who evaluated statements to determine whether the content reflected what was intended. Psychometric properties of all items were also evaluated as a function of demographic characteristics. PAI scores were compared with scores on structured interviews that tap severe psychiatric conditions, suicide potential, and general psychiatric symptoms. Correlations demonstrated evidence of convergent validity for screening feigned profiles, establishing clinical correlates of common disorders, and evaluating potential suicidal ideation. Scores on the alcohol and drug subscales of the PAI correlated significantly with scores on the alcohol scale composite and drug scale composite of the Addiction Severity Index (McLellan et al., 1992), respectively. Logistic regression found PAI scales were conceptually related to the domains of violence, psychosis, and personality disorder. Moreover, physical aggression and affective instability were related to violence and personality disorder, respectively.

Overall, scales of the PAI have been found to correlate with scales of other measures for assessment and diagnosis. The PAI manual contains information about the correlations of the individual scales with over 50 indices of psychopathology, and validity studies are summarized in the Interpretive Guide. More information on the validity of the PAI may also be found in Morey (1999).

Clinical Utility

High. The PAI is useful for screening clients, treatment planning, and describing forensic groups. Interpretation may be done in a straightforward and clinically meaningful manner. Additional norms are available for various aggressive and violent samples.

Research Applicability

Moderate. The PAI is a general screening tool, lengthy, and the majority of items are unrelated to anger, aggression, and violence. Thus it may not be the most efficient tool for research purposes, however, it does provide relevant information on anger, aggression, violence, and associated personality constructs.

Original Citation

Morey, L. C. (1991). *The Personality Assessment Inventory professional manual.* Odessa, FL: Psychological Assessment Resources.
Morey, L. C. (1996). *An interpretive guide to the Personality Assessment Inventory.* Odessa, FL: Psychological Assessment Resources.

Source

Psychological Assessment Resources, Inc., 16204 N. Florida Ave., Lutz, FL 33549.

Cost

The PAI comprehensive kit costs $295 on Psychological Assessment Resources (PAR). This kit includes the professional manual, 2 reusable item booklets, 2 administration folios, 25 hand-scored answer sheets, 25 profile forms, 25 critical items forms, and 1 professional report service answer sheet.

Alternative Forms

The PAI has been translated into Spanish, with a reported average alpha coefficient of .63 and a .71 average test–retest coefficient for a 2-week period.

References

McLellan, A. T., Cacciola, J., Kushner, H., Peters, R., Smith, I., Pettinati, H. (1992). The fifth edition of the Addiction Severity Index: Cautions, additions and normative data. *Journal of Substance Abuse Treatment,* 9(5), 461–480.
Morey, L. C. (1999). Personality Assessment Inventory. In M. E. Maruish (Ed.), *The use of psychological testing for treatment planning and outcomes assessment* (2nd ed., pp. 1083–1121). Mahwah, NJ: Lawrence Erlbaum Associates.

Point Subtraction Aggression Paradigm (PSAP)

Purpose

To measure aggressive behavior.

Population

Children, adolescents, and adults.

Background and Description

The Point Subtraction Aggression Paradigm (PSAP) is presented as an experimental game wherein participants are provided with response options. In the typical format, subjects sit in front of a panel that is equipped with two buttons. When participants press one button they receive points that can be exchanged for a reward. When participants press the alternate button points are subtracted from a fictitious opponent (a.k.a. "the point subtraction button"). Subjects are told that their "opponent" will also be able to subtract points from them. The frequency with which the subjects utilize the point subtraction button is used to measure levels of aggressive behavior. The PSAP can be modified to include escape or response options.

Administration

The PSAP requires a computer to run the program. The amount of time required is variable and can be set based on the assessment needed.

Scoring

The total number of points subtracted within a predetermined time frame can be used as a measure of aggression. The ratio of points earned to points subtracted can also be used as a measure of aggression.

Interpretation

Aggression is operationally defined as the intent to harm another. The ratio of points obtained to points subtracted is expected to covary with propensity for aggressive behavior.

Psychometric Properties

Reliability. Detailed information on the reliability of the PSAP is unavailable. However, it is believed to be a reliable measure because it has been used successfully in many diverse settings (Golomb, Cortez-Perez, Jaworski, Mednick, & Dimsdale, 2007).

Validity. The PSAP scores correlated significantly with Brown's History of Violence and the Overt Aggression Scale (pp. 131–133). According to Giancola and Chermack (1998), over 80 studies have used the PSAP to effectively distinguish between aggressive and nonaggressive individuals. For example, Cherek, Schnapp, Moeller, & Dougherty (1996) found violent individuals responded more aggressively (pushed the subtract button more frequently) than nonviolent individuals.

Clinical Utility

Limited. PSAP is a widely used assessments of aggression in basic research. The lack of normative data creates problems for routine clinical use.

Research Applicability

Moderate. The PSAP is a widely used measures of aggressive behavior in laboratory settings and has been used with a variety of ages and populations. Subjects are not required to respond aggressively during the testing paradigm and are given alternative response options, which lends to the utility of this measure as a less biased evaluation of aggressive behavior.

Original Citation

Cherek, D. R. (1992). *Manual for point subtraction aggression paradigm: A computer program to measure aggressive responding in human subjects under controlled laboratory conditions.* Houston, TX: University of Texas Health Science Center.

Source

Dr. Don R. Cherek, Department of Psychiatry, University of Texas-Houston, Health Science Center, 1300 Moursund Street, Houston, TX 77030, (713) 500-2500, Fax: (713) 500-2530, don.r.cherek@uth.tmc.edu

Cost

Please contact the source (above) for additional information on the PSAP.

Alternative Forms

A brief version of the PSAP has been adapted for use in research where group data are of interest as opposed to individual data. In the PSAP-FS, the methods of administration are the same but only the first session of the PSAP is used to collect data on an individual's aggressive responding, thus reducing the time necessary to administer the measure significantly. The PSAP-FS correlated with the Conflict Tactics Scale ($r=.27$, pp. 177–180) and the Statin Study Questionnaire-Conflict ($r=.26$) which requires participants to record episodes of aggressive/irritable behaviors that occurred in the previous 2 weeks while driving or on the telephone.

References

Cherek, D. R., Schnapp, W., Moeller, F. G., & Dougherty, D. M. (1996). Laboratory measures of aggressive responding in male parolees with violent and nonviolent histories. *Aggressive Behavior, 22,* 27–36.

Giancola, P. R., & Chermack, S. T. (1998). Construct validity of laboratory aggression paradigms: A response to Tedeschi and Quigley (1996). *Aggression and Violent Behavior, 3,* 237–253.

Golomb, B. A., Cortez-Perez, M., Jaworski, B. A., Mednick, S., & Dimsdale, J. (2007). Point Subtraction Aggression Paradigm: Validity of a brief schedule of use. *Violence and Victims, 22,* 95–103.

Problem-Solving Measure for Conflict (PSM-C)

Purpose

To assess the problem-solving skills of children in the contexts of peer, teacher–student, and parent–child conflict.

Population

Children.

Background and Description

Scoring and content of the Problem-Solving Measure for Conflict (PSM-C) were adapted from previously existing problem-solving measures (Allen, Chinsky, Larcen, Lochman, & Selinger, 1976; Lochman, Lampron, Burch, & Curry, 1985). The PSM-C is a 6-item measure of problem-solving skills. Items consist of stems, or stories, describing problematic situations and an outcome in which the problem is eliminated. Respondents are asked to provide the middle portion of the story, indicating a solution to the problem. Respondents are then asked to generate as many alternative solutions to the problems as possible.

Stories depict three interpersonal contexts for conflict (peer, teacher–student, and parent–child) and two levels of intent by the antagonist (frustration or hostile). In the frustration scenarios, the antagonist frustrates the child's wishes, but the antagonist's intent is ambiguous and not clearly hostile. In the hostile scenarios, the antagonist interacts with the child in a hostile and provocative way.

Administration

The PSM-C is estimated to take 25–35 min to complete.

Scoring

The PSM-C is scored across nine content categories: Verbal Assertion (i.e., verbal statements that are not aggressive), Direct Action (i.e., nonverbal, nonaggressive actions used to solve a problem), Physical Aggression (i.e., behaviors involving direct physical aggression against other characters), Help Seeking (i.e., solutions involving requests for help from someone else to solve the problem), Verbal Aggression (i.e., verbal statements of threats or insults, lying, or yelling),

Nonconfrontational (i.e., actions involving withdrawal from, escaping, or avoidance of the problem situation), Compromise (i.e., behaviors in which characters in the story share potential positive and negative outcomes), Bargaining (i.e., behaviors involving attempts to escape the potential negative consequences while maintaining as many positive consequences for the self), and Irrelevant (i.e., solutions not producing the stated outcome of the story).

Each of the nine content codes may be assessed across the three interpersonal contexts (peer, parent–child, teacher–student) and the two levels of intent (hostile or frustration). Additionally, scores for the total number of alternative solutions generated and the total number of protagonist solutions and nonprotagonist solutions (i.e., solutions initiated by someone other than the central character) may be calculated.

Interpretation

Scores are interpreted qualitatively, examining number and content of solutions across and within interpersonal contexts and level of intent.

Psychometric Properties

Reliability. Percent agreement and Kappa coefficients for total number of alternative solutions, protagonist solutions, nonprotagonist solutions, and content codes were assessed in several samples. Percent agreement ranged from 92.3 (total number of alternative solutions) to 99 (bargaining). Kappa ranged from .49 (bargaining) to .98 (physical aggression).

Validity. Research on the validity of the PSM-C has found situational effects for problem-solving skills across a sample of 38 aggressive and nonaggressive fourth and fifth graders. Across situations, nonaggressive children produced more verbally assertive responses in comparison to aggressive children.

Discriminant analyses were conducted. In one analysis, a model for aggressive children consisting of more direct action with teachers, fewer total alternative solutions in parent conflict, and more direct action in hostile situations correctly classified 74 % of all cases, 70 % of aggressive children and 78 % of nonaggressive children. In a second discriminant analysis, a model for aggressive children consisting of lower self-esteem, more direct action solutions with teachers, fewer total alternative solutions in parent conflicts, higher perceived cognitive competence, and lower perceived social competence correctly classified 79 % of individuals, 75 % of aggressive children and 83 % of nonaggressive children. Additionally, scores on the PSM-C have been shown to discriminate between teacher-identified aggressive and nonaggressive boys.

Clinical Utility

High. The PSM-C is a useful tool in identifying the predominant response set of children when confronted with hypothetical antagonistic or frustrating situations. Additionally, the PSM-C may be used as an aid to determine the need for problem-solving training and as a clinical outcome measure to assess the efficacy of problem-solving training.

Research Applicability

High. The PSM-C offers a means of examining the different ways in which children respond to situations involving antagonism and frustration.

Original Citation

Lochman, J. E., & Lampron, L. B. (1986). Situational social problem-solving skills and self-esteem of aggressive and nonaggressive boys. *Journal of Abnormal Child Psychology, 14,* 605–617.

Source

John E. Lochman, Department of Psychology, Box 870348, University of Alabama, Tuscaloosa, AL 35487, (205) 348-7678, Fax: (205) 348-8648, jlochman@as.ua.edu

Cost

Please contact the source (above) for additional information on the PSM-C.

References

Allen, G. J., Chinsky, J. M., Larcen, S. W., Lochman, J. E., & Selinger, H. V. (1976). Community psychology and the schools: A behaviorally oriented multilevel preventive approach. New York: Wiley.
Lochman, J. E., Lampron, L. B., Burch, P. R., & Curry, J. F. (1985). Client characteristics associated with treatment outcome for aggressive boys. *Journal of Abnormal Child Psychology, 13*, 527–538.

Propensity for Angry Driving Scale (PADS)

Purpose

To identify people who are likely to engage in hostile driving behaviors or acts of "road rage."

Population

People who are above the legal age required to obtain a license to drive an automobile.

Background and Description

Estimates suggest that road rage is a significant social problem. The Propensity for Angry Driving Scale (PADS) was developed to quantify the propensity to engage in aggressive driving. The PADS initially consisted of 27 driving scenarios, with each scenario having four possible responses. The intensity of each of the four responses was rated on the degree of emotional reaction and retaliation. Preliminary psychometric analysis resulted in the final version that contains 19 driving scenarios. Each scenario describes an aversive driving event and is accompanied by four potential responses.

Administration

The administration of the PADS is estimated to take 20 min.

Scoring

Scores for each response are given a number (mean and standard deviation) which was obtained during the development of the original scoring scheme.

Interpretation

Higher scores are indicative of a greater potential to engage in angry-driving behaviors.

Psychometric Properties

Norms. The original citation contains means and standard deviations for four samples: 51 undergraduates (15 males and 36 females), 318 safety professionals and industrial employees (189 males and 129 females), 38 undergraduate students (14 males and 24 females), and 96 undergraduates (41 males and 55 females).

Factor analysis. Factor analysis using the responses from 318 safety professionals and industrial employees (189 males and 129 females) revealed a single factor structure with item–factor loadings from .27 to .73.

Reliability. Test–retest reliability data were obtained for 38 undergraduate students (14 males and 24 females). The PADS had acceptable internal consistency with Cronbach's alphas .88 and .89 at time 1 and time 2, respectively. It also had a high test–retest reliability coefficient of .91.

Validity. Correlation analyses using responses from 96 undergraduate students (41 male and 55 females) found the PADS significantly related to the Buss–Durkee Hostility Inventory ($r = .40$, pp. 109–111) and the trait subscale of the State–Trait Anger Scale ($r = .40$, pp. 77–79). The PADS significantly correlated with gender ($r = .30$), anger ($r = .40$), hostility ($r = .40$), impulsivity ($r = .28$), obscene gestures ($r = .60$), and verbal confrontations ($r = .52$). Hierarchical regression indicated that the PADS significantly predicted both verbal confrontations and obscene gestures after controlling for anger and hostility. In a sample of 242 undergraduate students, the PADS was significantly related to scores on the Driving Anger Scale (DAS, pp. 53–55), a self-report measure of aggressive driving and a self-report measure of risky driving (Dahlen & Ragan, 2004).

Clinical Utility

Moderate. The PADS shows potential for clinical use in terms of screening for the propensity to engage in angry behavior associated with driving. The PADS could also be used to evaluate the effectiveness of interventions designed to decrease road rage. Normative data are needed for samples ticketed with aggressive driving violations.

Research Applicability

Moderate. The PADS could be used to study individual differences in angry driving and road rage. Prospective studies are needed to assess whether the PADS predicts proneness to angry driving.

Original Citation

DePasquale, J. P., Geller, E. S., Clarke, S. W., & Littleton, L. C. (2001). Measuring road rage: Development of the Propensity for Angry Driving Scale. *Journal of Safety Research, 32*, 1–16.

Source

DePasquale, J. P., Geller, E. S., Clarke, S. W., & Littleton, L. C. (2001). Measuring road rage:

Development of the Propensity for Angry Driving Scale. *Journal of Safety Research, 32*, 1–16.

Cost

Unavailable.

Alternative Forms

The PADS has been adapted for use in Australia. The Australian Propensity for Angry Driving Scale (Aus-PADS) contains 15 items and has acceptable internal consistency ($\alpha = .82$) (Leal & Pachana, 2008).

References

Dahlen, E. R., & Ragan, K. M. (2004). Validation of the Propensity for Angry Driving Scale. *Journal of Safety Research, 35*, 557–563.

Leal, N. L., & Pachana, N. A. (2008). Adapting the Propensity for Angry Driving Scale for use in Australian research. *Accident Analysis and Prevention, 40*, 2008–2014.

Rating Scale for Aggressive Behavior in the Elderly (RAGE)

Purpose

To assess aggressive behavior in geriatric inpatients.

Population

Geriatric inpatients on a psychiatric ward.

Background and Description

The Rating Scale for Aggressive Behavior in the Elderly (RAGE) was designed to measure aggressive behavior in psychogeriatric populations. The definition of aggression used to formulate items for the rating scale was, "an overt act, involving the delivery of noxious stimuli to (but not necessarily at) another organism, object or self, which is clearly not accidental" (Patel & Hope, 1992, p. 212). The notion of intentionality was not included because the authors felt it may not apply to an elderly population that may be cognitively impaired. This definition also allows for the inclusion of verbal aggression, which has been found to be common in the psychogeriatric population (Ware, Hope, & Fairburn, 1990).

Items were created from interviews with ward staff, observation of a psychogeriatric ward, and examining existing rating scales used in elderly populations. After initial examination, a 21-item rating scale was formed. Nineteen of the items refer to specific kinds of aggressive behavior, one item asks about the consequences of the aggressive behavior, and one item asks the rater to make an overall assessment of aggressive behavior. The ward nursing staff rate how frequently each of the 19 aggressive behavior items occurred during a 3-day observation period using a 4-point scale (0 = not once in the past 3 days, 3 = more than once every day in the past 3 days). The authors recommend that information for completing the RAGE is obtained from personal observations, ward notes, checklists, and discussions with other ward staff.

Administration

The RAGE is estimated to require up to 5 min to complete.

Scoring

Items are rated using a 4-point scale. A total score can be calculated by summing scores on the individual items.

Interpretation

Higher scores indicate greater occurrence of the specific aggressive behavior during the previous 3 days. A higher total score indicates greater frequency of general aggressive behavior during the previous 3 days.

Psychometric Properties

Factor analysis. A factor analysis with varimax rotation revealed five factors accounting for 69 % of the variance. Because two of the factors consisted of only one or two items, the factor analysis was repeated limiting it to three factors. The three factors were labeled: verbal aggression, physical aggression, and antisocial behavior.

Reliability. Internal consistency, as measured by Cronbach's alpha, was adequate ($\alpha = .89$). Test–retest reliability was assessed for three different time periods: 6 h, 7 days, and 14 days. Test–retest reliability for the 6-h time period ranged from .47 to .94 for individual items, with total score .91. Test–retest reliability for 7 days ranged from .48 to .93, with total score .84. Test–retest reliability for 14 days ranged from .50 to 1.00, with total score .88. Interrater reliability was assessed using the Kappa statistic. Kappas ranged from .41 to .92 for individual items, with an overall agreement of 86 % when a ward checklist was used in completing the RAGE ratings. When the ward checklist was not used in completing the ratings, kappas ranged from −.07 to .61 for individual items, with an overall agreement of 68 %. Split-half reliability, as measured by Guttman's split-half coefficient, was .88.

Validity. Content validity was assessed by correlating the individual items with the total scores. Seventeen of the items had correlations greater than .40, with 10 of the items correlating greater than .60. The RAGE total score rating was significantly related ($r = .86$) to the total number of recorded incidents of any type of aggressive behavior.

The RAGE has been found to be significantly related to the Cohen-Mansfield Agitation Inventory ($\rho = .73$; Cohen-Mansfield, 1986) and the Brief Agitation Rating Scale ($\rho = .72$; Finkel, Lyons, & Anderson, 1993). In a separate study of 26 psychogeriatric inpatients, the RAGE total score and subscales were found to significantly correlate with the Staff Observation and Aggression Scale (SOAS; pp. 153–155) and to facilitate the recording of aggressive behavior (Shah & De, 1997; Shah, Evans, & Park Ash, 1998).

Clinical Utility

Moderate. The RAGE has good psychometric properties and can be easily completed by any ward staff in a brief amount of time.

Research Applicability

Moderate. The RAGE has good psychometric properties and can be completed easily and quickly. It may be a useful tool in investigating correlates of aggressive behavior in elderly inpatients. It can also be used to assess the efficacy of potential treatments for aggressive behavior in the elderly.

Original Citation

Patel, V., & Hope, R. A. (1992). A rating scale for aggressive behavior in the elderly—The RAGE. *Psychological Medicine, 22*, 211–221.

Source

Dr. R. A. Hope, University Department of Psychiatry, Warneford Hospital, Oxford OX3 7JX.

Cost

Please contact the source (above) for permission to use the RAGE.

References

Cohen-Mansfield, J. (1986). Agitated behaviour in the elderly II. Preliminary results in the cognitively deteriorated. *Journal of the American Geriatrics Society, 34*, 722–727.

Finkel, S. I., Lyons, J. S., & Anderson, R. L. (1993). A Brief Agitation Rating Scale (BARS) for nursing home elderly. *Journal of the American Geriatrics Society, 41*, 50–52.

Shah, A., & De, T. (1997). The relationship between two scales measuring aggressive behavior among continuing-care psychogeriatric inpatients. *International Psychogeriatrics, 9*, 471–477.

Shah, A., Evans, H., & Park Ash, N. (1998). Evaluation of three aggression/agitation behaviour rating scales for use on an acute admission and assessment psychogeriatric ward. *International Journal of Geriatric Psychiatry, 13*, 415–420.

Ware, C., Hope, R. A., & Fairburn, C. G. (1990). A community-based study of aggressive behaviour in dementia. *International Journal of Geriatric Psychiatry, 5*, 337-342.

Revised Behavior Problem Checklist (RBPC)

Purpose

To assess externalizing and internalizing behavior problems.

Population

Children and adolescents.

Background and Description

The original Behavior Problem Checklist (BPC) was plagued by a limited initial item pool, resulting in three scales indexed by few items. The limited number of items created problems of reliability. The BPC, however, was still widely used, prompting revisions to strengthen the psychometric properties of the scale. To create the Revised Behavior Problem Checklist (RBPC), the item pool was increased to 150 items, with new items for the existing five scales taken from the literature or created. In preliminary analyses, items were cut if they failed to meet a 15 % level of endorsement, and the remaining items underwent factor analyses. The new scale retained the four broadband externalizing dimensions and the quantitative-dimensional model of the BPC.

The RBPC is a multidimensional measure of behavior pathology, consisting of 89 problem behaviors that are rated by teachers, parents, or anyone who has knowledge about the identified children. The RBPC consists of four major scales and two minor scales, accounting for 77 of the items. The remaining 12 items were retained for possible use with preschool children and to provide additional information for users. The six scales are representative of broad and narrower dimensions of child internalizing and externalizing behavior disorders. The four major scales are Conduct Disorder (CD; 22 items), Socialized Aggression (SA; 17 items), Attention–Problems–Immaturity (AP; 16 items), and Anxiety–Withdrawal (AW; 11 items). The two minor scales are Psychotic Behavior (PB; 6 items) and Motor Tension-Excess (ME; 5 items). Respondents rate each item using a 3-point scale (0 = not a problem, 1 = mild problem, and 2 = severe problem).

Administration

The RBPC is estimated to take 20–30 min to complete and may be completed by anyone who knows the identified child.

Scoring

Items for each scale are summed. The minimum score for each scale is 0. Maximum scores are as follows: Conduct Disorder (44), Socialized Aggression (34), Attention–Problems–Immaturity (32), Anxiety–Withdrawal (22), Psychotic Behavior (12), and Motor Tension-Excess (10).

Interpretation

Interpretation of scores may be done in several ways. Scores on each scale may be compared with means from an appropriate reference group. Such a comparison provides a relative index of the severity of the behavior and is used to determine behavioral deviance from the norm. A difference of 2 or more standard deviations from the mean of the reference group is considered significant. Normative data for parent and teacher ratings for a variety of normal and clinical samples, grades K through 12, are provided in the RBPC manual (Quay & Peterson, 1987).

Scores from different scales may be compared, allowing one to judge the relative severity of behavior dimensions within a child. These comparisons may be made in two ways. Pairwise comparisons may be made between T-scores of the scales, thus allowing a ranking of severity among dimensions to be obtained. An ipsative approach may also be used, minimizing the possibility of over-interpreting scale score differences. Significance levels for differences between scale scores are printed in Short (1991).

Psychometric Properties

Norms. Normative data for parent and teacher ratings for a variety of normal and clinical samples, grades K through 12, are provided in the RBPC manual. The authors also recommend the development of local norms.

Factor analysis. Using data from four samples (276 cases from two private psychiatric residential facilities, 198 cases of outpatients and inpatients, 114 cases from a private school for children with learning disabilities, and 172 cases from a community-sponsored school for children with developmental disabilities), a principal axis method extracted four major factors (Conduct Disorder, Socialized Aggression, Attention–Problems–Immaturity, and Anxiety–Withdrawal) and two minor factors (Psychotic Behavior and Motor Excess).

In a sample of kindergarten children, ages 5–6 years, a principal component analysis extracted five components for teachers (Conduct Disorder, Attention–Problems–Immaturity, Unmotivated-isolated, Anxiety–withdrawal, and

Psychotic Behavior) and six components for parents (Conduct Disorder, Attention Problems, Hyperactive-Impatient, Anxiety, Tense-Withdrawn, and Passive-Conforming). It should be noted that these factors are not the same as the factors produced in the original study.

Reliability. Complete psychometric properties are provided in the RBPC manual (Quay & Peterson, 1987). Across six samples, average intercorrelations between scales ranged from .12 to .52. Across three samples, the average Cronbach's alpha coefficient was .72 to .94. In a different study, Cronbach's alpha ranged from .48 to .90 in a community sample of males, .27–.86 in a community sample of females, .56–.93 in a clinic sample of males, and .72–.92 in a clinic sample of females. In a study focusing on the Anxiety–Withdrawal scale, Cronbach's alpha ranged from .74 to .89 across six samples. A mean interrater reliability coefficient of .72 was obtained for ratings made by the same rater at a 5-month interval. At 7, 12, and 17-month intervals, the mean interrater coefficient was .32 for different groups of teachers. Interrater reliability for combinations of 2 out of 10 staff members produced average scale interrater reliabilities ranging from .52 to .85.

Ratings among different raters have been consistently low, both in terms of raw score ratings and placement into categories (mildly deviant and highly deviant). Interrater reliabilities have been conducted for special education teachers, regular education teachers, and mental health professionals, behavior-disordered high school students and their teachers, two groups of teachers rating 120 secondary school students, parents and teachers rating third to fifth grade students, and two groups of teachers of middle school children. A different study found that combined parent and teacher ratings on RBPC externalizing factors of psychiatric outpatient boys, aged 6–12 years, were better at distinguishing externalizing and mixed disorders from internalizing disorders than individual parent or teacher ratings.

Test–retest scale reliabilities for teachers rating children in grades 1–6 for a 2-month interval ranged from .49 to .83. In an examination of the stability of RBPC scores in a sample of children from the kindergarten and first grade, few changes in scale means were found. Stability coefficients for a 5-month period for the same rater ranged from .50 to .75.

Validity. The authors of the RBPC stated that the concurrent, predictive, and construct validity established for the BPC might reasonably be assumed to generalize to the RBPC. The RBPC has been found to differentiate between normal children and children from clinical samples. In a sample of kindergarten children, ages 5–6 years, moderate correlations were found between RBPC teacher component scores and criterion measures (the SNAP rating scale, socioeconomic status, the Kaufman Assessment Battery for Children, and the Stanford Early School Achievement Test), providing support for the construct validity of the RBPC. Further evidence comes from data indicating that unpopularity with peers is related to aggression and inattentive/hyperactive behavior, and that there is an association between attentional problems and cognitive deficits (Hinshaw, Morrison, Carte, & Cornsweet, 1987).

Clinical Utility

High. The RBPC is useful for screening, aiding in making clinical diagnoses, classification, and as an outcome measure of treatment interventions for aggressive youth.

Research Applicability

High. The RBPC has been used as a criterion against which other measures have been compared and is useful for exploring the correlates and consequences associated with childhood aggression.

Original Citation

Quay, H. C. (1983). A dimensional approach to behavior disorder: The Revised Behavior Problem Checklist. *School Psychology Review, 12*(3), 244–249.

Source

Psychological Assessment Resources (PAR), 16204 N. Florida Ave, Lutz, FL 33549, 1-800-331-8378, Fax: 1-800-727-9329, http://www3.parinc.com/products/product.aspx?Productid=RBPC

Cost

The introductory kit, which includes the manual, 50 test booklets, and 50 profile sheets, may be purchased for $202 from PAR.

Alternative Forms

The RBPC has been translated into Spanish, with identical factors except for the Psychotic Behavior and small Conduct Disorder-Peers factor—suitable only for male children and adolescents.

References

Hinshaw, S. P., Morrison, D. C., Carte, E. T., & Cornsweet, C. (1987). Factorial dimensions of the Revised Behavior Problem Checklist: Replication and validation within a kindergarten sample. *Journal of Abnormal Child Psychology, 15*, 309–327.

Quay, H. C., & Peterson, D. R. (1987). *Manual for the Revised Behavior Problem Checklist*. Coral Gables: Authors.

Short, R. J. (1991). Interpreting scale score differences on the Revised Behavior Problem Checklist. *Educational and Psychological Measurement, 51*, 385–392.

Richardson Conflict Response Questionnaire (RCRQ)

Purpose

To measure direct and indirect aggression.

Population

Ages 13 years and older.

Background and Description

Research has indicated that school-age girls engage in more indirect aggression than school-age boys, but results in adult populations are less clear. Indirect aggression was defined in an equivalent manner to Buss' conceptualization of the nature of indirect aggression; indirect aggression, demonstrated verbally or physically, is a means of avoiding counterattack, consisting of behaviors aimed to harm and completed indirectly through other people or objects.

Items on the Richardson Conflict Response Questionnaire (RCRQ) were set in the context of anger to decrease confusion with prosocial motives; items are intended to reflect use for retaliation against or harm to the target. One item from the indirect aggression scale was developed by Huesmann (Zelli & Huesmann, 1993), and others were based on the direct/indirect aggression scales developed by Björkqvist, Österman, and Kaukiainen (1992). Most items reflecting direct aggression and filler items were taken from the Conflict Tactics Scale (pp. 177–180).

The RCRQ is a 28-item self-report measure of direct and indirect aggression carried out against a nonromantic partner. The measure consists of 10 items assessing indirect aggression, 10 items assessing direct aggression, and eight filler items. Items assessing direct aggression are included to enable comparisons between the frequency of use of indirect and direct aggression. Filler items reflect other strategies for dealing with conflict. The instructions ask participants to rate how often in the past year they engaged in an action when angry with a friend. Respondents rate each action on a 5-point scale, ranging from 1 ("never") to 5 ("very often"). Sample items follow.

- Made up stories to get them in trouble
- Yelled or screamed at them
- Didn't show that I was angry

Administration

The RCRQ is estimated to take 5–10 min to complete.

Scoring

Items from each scale (direct and indirect aggression scales) are summed, with scores ranging from 10 to 50 on each scale.

Interpretation

Higher scores indicate higher frequency of use of indirect or direct aggression.

Psychometric Properties

Reliability. Internal consistency was assessed using Cronbach's alpha. For the original scale, which consisted of seven indirect aggression items and seven direct aggression items, alpha values were .77 and .83, respectively. For the revised scale, consisting of ten indirect aggression items and ten direct aggression items, alpha values were .80 and .90, respectively.

Validity. The original items on the direct and indirect scales (14 items) were not significantly correlated ($r=.16$). Using the revised scale, consisting of 20 direct and indirect aggression items, the average correlation between the two scales was .42. This correlation was obtained using over 100 participants (ages 13–90 years) across eight studies. This average correlation provides evidence of the independence of the constructs of indirect and direct aggression. Additionally, self-reports and peer-reports of both direct and indirect aggression were moderately, but significantly, correlated (for direct aggression, $r=.60$ and for indirect aggression, $r=.48$), providing evidence for criterion validity.

Clinical Utility

Moderate. The RCRQ provides a useful means for assessing types of aggression used toward others. Instructions are flexible to allow the asses-sor to determine the period in which the aggression is assessed.

Research Applicability

Moderate. The RCRQ allows direct and indirect aggression to be independently assessed, providing a means for examining differences and similarities between the two constructs.

Original Citation

Green, L. R., Richardson, D. R., & Lago, T. (1996). How do friendship, indirect, and direct aggression relate? *Aggressive Behavior, 22,* 81–86.

Source

Deborah Richardson, Department of Psychology, Augusta State University, 2500 Walton Way, Augusta, GA 30904, (706) 729-2451, drichardson@aug.edu

Cost

Please contact the source (above) for permission to use the RCRQ.

Alternative Forms

The RCRQ is available in two versions, differing in whom the aggression is directed toward: same-gender target and opposite-gender target.

References

Björkqvist, K., Österman, K., & Kaukiainen, A. (1992). The development of direct and indirect aggressive strategies in males and females. In K. Björkqvist & P. Niemeal (Eds.), *Of Mice and Women: Aspects of Female Aggression* (pp. 51–64). San Diego, CA: Academic Press, Inc.

Zelli, A., & Huesmann, R. (1993). Information-processing and self-schemas in hostile biases: The role of beliefs about a violent world. *Aggressive Behavior, 19*, 73–74.

Right-Wing Authoritarianism Scale (RWA)

Purpose

To assess the authoritarianism attitudes of submission to authority, aggression, and conventionalism.

Population

Adults.

Background and Description

Right-wing authoritarianism was conceptualized as a personality trait reflective of three attitudes: authoritarian submission (i.e., submission to authority perceived as established and legitimate in society), authoritarian aggression (i.e., a general aggressiveness, directed against specific persons, and perceived as sanctioned by established authorities), and conventionalism (i.e., high degrees of adherence to social conventions, perceived as endorsed by the established society and its authorities). Initial items were developed from F-scale items (California F-scale; 1950) that covaried to a degree reflective of a unitary construct. Items consist of 30 attitudinal statements; half are worded to favor authoritarian attitudes (protrait items) and half are worded in opposition to authoritarianism attitudes (contrait items). Respondents indicate their degree of agreement or disagreement to each item on a 9-point scale, ranging from −4 ("very strongly disagree") to 4 ("very strongly agree").

Administration

The RWA is estimated to take 5–10 min to complete.

Scoring

Contrait items are reverse scored. Responses to items are summed to produce a single score. Scores on the RWA range from 30 to 270. Neutral answers ("0") are assigned a score of "5"; thus, a respondent who indicates neutrality to all items will receive a score of 150.

Interpretation

Scores greater than 150 reflect increasing degrees of adherence to authoritarianism attitudes.

Psychometric Properties

Factor analysis. Original data indicated that one factor, on which nearly all scale items loaded, accounted for 23.3 % of the total variance. In a sample of 339 undergraduate students, a principal axis analysis of the 30 items, followed by varimax and promax rotations, produced two factors: one for protrait items and one for contrait items. These two factors correlated at .40, suggesting the presence of a single, higher order factor. In a sample of 269 undergraduate, white South-African students, a principal factors analysis with oblique rotation and orthogonal varimax solution produced a two-factor fit with all but six items loading significantly on the first factor. These two factors did not have a content-based interpretation. Seven of the nine items loading on the second factor were contrait items, suggesting two factors based upon wording (protrait or contrait). These two factors correlated at .47, again suggesting the presence of a single general factor underlying the items of the RWA.

Reliability. Initial coefficient alphas were reported to range from .85 to .89, with test–retest reliabilities of .95 for a 1-week period and .85 for a 28-week period. Cronbach's alpha coefficients were .86 in a sample of 339 undergraduate students and .93 in a sample of 269 undergraduate, white South-African students.

Validity. The RWA correlates .59 with measures of conformity and .57 with measures of conservatism. Other studies have found scores on the RWA to correlate with acceptance of parents' religious values, self-ratings on liberalism and conservatism, support for government censorship of political material, use of government detention without a trial, opposition to peaceful protest of the government by political opponents, and measures of prejudice or discrimination. Individuals scoring high on the RWA also tend to make harsher judgments, are more punitive toward those failing to conform to legitimate authority, and place more emphasis on values of power, conformity, tradition, and security. Individuals scoring low on the RWA typically endorse more universalistic values such as those concerned with pleasure, stimulation, and self-direction.

Clinical Utility

Moderate. The RWA can be used to assess the strength of authoritarianism attitudes held by an individual, which may lead to acts of aggression or violence.

Research Applicability

High. The RWA has adequate to good psychometric properties and is a time-efficient measure to be used when researching correlates of authoritarianism beliefs.

Original Citation

Altemeyer, B. (1981). *Right-wing authoritarianism.* Winnipeg, MB: University of Manitoba Press.

Source

Robert Altemeyer, Department of Psychology 206 Chancellor's Hall, 177 Dysart Rd, University of Manitoba, Winnipeg, MB R3T 2N2, altemey@cc.umanitoba.ca

Cost

Please contact the source (above) for permission to use the RWA.

Alternative Forms

The RWA has been adapted for use in Italy.

A short version of the RWA was created by using exploratory and confirmatory factor analyses. The 14-item short scale RWA has two dimensions: authoritarian aggression and submission and conservatism. It has good internal consistency with Cronbach's alphas ranging from .77 to .85 for the total score and .72 to .75 for the subscales. It was found to be significantly related to the original RWA ($r = .97$), blatant prejudice ($r = .63$), and subtle prejudice ($r = .50$). A full listing of the items can be found in Manganelli Rattazzi, Bobbio, and Canova (2007).

Reference

Manganelli Rattazzi, A. M., Bobbio, A., & Canova, L. (2007). A short version of the Right-Wing Authoritarianism (RWA) Scale. *Personality and Individual Differences, 43*, 1223–1234.

Sentences

Purpose

To explore attributional biases in ambiguous situations.

Population

Adults.

Background and Description

Research has suggested that reactive aggression and sensitivity to hostile cues may be indicative of hostile attributions, which are related to quick decision making and the tendency to ignore relevant cues. Methodological shortcomings, however, exist in these studies (e.g., a confound of social desirability), and many of these studies have been conducted with children. The use of sentences is an information-processing task, independent of self-report measures, that eliminates some of the previous methodological difficulties.

Seventy sentences are administered, 36 unambiguous, neutral filler sentences interspersed randomly among 24 ambiguous sentences. Of the 24 ambiguous sentences, 12 of these are interpretable in either a violent threatening or a neutral manner (e.g., "The painter drew the knife."). The remaining 12 are interpretable in either a social anxiety threatening or a neutral manner (e.g., "Mark's speech made everyone giggle"). Respondents are presented with a sentence and are forced to choose, from two options, the last word of each sentence. The last word creates either a violent threatening or neutral sentence, or an anxiety threatening or neutral sentence. Respondents then complete a recognition memory task in which they are presented with two disambiguated versions of each of the ambiguous sentences. These sentences remain consistent with interpretation as either threatening or nonthreatening. Respondents indicate whether each disambiguated sentence was consistent with the meaning of previously shown sentences. Then, respondents indicate the degree of confidence in their decision on a 5-point Likert-type scale, ranging from 1 ("not at all confident") to 5 ("highly confident").

Administration

In the first task, each sentence is presented on a computer screen for 4 s and then followed by two words. The next sentence appears on the screen after a choice between the two words has been made by pressing a key on the keyboard. If the respondent fails to respond within 10 s, the next sentence is presented and the item is scored as invalid. For the memory recognition task, each of the 48 items is shown on the computer screen, one every 10 s. Respondents indicate whether each sentence has the same meaning as a previous sentence by pressing a key on the keyboard. Each sentence appears for a maximum of 5 s. After 8.5 s, respondents indicate the level of confidence in their choice.

Scoring

The number of violent threatening, neutral, and anxiety threatening responses are calculated.

Interpretation

Higher frequencies of violent threatening or anxiety threatening responses indicate that the individual interprets situations as more violent or anxiety threatening, respectively.

Psychometric Properties

Reliability. No reliability data were reported.

Validity. The face validity of this procedure was determined by six independent judges who evaluated the plausibility of each sentence and determined whether the disambiguated sentences were similar in meaning to their original counterparts. Violent and nonviolent offenders endorsed more ambiguous sentences as violent and threatening than non-offenders. The endorsement of violent threat sentences was also related to the total hostility score on the Hostility and Direction of Hostility Questionnaire (Caine, Foulds, & Hope, 1967).

Clinical Utility

Limited. Although the procedure may provide insight into attributional biases of individuals, it is a lengthy procedure and lacks interpretive meaning on an individual basis.

Research Applicability

Moderate. Although lengthy and requiring considerable amounts of equipment and some computer expertise, the procedure is useful for examining common attributional biases in various populations.

Original Citation

Copello, A. G., & Tata, P. R. (1990). Violent behavior and interpretative bias: An experimental study of the resolution of ambiguity in violent offenders. *British Journal of Clinical Psychology, 29*, 417–428.

Source

A list of sentences used may be obtained from Dr. Alex G. Copello, Clinical Director, Birmingham and Solihull Substance Misuse Services and Senior Lecturer, School of Psychology, University of Birmingham, Edgbaston, Birmingham B15 2TT, UK, Phone: 0121 414 7414, a.g.copello@bham.ac.uk

Cost

Please contact the source (above) for permission to use the Sentences measure.

Reference

Caine, T. M., Foulds, G. A., & Hope, K. (1967). *Manual of the Hostility and Direction of Hostility Questionnaire*. London: University of London Press.

Situations–Reactions Hostility Inventory (SRHI)

Purpose

To assess types of situations which are typically emotion provoking and the types and intensity of responses to these situations.

Population

Adults.

Background and Description

Much of the content and format of the Situations–Reactions Hostility Inventory (SRHI) was adapted from the work of Endler and Hunt (1968). Some of the situations presented are identical to those developed by Endler and Hunt, whereas others were developed from known events that preceded aggressive behavior in the hospital.

The SRHI is a 14-item, self-report measure of potentially provoking situations and possible responses to these situations. The SRHI is in the form of a booklet, consisting of instructions and an example, followed by descriptions of 14 situations and 12 possible responses to each situation. Items depict situations ranging from mildly annoying to highly threatening that are assumed to predict aspects of frustration, threat, attack, or pain that may precede displays of anger or aggression.

The 14 situations are grouped into two categories based upon content: attack and frustration. Situations in the attack category depict events in which an individual's physical or psychological well-being is challenged through criticism, assault, or threat of harmful consequences. Situations in the frustration category depict events in which the individual's anticipated goal or reward is prevented.

The 12 reactions consist of covert and overt responses, which are typically linked to anger arousal and aggression. Reactions include feelings of anger and tension, physiological reactions, and verbal and physical aggression. Reactions are grouped into three categories: aggression, anger, and arousal. Reactions in the aggression category are reflective of extrapunitive aggression or the desire to hurt and/or engage another in injurious behavior. Reactions in the anger category reflect experiences of anger arousal. Reactions in the arousal category reflect an increase in autonomic and somatic activity.

Respondents are asked to rate, on a 5-point scale ranging from 0 ("not at all") to 4 ("very much"), the intensity of their reactions to the described situation. Sample situations are as follows.

- You have just been blamed for something you didn't do.
- You accidentally spill hot tea over yourself.
- Someone calls you a dirty name.
  The following are samples of reactions:
- You lash out.
- Lose your temper.
- Feel tense.

Administration

The SRHI is estimated to take 10–15 min to complete.

Scoring

Mean intensity ratings are created for each situation. Mean intensity ratings for attack situations and frustration situations are summed to produce scores for attack and frustration. Responses to reactions in the anger, arousal, and aggression categories are summed to create a total score for each category. The mean intensity rating for each category is obtained by dividing the total score by the number of responses in that category.

Interpretation

Higher scores for the type of situation (attack or frustration) indicate a higher degree of response to those types of situations. Higher intensity ratings for type of response (arousal, aggression, or arousal) indicate higher levels of intensity when exhibiting that type of response in provoking situations.

Psychometric Properties

Factor analysis. Separate principal components analyses were performed on situations and

responses. Before rotation, a general component was found to underlie all situations. Rotation produced two components: attack and frustration. For the responses, a general angry aggression factor was produced before rotation. After rotation, three factors emerged: aggression, anger, and arousal.

Reliability. No reliability statistics have been reported.

Validity. Psychopathic individuals were found to react more strongly to situations that involve attack than non-psychopathic individuals. Withdrawn subjects, whether psychopathic or not, were also found to react more strongly to situations than more sociable individuals. Individuals also responded more strongly to attack situations than frustration situations.

Clinical Utility

Moderate. The SRHI provides a means of examining types of situations typically provoking to an individual, as well as common responses and the intensity of these responses. Thus, the SRHI may be useful as an outcome measure in assessing treatment effectiveness. Lack of reliability and validity data; however, make interpretation of the SRHI difficult.

Research Applicability

Limited. Lack of reliability and validity data make it difficult to interpret scores in comparison with other measures and constructs.

Original Citation

Blackburn, R., & Lee-Evans, J. M. (1985). Reactions of primary and secondary psychopaths to anger-evoking situations. *British Journal of Clinical Psychology, 24*(2), 93–100.

Source

Ronald Blackburn, University of Liverpool, Department of Clinical Psychology, The Whelan Building, Quadrangle, Brownlow Hill, Liverpool, L69 3GB, UK, ronb@liverpool.ac.uk

Cost

Please contact the source (above) for permission to use the SRHI.

Reference

Endler, N. S., & Hunt, J. M. (1968). S-R inventories of hostility and comparisons of the proportions of variance from persons, responses, and situations for hostility and anxiousness. *Journal of Personality and Social Psychology, 9*, 309–315.

Staff Observation Aggression Scale (SOAS)

Purpose

To monitor the degree and frequency of aggressive, violent, and assaultive acts in psychiatric inpatients.

Population

Inpatients on psychiatric wards.

Background and Description

The Staff Observation Aggression Scale (SOAS) was developed as a means of operationalizing and assessing causes of aggressive acts and as a systematic observational system allowing for the differentiation between aggressive events. The SOAS is an incident-based measure used by nurses on psychiatric wards for the systematic observation and reporting of verbal and physical aggression toward others and property damage committed by inpatients. The SOAS report form consists of three components: patient identification, short instructions for the observer, and a report section. The report section consists of five columns, with specific alternatives listed in each column, designed to assess differential aspects of the aggressive events. The columns assess provocation, means used by the patient, aim of aggression, consequence(s) for victim(s), and behaviors used to stop aggression. Observers check the appropriate item(s) observed for each column. Scoring for each criteria ranges from 0 to 4 points (0 = no means, no aim, no resulting injury/damage and 4 = highest score on each item). Items are operationally defined in the scoring criteria. Items on the "means" and "aims" columns can receive scores from 1 to 4; it is assumed that an event without identifiable means or aims cannot be recognized by an observer.

Administration

The SOAS can be completed by the nursing staff after observing aggressive events. The measure takes approximately 5 min to complete.

Scoring

Items are scored according to the criteria given in the original citation. An individual aggression frequency is calculated by finding the quotient of the total number of aggressive events divided by the number of observation days. The global severity scale score is the sum of the three core items (means, aims, and result). Scores on the global severity scale range from 0 to 12 points.

Interpretation

Aggressive events on the global severity scale are categorized as mild (2–5 points), moderate (6–8 points), and severe (9 or more points).

Psychometric Properties

Reliability. In one study, four aggressive events were described to 12 staff members who were not trained or familiar with the SOAS. The interclass coefficient for the total SOAS score was .96. In a second sample, simultaneous, independent ratings of aggressive behavior were observed and recorded during a 2-week period. Although interrater reliabilities could not be calculated due to lack of consistent records of recorded events by the same observers, total scores and items per category differed by no more than 1 point.

In a third sample, 123 patients were observed for 24 weeks. For interrater reliability Pearson's correlation was .87 and the Kappa value for the total scores was .61, indicating that the SOAS has fair to good interrater reliability.

Validity. The SOAS has been shown to differentiate between aggressive acts in demented, acute schizophrenic, and acute non-schizophrenic patients. Additionally, studies have shown that use of the SOAS reduces aggressive behavior on inpatient wards, suggesting that the SOAS may help staff to identify precipitating factors of aggressive acts and to make necessary changes to prevent these acts (see also Nijman, Allertz, Merckelbach, Joost, L. à Campo, & Ravelli, 1997).

Validity of the severity scores was examined by comparing the scores with the Visual Analogue Scale (VAS). A significant correlation of .38 was obtained. Predictive validity was examined by correlating SOAS scores with scores on the Brief Psychiatric Rating Scale (Overall & Gorham, 1972). Results indicated that the highest correlation ($r=.58$) was between the hostility scale of the Brief Psychiatric Rating Scale and serious violence on the SOAS. The best prediction model, stable for a period of within 8 days, was high scores of hostility and anxiety combined with low scores of grandiosity.

Additionally, the scores on the SOAS have been compared with scores on the Rating Scale for Aggressive Behavior in the Elderly (RAGE, pp. 141–143). Results revealed correlations ranging from .17 to .85, all of which were significant.

Clinical Utility

High. The SOAS is used by nursing staff that are in a prime position for making observations because they have the most contact with patients. Additionally, the SOAS is quick and easy to learn, administer, and to integrate into the routines of the inpatient ward (e.g., scoring is separate from the observation so that it does not interfere with the observation or other duties). A drawback of the SOAS is that self-injurious behavior is not included.

Research Applicability

High. The SOAS is simple to complete and to score. It has been used to assess provocation, means, targets, and consequences of aggressive acts, as well as to examine characteristics of patients who engage in similar aggressive acts. Additionally, the measure distinguishes between components of an aggressive act and the severity of the act, allowing it to be used to examine patterns of aggression and as an outcome measure. The SOAS is limited in that "aims" of the aggression is conceptualized only in terms of who or what the aggression is aimed at, and the severity ratings are based upon a hierarchy of injuries.

Original Citation

Palmstierna, T., & Wistedt, B. (1987). Staff Observation Aggression Scale, SOAS: Presentation and evaluation. *Acta Psychiatrica Scandinavica, 76*(6), 657–663.

Source

Tom Palmstierna, M. D., Department of Clinical Neuroscience, Karolinska Institute, Division of Forensic Psychiatry, Stockholm, Sweden, tom.palmstierna@ki.se

Cost

Please contact the source (above) for permission to use the SOAS.

Alternative Forms

The SOAS-R contains an option to record auto-aggressive behavior (e.g., self-mutilation and suicide attempts), two new measures for stopping aggression (seclusion and physical restraints) were added, and scoring was slightly revised (Nijman, Muris, Merckelbach, Palmstierna, Wistedt, Vos, et al., 1999).

A Dutch version of the SOAS also has been created.

The SOAS-E is an extended version of the SOAS that includes additional categories for recording warning signals that precede violent incidents. This allows for a more detailed characterization of the aggressive incident (Hallsteinsen, Kristensen, Dahl, & Eilertsen, 1997).

References

Hallsteinsen, A., Kristensen, M., Dahl, A. A., & Eilertsen, D. E. (1997). The extended Staff Observation Aggression Scale (SOAS-E): Development, presentation and evaluation. *Acta Psychiatrica Scandinavica, 97*, 423–426.

Nijman, H. L. I., Allertz, W. F. F., Merckelbach, H. L. G. J., Joost, L. M. G., à Campo, J. L. M. G., & Ravelli, D. P. (1997). Aggressive behaviour on an acute psychiatric admissions ward. *European Journal of Psychiatry, 11*(2), 106–114.

Nijman, H. L. I, Muris, P., Merckelbach, H. L. G. J., Palmstierna, T., Wistedt, B., Vos, A. M., et al. (1999). The Staff Observation Aggression Scale—Revised (SOAS-R). *Aggressive Behavior, 25*, 197–209.

Overall, J. E., & Gorham, D. R. (1962). The brief psychiatric rating scale. *Psychological Reports, 10*, 799–812.

Measures of Violence

5

Quick-View Table for Measures of Violence

The quick-view table in this chapter provides easy access to basic descriptive information on each of the measures reviewed. The goal is to provide enough information to allow for an estimate of the likelihood that reading additional information about a particular measure would prove fruitful. Table entries are organized alphabetically and provide the name of the measure, the purpose for which the measure was developed, and the target population. The tables also provide information on the method of assessment, the amount of time involved, and the page number where additional information is available.

Quick-View Table for Measures of Violence

Name	Purpose	Population	Method	Time	Page #
Abuse Assessment Screen	To screen for domestic violence in pregnant women	Pregnant women	Self-report questionnaire	1–5 min	162
Abusive Behavior Inventory	To measure physical and psychological abuse of women committed by their partners	Adults	Self-report questionnaire	15–20 min	164
Acceptance of Interpersonal Violence	To measure the degree to which one accepts the use of interpersonal violence in a relationship	Adults	Self-report questionnaire	1–2 min	166
Accountability Scale	To assess dysfunctional attitudes related to intimate partner violence	Adults	Self-report questionnaire	5 min	168
Child Abuse Potential Inventory	To screen for the potential for physical abuse of a child	Parents or primary caregivers	Self-report questionnaire	30–45 min	170

(continued)

G.F. Ronan et al., *Practitioner's Guide to Empirically Supported Measures of Anger, Aggression, and Violence*, ABCT Clinical Assessment Series, DOI 10.1007/978-3-319-00245-3_5,
© Springer International Publishing Switzerland 2014

(continued)

Name	Purpose	Population	Method	Time	Page #
Childhood Trauma Questionnaire	To assess a broad range of traumatic experiences in childhood	Adults and adolescents	Retrospective self-report questionnaire	10–15 min	172
Children's Report of Exposure to Violence	To assess exposure to community violence	Preadolescents to adolescents	Self-report questionnaire	10 min for individual administration, 20 min for group administration	173
Composite Abuse Scale	To assess the frequency and consequences of physical, sexual, and emotional abuse	Adults	Self-report questionnaire	25–30 min	175
Conflict Tactics Scale	To assess the strategies partners use for resolving conflicts	Adults in marital, cohabiting, or dating relationships	Self-report questionnaire	10–15 min	177
Criminal Sentiments Scale Modified	To quantify the attitudes of convicted criminals.	Convicted criminals of all ages	Self-report questionnaire	8–12 min	180
Danger Assessment Instrument	To help battered women assess their risk of being killed by their spouse	Adult women	Self-report questionnaire	10 min	181
Date Rape Decision-Latency Measure	To measure the ability of college males to determine when a man should terminate unwanted sexual advances toward a woman	College-age males	Decision-latency method	Up to 6 min and 30 s	183
Deviant Peers	To determine the level of exposure a child or adolescent has to deviant peers	Children and adolescents	Questionnaire	3–5 min	185
Domestic Violence Inventory	To assess the risk and needs of perpetrators of physical, emotional, and verbal abuse	Adults	Self-report questionnaire	30–40 min	186
Domestic Violence Myth Acceptance Scale	To assess the degree to which an individual accepts myths about domestic violence as true	Adults	Self-report questionnaire	10–15 min	188
Dominance Scale	To assess three forms of dominance perceived as risk factors for intimate partner violence	Adults	Self-report questionnaire	10 min	190
Feelings and Acts of Violence Scale-Short Form	To measure the risk of violence	Adults	Self-report questionnaire	3–5 min	191

(continued)

(continued)

Name	Purpose	Population	Method	Time	Page #
Firestone Assessment of Violent Thoughts	To assess negative thoughts about self and others	Ages 17 and older	Self-report questionnaire	15 min	193
Historical–Clinical–Risk Assessment	To assess the risk of future violence in mentally ill, personality disordered, and forensic populations	Adults with a history of violence and likelihood of mental illness or personality disorder	Semistructured interview	Varies, average 90 min for interview, 2½ to 3 h for total completion time (including scoring and review of collateral information)	194
Index of Spouse Abuse	To measure frequency and severity of intimate partner violence	Adult women suspected of experiencing intimate partner violence	Self-report Questionnaire	5 min	196
Interview Schedule for Violent Events	To qualitatively and quantitatively assess physical attacks and the situation in which they occurred	Adult women	Interview	Varies	199
Level of Service Inventory-Revised	To assess offenders for criminal risk and need for treatment	Ages 16 and older	Semistructured interview	30–45 min	200
Levenson Self-Report Psychopathy Scale	To assess primary and secondary psychopathic traits in noninstitutionalized individuals	Noninstitutionalized samples	Self-report questionnaire	15–20 min	202
Maudsley Violence Questionnaire	To assess thoughts related to violent behavior	Ages 16 and older	Self-report questionnaire	10–15 min	204
Multidimensional Measure of Emotional Abuse	To assess emotional abuse that occurs in the context of dating relationships	Adults in dating relationships	Self-report questionnaire	10–15 min	206
My Exposure to Violence	To assess child and youth exposure to violence	Children to young adults	Structured interview	30–45 min	208
Pride in Delinquency Scale	To assess the degree of shame and pride associated with participation in specific criminal behaviors	Adolescents and adults	Self-report questionnaire or structured interview	15 min	210
Propensity for Abusiveness Scale	To measure propensity for abusiveness in males against female partners	Adults	Self-report questionnaire	15–20 min	211

(continued)

(continued)

Name	Purpose	Population	Method	Time	Page #
Proximal Antecedents to Violent Episodes Scale	To identify events that are likely to elicit partner violence committed by males	Adult males	Self-report questionnaire	10 min	213
Psychological Maltreatment Inventory	To retrospectively rate an individual's negative experiences with their parents	Adults	Retrospective self-report questionnaire	5–10 min	215
Psychological Maltreatment of Women Inventory	To quantify the psychological maltreatment experienced by women in intimate relationships	Adults	Self-report questionnaire	10–15 min	216
Psychological Maltreatment Rating Scales	To code dimensions of psychological abuse and neglect in parent–child interactions	Parents interacting with their 5–9 year old children	Independent raters code a parent–child interaction	15 min	218
Psychopathy Checklist-Revised	To assess antisocial behavior	Adults	Semistructured interview and file review	90 min for interview, 2½–3 h total completion time (including scoring and review of collateral information)	220
Rape Conformity Assessment	To assess potential to commit rape	Adult males	Small-group discussion on responses to multiple-choice questions	35–45 min	222
Rape Myth Acceptance Scale	To assess the degree to which an individual adheres to false information about rape, rapists, and rape victims	Adults	Questionnaire	4–7 min	224
Relationship Conflict Inventory	To assess the process and content of conflict in relationships	Adults	Self-report questionnaire	40–45 min	226
Risk of Eruptive Violence Scale	To measure the general tendency to act violently and/or erupt into "sudden and unexpected episodes of violence"	Adolescents and adults	Self-report questionnaire	8 min	227
Sensational Interests Questionnaire	To assess sensational interests (i.e., "potentially pathological interests of a lurid, morbid, or violent kind")	Adults	Self-report questionnaire	5–10 min	229
Seventh Grade Inventory of Knowledge and Attitudes	To measure adolescents' knowledge and attitudes about relational abuse	Adolescents	Self-report questionnaire	35–45 min	231

(continued)

(continued)

Name	Purpose	Population	Method	Time	Page #
Severity of Violence Against Men Scales	To measure how serious, aggressive, abusive, violent, and threatening an act is when a woman does the act to a man	Adult men	Self-report questionnaire	10–15 min	233
Severity of Violence Against Women Scales	To measure how serious, aggressive, abusive, violent, and threatening an act is when a man does that act to a woman	Adult women	Self-report questionnaire	10–15 min	235
Sex Inventory	To assess various aspects of sexuality, including sex interests, drives, attitudes, adjustment, conflict, cathexes, controls, and sociopathic tendencies	Adults	Self-report questionnaire	45–60 min	237
Sexual Adjustment Inventory	To assess attitudes and behaviors of accused or convicted sexual offenders	Accused or convicted adult sexual offenders	Self-report questionnaire	1 h	239
Sexual Experiences Survey	To assess sexual aggression and victimization from a dimensional viewpoint	Adults	Self-report questionnaire	10–15 min	241
Spousal Assault Risk Assessment	To assess risk factors associated with re-assault in individuals committing spousal assault	Adults	Checklist completed by mental health professionals with information obtained via interviews, self-report measures, collateral contacts and file reviews	Varies	243
Stalking Victimization Survey	To assess various aspects of stalking	Adults	Self-report questionnaire	5–10 min	246
Statistical Information on Recidivism	To predict the likelihood of recidivism of released offenders	Adult, non-native males	Semistructured interview and file review	Varies depending on the depth of information provided by the respondent and amount of information contained in the respondent's files	247
Subtle and Overt Psychological Abuse of Women Scale	To measure psychological abuse	Adult women	Self-report questionnaire	10–15 min	249

(continued)

(continued)

Name	Purpose	Population	Method	Time	Page #
Tolerance Toward Violence Scale	To measure tolerance toward violence	Adults	Self-report questionnaire	10 min	251
Victimization Screening Form	To assess the risk of future injury at the time of adolescent health maintenance visits	Adolescents	Brief interview	30 s to 1 min	253
Video Camera Surveillance	To more reliably characterize and classify violent assaults	Adult inpatients	Video recording and subsequent coding of events by clinic staff	Varies	254
Violence and Suicide Assessment Form	To assess suicide and violence risk in the psychiatric emergency room	Adult emergency room patients	Interview and questionnaire completed by patient's clinician	Varies	256
Violence Risk Appraisal Guide	To assess risk of violent recidivism	Adult offenders	File review	Varies depending on the amount of information contained in the respondent's files	258
Violence Scale	To measure aggression and violent behaviors in hospital settings	Adult psychiatric inpatients	Behavioral rating scale completed by ward staff	10–20 min	260

Abuse Assessment Screen (AAS)

Purpose

To screen for domestic violence in pregnant women.

Population

Adult women.

Background and Description

The Abuse Assessment Screen (AAS) was developed by the Nursing Research Consortium on Violence and Abuse to screen for the occurrence of domestic violence in pregnant women. The authors viewed the assessment of violence during pregnancy as essential and possible because most pregnant women consistently interact with the healthcare system. Questions were developed to encourage a nonjudgmental, gentle, but direct approach.

The AAS contains three items to identify remote and recent occurrence of domestic violence, as well as fear of the abuser. Although the measure was developed for use with pregnant women, nonpregnant women can be assessed by omitting the question about violence experienced while pregnant. Items assess the frequency, severity, and location of injury. A body map is provided to help women identify the site of injury. Sample items are reprinted below.

- Since you've been pregnant, have you been hit, slapped, kicked, or otherwise physically hurt by someone?
  Yes   No
- Within the last year, has anyone forced you to have sexual activities?
  Yes   No

Administration

The AAS takes approximately 1–5 min to administer.

Scoring

No total score is available. Indications of the presence of abuse should be followed up to assess the frequency and severity of abuse. Follow-up responses are coded using a scale that measures level of threat (i.e., threat of abuse included use of a weapon) and degree of abuse (i.e., wound from a weapon).

Interpretation

Items are used to screen for abuse. Items that are positively endorsed should result in additional queries. If abuse is present, then additional information and an appropriate referral should be provided.

Psychometric Properties

Reliability. Test–retest reliabilities were calculated using scores from 48 women who completed the AAS twice during the same trimester. Results indicated an 83 % agreement rate. The procedure was repeated using a second sample of 40 women and resulted in a 98 % agreement rate.

Validity. To increase content validity, the AAS was reviewed by Anglo, African American, and Hispanic nurse researchers who worked with victims of abuse. To establish criterion validity, the AAS was compared to the Conflict Tactics Scale (CTS, pp. 177–180), the Index of Spouse Abuse

(pp. 196–198), and the Danger Assessment Instrument (DA, pp. 181–183). Correlations between the AAS and the above measures ranged from .29 (CTS, Severe Violence) to .39 (DA). Correlations between frequency of abuse and each of the above measures ranged from .13 (CTS, Verbal Aggression) to .37 (CTS, Severe Violence). Responses to the AAS item "Since you've been pregnant, have you been hit, slapped, kicked or otherwise physically hurt by someone?" were compared to responses on the DA item "Have you ever been beaten while you were pregnant?" Results indicated a 96 % agreement rate between the two items.

Criterion validity was examined by comparing the AAS to a routine social service interview in a hospital setting using a sample of 334 women. The routine social interviews obtained information about social history (including domestic violence), health behaviors, and psychological risks. Categories compared were history of domestic violence, recent abuse, battering during pregnancy, and sexual abuse. For each of these categories, the AAS detected higher rates of violence than the routine social service interview (Norton, Peipert, Zierler, Lima, & Hume, 1995).

Clinical Utility

Moderate. The AAS may be useful as a screener in inpatient and outpatient healthcare facilities to identify pregnant women who are abused. Information gained from the AAS can be used to facilitate follow-up assessment or to identify women in need of information concerning domestic violence. However, there is concern that the AAS should not be used in isolation as a screening measure as it may miss identifying a considerable number of victims (Reichenheim & Moraes, 2004).

Research Applicability

High. The AAS has been successfully used as a screener for abuse in pregnant women who were then evaluated for psychological and behavioral responses to birth outcomes (D'Avolio et al.,

2001). It has also been used to examine opportunities and keys to implementing a screening program. The AAS can also be used to assess changes in abuse throughout pregnancy.

Original Citation

Parker, B., & McFarlane, J. (1991). Identifying and helping battered pregnant women. *American Journal of Maternal Child Nursing, 16*(3), 161–164.

Source

Dr. Barbara Parker, University of Virginia School of Nursing, P.O. Box 800826, Charlottesville, VA, 22908-0826, (434) 982-1976, Fax: (434) 982-1809, bjp8c@Virginia.edu

Cost

The AAS may be obtained from the Nursing Network on Violence Against Women, International website NNVAWI.ORG.

Alternative Forms

A Chinese version is available. The AAS has also been translated into Spanish, Haitian French Creole, and Brazilian Portuguese (Pearce, Hawkins, Kearney, Peyton, Dwyer, Haggerty, et al., 2003; Tiwari, Fong, Chan, Leung, Parker, & Ho, 2007).

References

D'Avolio, D., Hawkins, J. W., Haggerty, L. A., Kelly, U., Barrett, R., Durno Toscano, S. E., et al. (2001). Screening for abuse: Barriers and opportunities. *Health Care for Women International, 22*, 349–362.

Norton, L. B., Peipert, J. F., Zierler, S., Lima, B., & Hume, L. (1995). Battering in pregnancy: An assessment of two screening methods. *Obstetrics and Gynecology, 85*, 321–325.

Pearce, C. W., Hawkins, J. W., Kearney, M., Peyton, C. E., Dwyer, J., Haggerty, L. A., et al. (2003). Translation

of domestic violence instruments for use in research. *Violence Against Women, 9*, 859–878.

Reichenheim, M. E., & Moraes, C. L. (2004). Comparison between the Abuse Assessment Screen and the revised Conflict Tactics Scale for measuring physical violence during pregnancy. *Journal of Epidemiology and Community Health, 58*, 523–527.

Tiwari, A., Fong, D. Y. T., Chan, K. L., Leung, W. C., Parker, B. & Ho, P. C. (2007). Identifying intimate partner violence: Comparing the Chinese Abuse Assessment Screen with the Chinese Revised Conflict Tactics Scales. *BJOG, 114*, 1065–1071.

Abusive Behavior Inventory (ABI)

Purpose

To measure physical and psychological abuse of women committed by their partners. The scale was originally designed for use in clinical settings to evaluate programs for battering men.

Population

Adults.

Background and Description

The Abusive Behavior Inventory (ABI) differs from other measures of abuse in that it considers violence outside the context of family conflict. The ABI was initially developed to assess outcomes of a domestic abuse program and the content of the inventory was developed based on collaborations between battered women and the staff of a program that provided services to men who battered women. It reflects a feminist perspective that views physical abuse as a means to establish power and control over the victim. The authors identified 20 psychological abuse items from the following categories of the curriculum: emotional abuse, isolation, intimidation, threats, use of male privilege, and economic abuse. The remaining 10 items reflect physical abuse.

Males and females can respond to the ABI. The 30 items assess the frequency of physically and psychologically abusive behaviors that occurred during the past 6 months. The authors suggest that this time frame can be modified as needed. Subjects rate the frequency on a Likert-type scale, ranging from 1 ("never") to 5 ("very frequently"). Sample items are listed below:

- Used the children to threaten you (ex. told you that you would lose custody, said he would leave town with the children).
- Slapped, hit, or punched you.

Administration

The ABI requires approximately 15–20 min to complete.

Scoring

The 20 psychological abuse items are summed, and the total score is divided by 20 to reflect the average frequency of the occurrence of psychological abuse (1 = "no psychological abuse", 5 = "very frequent psychological abuse"). Similarly, the 10 physical abuse items are summed, and the total score is divided by 10 to reflect the average frequency of the occurrence of physical abuse (1 = "no physical abuse", 5 = "very frequent physical abuse").

Interpretation

Higher scores are reflective of greater frequency of abuse.

Psychometric Properties

Factor analysis. Items were correlated with scores on each subscale (using corrected item–total correlations) and other variables (e.g., age and household size). Analyses indicated that for men, all items on the physical abuse subscale had the highest correlations with the total score on the

physical subscale, but 7 of 20 items on the psychological abuse subscale had higher correlations with the total score on the physical abuse subscale than the psychological abuse subscale. For women, 2 items from the physical abuse subscale and 3 items from the psychological abuse subscale correlated higher with the total score on the psychological abuse and physical abuse subscales, respectively. Thus, the current item assignments are questionable.

Reliability. A sample of 100 males and 78 females, who were grouped as abusers, abused, non-abusers, or non-abused was used for reliability analyses. Cronbach's alpha coefficients for both the psychological and physical abuse subscales were calculated for each group. Cronbach's alpha ranged from .70 (physical abuse subscale, non-abused group) to .92 (psychological abuse subscale, non-abused group), indicating that the ABI subscales have adequate internal consistency.

Validity. The authors examined the extent to which the ABI distinguished between groups of people with known levels of abusive relationships. The authors found significant mean differences between people in abusive relationships (scores were more than 25 % higher) and those in non-abusive relationships. Additionally, scores on the ABI accounted for the most variance in differences between the two groups (approximately 25 %) when compared with age and education.

The ABI scores were compared with variables believed to be associated with abuse (e.g., clinical assessment of abuse, client assessment of abuse, and previous arrest for domestic abuse) to establish convergent validity. The ABI scores were compared with variables believed to be unassociated with abuse (e.g., age and household size) to establish divergent validity. Analyses revealed that scores on the ABI were correlated substantially higher with variables believed to be associated with abuse than with those believed to be unassociated.

Clinical Utility

High. The ABI is useful in determining levels of physical and psychological abuse experienced by an individual. Additionally, the ABI is useful as an outcome measure for batterers. The ABI can be modified to fit various time frames (e.g., past year as opposed to past 6 months).

Research Applicability

High. The ABI has been used in several studies to examine correlates of physical and psychological abuse. For example, Neufeld, McNamara, and Ertl (1999) found that physical and/or psychological abuse was correlated with length of longest relationship in past 6 months, histories of greater numbers of sexual partners, histories of greater numbers of emotional partners, higher estimates of male partner control, and greater numbers of emotional partners in past 6 months. Mills and Malley-Morrison (1998) examined the relationship between level of emotional commitment and frequency of abusive behaviors, acceptability of abusive behaviors, and causal attributions. They found that individuals that were more committed blamed their partners significantly less for abusive behaviors than less committed individuals.

Original Citation

Shepard, M. F., & Campbell, J. A. (1992). The Abusive Behavior Inventory. *Journal of Interpersonal Violence, 7*, 291–305

Source

Melanie F. Shepard, 220 Bohannon Hall, 1207 Ordean Court, University of Minnesota, Duluth, Duluth, MN 55812, (218) 726-8859, Fax: (218) 726-7185, mshepard@d.umn.edu

Cost

Contact the source (above) for permission to use the ABI.

Alternative Forms

Forms are available for males and females.

References

Mills, R. B., & Malley-Morrison, K. (1998). Emotional commitment, normative acceptability, and attributions for abusive partner behaviors. *Journal of Interpersonal Violence, 13*, 682–699.
Neufeld, J., McNamara, J. R., & Ertl, M. (1999). Incidence and prevalence of dating partner abuse and its relationship to dating practices. *Journal of Interpersonal Violence, 14*, 125–137.

Acceptance of Interpersonal Violence (AIV)

Purpose

To measure the degree to which one accepts the use of interpersonal violence in a relationship.

Population

Adults.

Background and Description

A large pool of items was initially developed to examine sexual attitudes. The Acceptance of Interpersonal Violence (AIV) is one of the four resulting scales designed to examine attitudinal correlates of rape myth acceptance. The other three scales are Sex Role Stereotyping, Sexual

Conservatism, and Adversarial Sexual Beliefs. Item analyses were conducted to identify the best items; these items make up the current version of the AIV.

The AIV is a 6-item self-report measure. Respondents rate the degree to which they agree with each item statement using a 7-point Likert-type scale, ranging from strongly agree to strongly disagree. Three of the items are reverse scored and 5 of the items specifically reflect violence toward women. Sample items follow:

- Sometimes the only way a man can get a cold woman turned on is to use force.
- A man is never justified in hitting his wife.

Administration

The AIV is estimated to take 1–2 min to complete.

Scoring

Some items are reversed scored. A total score is obtained from summing items.

Interpretation

Higher scores are indicative of a greater degree of acceptance of interpersonal violence toward women.

Psychometric Properties

Factor analysis. The AIV was initially conceptualized as a unidimensional scale designed to measure beliefs about violence toward women. A principal components analysis with varimax rotation was conducted on data from 386 men. The results suggested a two-factor solution; the first factor was labeled Sexual Violence (SV) and the second factor was labeled Intimate Partner Violence (IPV). A confirmatory factor analysis was conducted on a separate sample of 386 men and confirmed the adequacy of the two-factor model (Ogle, Noel, & Maisto, 2009).

Reliability. Item–total correlations ranged from .21 to .40. Internal consistency, calculated using Cronbach's alpha, was reported as .59. In two other samples of 21 and 86 respondents, alpha was .59 and .48, respectively. Test–retest reliability over a 2-week interval was .56 for a sample of 86 respondents. In a sample of 386 men, Cronbach's alpha was .63 and .36 for the SV and IPV subscales, respectively (Ogle et al., 2009).

Validity. The AIV correlated .56 with a measure of sexual coercion. Scores on the AIV were found to predict rape myth acceptance and have been found to have a stronger relationship (than the other attitudinal scales developed by Burt) with sexual aggression, as measured by the Sexual Experiences Survey (pp. 241–243). Other studies have found scores on the AIV to be significantly correlated with scores on the Rape Conformity Assessment, Attraction to Sexual Aggression, Adversarial Sexual Beliefs, and Rape Myth Acceptance (pp. 224–226) measures.

Clinical Utility

Limited. The AIV provides information on attitudes individuals hold toward the acceptability of violence in intimate relationships but provides little insight into the origination of such beliefs or their effect on behavior. The AIV is easy to administer and has demonstrated predictive validity, however, the reliability coefficients are generally less than .60.

Research Applicability

Moderate. The AIV requires little time to complete and might be useful in exploring attitudinal correlates of interpersonal violence.

Original Citation

Burt, M. R. (1980). Cultural myths and supports for rape. *Journal of Personality and Social Psychology, 38*, 217–230.

Source

Martha R. Burt, Urban Institute, 2100 M ST NW, Washington, DC 20037-1264, (202) 261-5709, mburt@urban.org

Cost

Contact the source (above) for permission to use the AIV.

Reference

Ogle, R. L., Noel, N. E., & Maisto, S. A. (2009). Assessing acceptance of violence toward women: A factor analysis of Burt's Acceptance of Interpersonal Violence Scale. *Violence Against Women, 15,* 799–809

Accountability Scale (AS)

Purpose

To measure dysfunctional attitudes pertaining to abuse that may be targets for change.

Population

Male and female perpetrators of domestic violence.

Background and Description

Accountability in relation to intimate partner violence is the notion that an individual acknowledges past involvement in domestic violence and accepts responsibility for his/her actions (Costa, Canady, & Babcock, 2007). Some researchers have proposed that increasing accountability and changing negative attitudes may be crucial in changing violent behavior. There were no previously existing measures of accountability, which precluded research into the construct and its implications for treatment outcome. The Accountability Scale (AS) was designed to provide such a measure of accountability. It was created based on the clinical work of Barbara Hart (1988) and the Pennsylvania Coalition Against Domestic Violence.

The AS is an 11-item self-report questionnaire. Respondents rate how much they agree with each statement using a 4-point Likert style scale ranging from 1 (disagree strongly) to 4 (agree strongly). Sample items follow.
- I realized that my pattern of abusive control harmed him/her.
- My behavior was caused by stress, alcohol, or other outside factors.

Administration

The AS requires approximately 5 min to complete.

Scoring

Some items are reverse scored.

Interpretation

Higher scores on the Acknowledging Harm subscale indicate greater acknowledgment of the consequences of one's violent actions. High scores on the Internalizing Responsibility subscale indicate acceptance of one's violent actions and lack of attributing one's behavior to external circumstances. In contrast, low scores on this subscale indicate externalizing blame for one's violent behavior.

Psychometric Properties

Factor analysis. The original version of the AS contained 17 items and was administered to 108 men and women in treatment for intimate partner violence. Data were subjected to principal components analysis with varimax rotation. Examination of a scree plot suggested a two-factor solution. Two items were eliminated that either loaded highly on both factors or did not load highly on either factor. The first factor was labeled Acknowledging Harm and the second factor was labeled Internalizing Responsibility.

The 17-item version of the AS was also administered to a community sample of 109 couples who reported a history of domestic violence. A confirmatory factor analysis was performed to verify the two-factor solution identified in the clinical sample. The two-factor solution fit the data with only one item loading on a different factor. Four items were subsequently eliminated to increase the interpretability of the factors. The two factors were negatively correlated.

Reliability. Internal consistency estimates were calculated for the initial 15-item version of the AS. Cronbach's alpha was .71 for the Acknowledging Harm subscale, .60 for the Internalizing Responsibility subscale, and .80 for the total scale.

Internal consistency estimates were calculated for the 11-item version of the AS administered to a community sample. Cronbach's alpha was .80 for the Acknowledging Harm subscale and .66 for the Internalizing Responsibility.

Validity. The 15-item version of the AS was administered to a clinical sample and was correlated with the University of Rhode Island Change Assessment-Domestic Violence (URICA-DV; Levesque, Gelles, & Velicer, 2000) to examine convergent validity. The Acknowledging Harm subscale was significantly, positively correlated with the Contemplation, Maintenance, Action, and Readiness to Change subscales of the URICA-DV and negatively correlated with the Precontemplation subscale. The Internalizing Responsibility subscale was not significantly correlated with any of the URICA-DV subscales.

The 11-item version of the AS was administered to a community sample along with conceptually related and unrelated measures to examine convergent and discriminant validity. The Acknowledging Harm subscale was significantly correlated with conceptually related constructs including male-to-female violence ($r=.45$) and marital satisfaction ($r=-.27$). The Internalizing Responsibility subscale was also significantly correlated with related constructs including perspective taking ($r=.30$) and male-to-female violence ($r=-.47$). The Internalizing Responsibility subscale was related to socially desirable responding ($r=.26$), as was the Acknowledging Harm subscale ($r=-.33$). Discriminant validity was demonstrated for both subscales.

Clinical Utility

Moderate. Data from preliminary studies suggest the AS has acceptable psychometric properties and may be useful in clinical and community settings to assess attitudes related to abuse that may be targets for treatment.

Research Applicability

Moderate. The AS is a brief, easy-to-administer measure that may yield useful information for researching attitudes about past violent behavior and implications for batterer treatment programs. Preliminary studies suggest the scale has acceptable psychometric properties, but further research is necessary.

Original Citation

Costa, D. M., Canady, B., & Babcock, J. C. (2007). Preliminary report on the Accountability Scale: A change and outcome measure for intimate partner violence research. *Violence and Victims, 22,* 515–531.

Source

Julia C. Babcock, Department of Psychology, The University of Houston, 126 Heyne Building, Houston, TX 77204, (713) 743-8500, jbabcock@ uh.edu

Cost

Please contact the source (above) for permission to use the AS.

Child Abuse Potential Inventory (CAP)

Purpose

To screen for the potential for physical abuse of a child.

Population

Parents or the primary caregivers actively involved with the child.

Background and Description

The Child Abuse Potential Inventory (CAP) was developed to aid child protection service workers in screening parents suspected of physical child abuse. Psychiatric and interpersonal factors related to the etiology of physical abuse guided the development of individual items. The original version contained 334 items. The revised version contains 160 items that are organized into seven abuse scales (distress, rigidity, unhappiness, problems with child and self, problems with family, problems with others, total physical child abuse), three validity scales (lie scale, random response scale, inconsistency scale), and three response distortion indices (faking-good, faking-bad, random response). Items are rated using an agree or disagree format.

Administration

The CAP can be administered in an individual or group setting, and is estimated to require 30–45 min to complete.

Scoring

Scoring is determined by examining the 10 scales (one primary, six factor, and three validity) and involves computations with weighted scores. Both hand and computer scoring systems are available.

Interpretation

Scores are interpreted individually for each scale. Both a scoring and an interpretative manual are available.

Psychometric Properties

Norms. Original data obtained during the development of the instrument were evaluated in a small ($N=38$) and relatively homogeneous sample of department of social service clients. Data from a sample of 2,610 participants representing control, at-risk, neglect, and abuse groups were also collected.

Factor analysis. Seven factors have been identified: distress, rigidity, child with problems, problems from family and others, unhappiness, loneliness, and negative concept of child and self. Following a principal axis factoring with oblique rotations, the following dimensions were most predictive of abuse: loneliness; rigidity; problems with self, friends, and other things; and lack of social and self control (Milner & Wimberley, 1979).

Reliability. Reliability information has been demonstrated for both internal consistency and temporal stability. Corrected split-halves and KR-20 internal consistency estimates for the 77-item physical abuse scale are high and range from .91 to .96 for controls and .95 to .98 for abusers. Lower internal consistency estimates have been produced for factor and validity scales, with abuser estimates generally higher than those for controls. The temporal stability estimate for the revised CAP over a period of one week was .90.

Validity. Content validity was considered when generating items based on psychiatric and interactional models of child abuse, as well as the judgments of knowledgeable professionals. Numerous studies have found expected relationships between performance on the CAP and constructs known or thought to be related to child abuse. CAP scores have also been shown to decrease following treatment for child abuse. Factor analysis has resulted in six subscales consistent with child abuse. Available data support expectations that, using 215 points as a cut off, correct identification of active, non-treated, moderate to severe physical abusers in a high risk population will be near the 80 % level and that correct identification of controls will be near or above the 90 % level. The previously mentioned percentages may rise to a level identifying 88 % of physical abusers and 100 % of controls with Milner's recommended interpretation procedure (i.e., rounded, weighted scores and valid protocol only responses for more than 90 % of items, totals prorated for missing responses, and acceptable response distortion indexes). In recent studies, individual correct classification rates based on discriminate analysis have been in the mid-80 % to the low 90 % range (i.e., Caliso & Milner, 1992; Milner, Gold, & Wimberley, 1986; Milner & Williams, 1980; Milner & Robertson, 1989). Finally, adequate longitudinal predictive validity has been demonstrated for the abuse scale.

Clinical Utility

High. The CAP has been often used in a number of clinical settings and has been demonstrated to discriminate well between abusers and non-abusers.

Research Applicability

High. The CAP has been extensively used within a number of research studies and is one of the most widely used measures of child abuse potential.

Original Citation(s)

Milner, J. S. (1986). The *Child Abuse Potential Inventory: Manual* (2nd ed.). Webster, NC: Psytec.
Milner, J. S. (1990). An *interpretive manual for the Child Abuse Potential Inventory.* Webster, NC: Psytec.

Milner, J. S., & Wimberley, R. C. (1979). An inventory for the identification of child abusers. *Journal of Clinical Psychology, 35*, 95–100.

Source

Psychological Assessment Resources, 16204 N Florida Ave, Lutz, FL 33549, 1-800-331-8378

Cost

The CAP Introductory Kit costs $180 from Psychological Assessment Resources (PAR).

Alternative Forms

Dutch and Spanish versions are available (de Paul Ochotorena, Arruabarrena, & Milner, 1991). A brief, 24-item version of the CAP (BCAP) has been developed that has demonstrated adequate internal consistency ($\alpha=.89$) and significant correlations with scores on the Abuse risk score of the CAP ($r=.96$; Ondersma, Chaffin, Mullins, & LeBreton, 2005).

References

Caliso, J. A., & Milner, J. S. (1992). Childhood history of abuse and child abuse screening. *Child Abuse and Neglect, 16*(5), 647–659.
de Paul Ochotorena, J., Arruabarrena, I., & Milner, J. S. (1991). Validation of the Spanish version of the Child Abuse Potential Inventory for use in Spain. *Child Abuse and Neglect, 15*(4), 495–504.
Milner, J. S., Gold, R. G., & Wimberley, R. C. (1986). Prediction and explanation of child abuse: Cross-validation of the Child Abuse Potential Inventory. *Journal of Consulting and Clinical Psychology, 54*(6), 865–866.
Milner, J. S., & Robertson, K. R. (1989). Inconsistent response patterns and the prediction of child maltreatment. *Child Abuse and Neglect, 13*, 59–64.
Milner, J. S., & Williams, P. P. (1980). Prediction and explanation of child abuse. *Journal of Clinical Psychology, 36*(4), 875–884.
Ondersma, S. R., Chaffin, M. J., Mullins, S. M., & LeBreton, J. M. (2005). A brief form of the Child Abuse Potential Inventory: Development and validation. *Journal of Clinical Child and Adolescent Psychology, 34*(2), 301–311.

Childhood Trauma Questionnaire (CTQ)

Purpose

To provide a brief, reliable, and valid assessment of a broad range of traumatic experiences in childhood.

Population

Adolescents and adults.

Background and Description

The Childhood Trauma Questionnaire (CTQ) was developed to expand upon several commonly used methods for obtaining information regarding histories of childhood trauma and to compare the impact of specific forms of trauma. The CTQ is a retrospective 70-item self-report questionnaire of child abuse, child neglect, and related aspects of the child-rearing environment. Items on the CTQ begin with the phrase "When I was growing up" and are rated on a 5-point Likert-type scale according to the frequency with which experiences occurred. Response options range from "never true" to "very often true."

Administration

The administration of this instrument is estimated to require 10–15 min.

Scoring

Items are summed to produce a total score.

Interpretation

Higher scores indicate a significant history of child abuse and neglect.

Psychometric Properties

Norms. Norms were developed from 286 drug or alcohol dependent patients. Forty of these patients were administered the questionnaire again after a 2–6 month interval.

Factor analysis. A principal components analysis yielded four factors: Physical and Emotional Abuse; Emotional Neglect; Sexual Abuse; and Physical Neglect. Subsequent factor analyses suggested a five-factor model provided a better fit wherein physical and emotional abuse were separated into distinct factors (as cited in Scher, Stein, Asmundson, McCreary, & Forde, 2001).

Reliability. Cronbach's alpha for the factors ranged from .79 to .94. The CTQ demonstrated acceptable test–retest reliability over a 2–6 month interval (intraclass correlation .88), as well as convergence with the Childhood Trauma Interview. This convergence suggests that reports of child abuse and neglect were stable across instruments.

In a sample of 44 patients enrolled in a treatment study for past childhood abuse, internal consistency of the subscales ranged from $\alpha = .82$ to .94. Test–retest reliability was adequate to good for most subscales over a period of 29 weeks and ranged from $r = .62$ to .92 (Paivio, 2001).

Validity. The CTQ demonstrated convergent validity with the Childhood Trauma Interview. Discriminant validity was demonstrated by the CTQ being largely unrelated to measures of verbal intelligence and social desirability. CTQ scores were significantly correlated with PTSD diagnoses, symptom severity (as measured by the PTSD Symptom Severity Interview, PSS-I; Foa, Riggs, Dancu, & Rothbaum, 1993), and Impact of Event Scale scores (IES; Horowitz, 1986) in a sample of 44 patients seeking treatment for past childhood abuse (Paivio, 2001).

Clinical Utility

Moderate. The CTQ has not been widely investigated and has limited norms. However, the short form of the CTQ has been used as a screening measure in a variety of clinical settings and has demonstrated acceptable psychometric properties.

Research Applicability

Moderate. The measure has promise for further research due to its ease of use and brevity. Also, the measure uses continuous scores regarding trauma experiences and may prove to be a good screening measure.

Original Citation

Bernstein, D. P., Fink, L., Handelsman, L., Foote, J., Lovejoy, M., Wenzel, K., Sapareto, E., & Ruggiero, J. (1994). Initial reliability and validity of a new retrospective measure of child abuse and neglect. *American Journal of Psychiatry, 151*(8), 1132–1136.

Source

Dr. David Bernstein, Maastricht University, PO Box 616, 6200 MD Maastricht, The Netherlands, d.bernstein@maastrichtuniversity.nl

Cost

Contact the author (above) for permission to use.

Alternative Forms

A short form of the CTQ (CTQ-SF) has been developed. The CTQ-SF is a 28-item measure designed to be used as a screening instrument for abuse histories in clinical and community groups. The CTQ-SF has five subscales that demonstrated acceptable levels of internal consistency with alphas ranging from .81 to .95. There is also evidence of criterion validity with CTQ-SF scores significantly correlating with therapist ratings of patient abuse and neglect (Bernstein, Stein, Newcomb, Walker, Pogge, & Ahluvalia, 2003).

The CTQ-SF has also been translated into several other languages including Dutch, Persian, and Swedish (Garrusi & Nakhaee, 2009; Gerdner & Allgulander, 2009; Thombs, Bernstein, Lobbestael, & Arntz, 2009).

References

Bernstein, D. P., Stein, J. A., Newcomb, M. D., Walker, E., Pogge, D., & Ahluvalia, T. (2003). Development and validation of a brief screening version of the Childhood Trauma Questionnaire. *Child Abuse & Neglect, 27*, 169–190.

Foa, E. B., Riggs, D. S., Dancu, C. V., & Rothbaum, B. O. (1993). Reliability and validity of a brief instrument for assessing posttraumatic stress disorder. *Journal of Traumatic Stress, 6*, 459–473.

Garrusi, B., & Nakhaee, N. (2009). Validity and reliability of a Persian version of the Childhood Trauma Questionnaire. *Psychological Reports, 104*, 509–516.

Gerdner, A., & Allgulander, C. (2009). Psychometric properties of the Swedish version of the Childhood Trauma Questionnaire – Short Form (CTQ-SF). *Nordic Journal of Psychiatry, 63*, 160–170.

Horowitz, M. D. (1986). *Stress response syndromes* (2nd ed.). Northvale, NJ: Jason Aronson.

Paivio, S. C. (2001). Stability of retrospective self-reports of child abuse and neglect before and after therapy services for child abuse issues. *Child Abuse and Neglect, 25*, 1053–1068.

Scher, C. D., Stein, M. B., Asmundson, G. J., McCreary, D. R., & Forde, D. R. (2001). The Childhood Trauma Questionnaire in a community sample: Psychometric properties and normative data. *Journal of Traumatic Stress, 14*, 843–857.

Thombs, B. D., Bernstein, D. P., Lobbestael, J., & Arntz, A. (2009). A validation study of the Dutch Childhood Trauma Questionnaire – Short Form: Factor structure, reliability, and known-groups validity. *Child Abuse and Neglect, 33*, 518–523.

Children's Report of Exposure to Violence (CREV)

Purpose

To assess exposure to community violence.

Population

Preadolescents to adolescents.

Background and Description

The Children's Report of Exposure to Violence (CREV) was developed to study possible reasons for the rapidly escalating incidence of violent crimes being committed against children. The goal was to assess the effects of direct exposure to overt violence, as well as the effects of indirect exposure through sources such as the media and hearsay reports. Exposure to community violence is assessed within four different contexts: media, hearsay reports, direct witnessing, and direct victimization. The survey, consisting of 32 items, begins with a brief query for background information followed by 29 items asking subjects to provide a frequency rating to questions. The frequency ratings are followed by three additional questions asking the subject to write in any other instances of having been told, having seen, or having experienced other violent situations in real life that were not covered by the previous questions. The frequency ratings are partitioned along a 5-point scale utilizing written descriptors (Never, One Time, A Few Times, Many Times, and Every Day). Children are asked to place an "X" beneath the descriptor that most accurately reflects their answer to the particular item.

Administration

The CREV can be administered to a group or individually. Individual administration requires approximately 10 min, whereas group administration requires about 20 min. Depending on the age and maturity of the child, they can be allowed to complete the CREV at their own pace or be guided through the instrument by the administrator. For children who have difficulty reading, the test questions can be read to them.

Scoring

A Total Score, ranging from 0 to 116, is obtained by summing the 29 item scores. A numerical value can also be assigned to each of the scales (Media Scale, Reported Scale, Witnessed Scale, and Victim Scale) and Subscale scores (Reported Stranger Subscale, Reported Familiar Subscale, Witnessed Stranger Subscale, Witnessed Familiar Subscale).

Interpretation

According to the authors, the magnitude of the CREV Total Score is the best indicator of the degree to which the subject has been exposed to violence. Exploratory factor analysis revealed that, despite the presence of four scales in the CREV, only two distinct factors emerged. These factors were labeled as "Direct Exposure" which was composed of the Reported and Witnessed Scales and "Media Exposure" which was composed of the Media Scale. The content areas for the Victim Scale did not consistently load on 1-factor. These findings should be taken into account when interpreting the current scales of the CREV. Factor scores (Direct Exposure Factor and Indirect/Media Exposure Factor) can be derived from summing the responses to the appropriate items.

Psychometric Properties

Reliability. Test–retest reliability for the CREV was determined on a small subsample of the original subjects ($n=42$) who were retested 2 weeks after the original test date. The Pearson correlation coefficient was .75 for the CREV Total Score, .78 for the Direct Exposure factor (Reported Scale + Witnessed Scale), and .52 for the Media Exposure factor (Media Scale). Gender and age differences in the reliabilities were not notable except for individuals in the 13–15 year age group whose retest results were less reliable on the Media Exposure Factor than those of other groups ($r=.25$). Cronbach's alpha was used to assess internal consistency. Coefficient alpha for the Direct Exposure factor items was .93, for the Media Exposure factor items was .75, and for the Total Score was .75.

Validity. Relating to construct validity of the CREV, exploratory factor analysis suggested that the four scales initially designed for the CREV were actually best explained by two factors, a Direct Exposure factor (comprising the Reported and Witnessed Scales) and a Media Exposure factor (comprised of the Media Scale). The content of the Victim Scale did not significantly load on either of these factors and it was noted by the authors that in the study sample, relatively few subjects reported high levels of victimization resulting in a restricted range of responses for these items.

Additional evidence supporting the validity of the CREV came from a sample of 64 urban youth. In this study, high CREV scores were associated with greater sleep disturbance and higher resting heart rate and pulse as hypothesized (Cooley-Quille & Lorion, 1999).

Clinical Utility

Moderate. The CREV provides a relatively quick, easy-to-administer, and interpret method for assessing the amount of exposure to community violence children have experienced. Lack of normative data make interpreting levels of exposure difficult.

Research Applicability

Moderate. The factors resulting from the CREV are of theoretical interest and possess relatively good psychometric properties. The CREV can be administered in an individual or group format and requires minimal training to use correctly.

Original Citation

Cooley, M. R., Turner, S. M., & Beidel, D. C. (1995). Assessing community violence: The children's report of exposure to violence. *Journal of the American Academy of Child and Adolescent Psychiatry, 34*(2), 201–208.

Source

Michelle Cooley-Quille, Ph.D., School of Public Health, Johns Hopkins University, The Candler Building, 111 Market Place, Suite 850, Baltimore, MD 21202, (410) 347-3203, Fax: (310) 822-9231

Cost

Contact the source (above) for permission to use the CREV.

Reference

Cooley-Quille, M., & Lorion, R. (1999). Adolescents' exposure to community violence: Sleep and psychophysiological functioning. *Journal of Community Psychology, 27*, 367–375.

Composite Abuse Scale (CAS)

Purpose

To assess the frequency and consequences of physical, sexual, and emotional abuse.

Population

Adults.

Background and Description

The Composite Abuse Scale (CAS) defines domestic abuse as partner abuse within heterosexual relationships. Items were based on a review of the content contained in the Conflict Tactics Scale (CTS, pp. 177–180), Measure of Wife Abuse [(Rodenberg & Fantuzzo, 1993), Index of Spouse Abuse (pp. 196–198), and the Psychological Maltreatment of Women Inventory (pp. 216–218)]. Items were formatted to be first-person, past tense, gender neutral, and culturally appropriate. The 74 items relate to physical, sexual, and emotional abuse. Respondents rate the amount of abuse (one, a little, some, moderate, great) and the frequency of abuse in the past year (daily, once per week, once per month, several times, only once).

Administration

The CAS is estimated to take 25–30 min to complete.

Scoring

Item scores are summed to produce scale scores.

Interpretation

Higher scores are indicative of a greater amount and/or frequency of abuse.

Psychometric Properties

Factor analysis. A principal components analysis produced a best-fit solution with four factors: Severe Combined Abuse (SCA), Emotional Abuse (EA), Physical Abuse (PA), and Harassment (H). These factors are used to represent four dimensions of abuse. The four factor model was found in another study that used a sample of 1,836 women (Hegarty, Bush, & Sheehan, 2005).

Reliability. All item–total correlations were higher than .60. Cronbach's alpha for the SCA, EA, PA, and H scales were .95, .92, .95, and .91, respectively.

Validity. Content validity was established through selecting items from a review of other available measures. Face validity was established by having items reviewed by Australian domestic violence researchers and domestic violence workers and victims. Criterion validity was examined by correlating the four dimensions of the CAS with Verbal Aggression, Minor Violence, and Severe Violence subscales of the CTS. With the exception of a Pearson correlation of .46 between the SCA scale and the Verbal Aggression scale of the CTS, correlations ranged from .61 to .93.

Clinical Utility

Moderate. The psychometric properties of the CAS have been established only for a selective sample and cannot be generalized to the community. Additional research and normative data are needed prior to the widespread clinical use of the scale.

Research Applicability

Moderate. The CAS allows for a thorough assessment of aspects of physical, emotional, and sexual abuse. Separate scores for amount and frequency of abuse can be useful for determining correlates of each component.

Original Citation

Hegarty, K., Sheehan, M., & Schonfeld, C. (1999). A multidimensional definition of partner abuse: Development and preliminary validation of the Composite Abuse Scale. *Journal of Family Violence, 14*, 399–415.

Source

Kelsey Hegarty, University of Melbourne, Department of General Practice, 200 Berkeley Street, Carlton Victoria 3053, Australia, Phone: +61 3 8344 4992, Fax: +61 3 9347 6163, k.hegarty@unimelb.edu.au

Cost

Please contact the source (above) for permission to use the CAS.

Alternative Forms

A short form of the CAS was created that contains 30 items. The items were chosen for the short form from the original CAS to maximize internal consistency reliability. The four scales had Cronbach's alphas .87 or higher in a sample of 427 women. Evidence of convergent and discriminant validity exists as the CAS-short form was found to correlate with self-ratings of abuse, thus demonstrating evidence of convergent validity, and was not found to be associated with education level, thus demonstrating evidence of divergent validity.

References

Hegarty, K., Bush, R., & Sheehan, M. (2005). The Composite Abuse Scale: Further development and assessment of reliability and validity of a multidimensional partner abuse measure in clinical settings. *Violence and Victims, 20,* 529.

Rodenberg, F., & Fantuzzo, J. (1993). The measure of wife abuse: Steps toward the development of a comprehensive assessment technique. *Journal of Family Violence, 8,* 203–217.

Conflicts Tactics Scales-Revised (CTS2)

Purpose

To assess the strategies partners use for resolving conflicts.

Population

Adults in marital, cohabiting, or dating relationships.

Background and Description

The Conflict Tactics Scale was based on the assumption that conflict is inevitable in human interactions, but the tactics used to deal with conflict are not inevitable. The CTS2 is an updated and expanded version of the original Conflict Tactics Scale. Scale names were changed, items were added, and new scales were developed. The Verbal Aggression Scale was changed to Psychological Aggression and the Violence Scale was changed to Physical Assault. A Negotiation Scale replaced the Reasoning Scale, and two new scales (Sexual Coercion and Injury) were added.

The 39-item CTS2 samples concrete acts used to deal with conflict. Each item asks the respondent to indicate the frequency with which they use each tactic and then to indicate the frequency with which their partner uses the tactic. Thus, the total 78 questions provide information about the respondent both as a victim and as an aggressor in the relationship. The CTS2 consists of five scales, three primary scales (Negotiation, Psychological Aggression, and Physical Assault) and two collateral scales (Sexual Coercion and Injury). Items from the scales are interspersed to reduce response sets and to minimize demand characteristics. The Negotiation scale reflects actions used to settle disagreements through discussion and consists of six items: three refer to cognitive strategies and three refer to emotional strategies. Psychological aggression consists of eight items: four items measure minor acts of psychological aggression and four assess severe acts of psychological aggression. Physical Assault measures physical violence and consists of 12 items: five items sample minor acts of violence and seven items sample major acts of violence. The 7-item Sexual Coercion scale measures behaviors meant to compel the partner to engage in unwanted sexual activity, ranging from verbal insistence to physical force. The 7-item Injury scale assesses partner-inflicted physical injury (i.e., bone or tissue damage, need for medical attention, and pain continuing for one day or more). Items are written at a sixth grade reading level and respondents indicate how often each act occurred in the previous year, but the instructions can be modified to assess other referent periods or specific situations. Responses are made using eight categories, ranging from 0 to 7.

Administration

The CTS2 is estimated to take 10–15 min to complete.

Scoring

Scores are calculated for the five scales by summing the values assigned to each category. To calculate scale and subscale scores, category numbers (0–6) may be summed. The authors, however, recommend summing the midpoints for the response categories chosen by the respondent. For response categories 0, 1, and 2, midpoints are 0, 1, and 2, respectively. For category 3 (3–5 times), the midpoint is 4. For category 4, the midpoint is 8. The midpoint of category 5 is 15, and the midpoint of category 6 is recommended as 25.

The authors recommend two scoring possibilities for category 7 ("Not in the past year, but it did happen before"). If scores for the previous year are desired, this category is scored as 0. If the examiner is interested in whether the assault ever occurred, this response is scored as 1.

Prevalence and chronicity variables may also be created for the physical assault, sexual coercion, and physical injury scales. Prevalence is scored 0 or 1 if no acts or one or more acts in the scale occurred, respectively. Chronicity is the number of times all acts in a scale occurred for reported acts.

Interpretation

Higher scores indicate higher frequencies of occurrences of the behaviors endorsed.

Psychometric Properties

Factor analysis. A confirmatory factor analysis of data from a sample of 295 women supported the existence of a 5-factor solution. The 5-factor structure was also supported by data from a factor analysis conducted on a sample of 359 incarcerated women, suggesting that the scale works for an incarcerated female population as well as a community sample (Lucente, Fals-Stewart, Richards, & Goscha, 2001).

Reliability. Internal consistency was measured using Cronbach's alpha coefficient. In a sample of college students, alpha coefficients ranged from .79 to .95. In a female sample wherein category numbers were used as item scores and the authors' suggested midpoint scoring system was used, alphas were as follows: .84 and .86 (negotiation), .70 and .77 (psychological aggression), .66 and .74 (minor psychological aggression), .49 and .63 (severe psychological aggression), .67 and .78 (physical assault), .62 and .75 (minor physical assault), and .43 and .57 (severe physical assault). In a sample of incarcerated women, self-as-victim scores resulted in alphas ranging from .62 (sexual coercion) to .91 (negotiation).

Validity. Validity of the Conflict Tactics Scale was well established. Because the CTS2 is an extension of the original Conflict Tactics Scale, much of the validity of the original CTS will likely extend to the CTS2.

Support for the construct validity of the CTS2 comes from correlations among scales of the CTS2 and differential correlations between men and women. The psychological aggression and physical assault scales were more highly correlated with the sexual coercion scale in men than women. The physical assault and injury scales were correlated more highly in men than in women. The sexual coercion and injury scales correlated more highly in men than in women as well. Additionally, high correlations were found between psychological aggression and physical assault, and social integration was negatively correlated with physical assault.

Separating responses into aggressor or victim responses, the physical assault scale correlated positively with all other scales for both aggressor and victim responses. All scales correlated significantly with each other for aggressor and victim responses except the following: aggressor responses for the injury subscale did not correlate with aggressor responses for sexual coercion and aggressor negotiation did not correlate with victim injury.

Support for the discriminant validity of the CTS2 was also found. Researchers found nonsignificant or low correlations between the negotiation and sexual coercion scales, and the negotiation and injury scales. Higher prevalence and chronicity rates were found in a sample of incarcerated women compared to a sample of college women.

Aggressor responses to physical assault, negotiation, and sexual coercion, and victim responses to physical assault, sexual coercion and injury were correlated with the scores on the Abusive Behavior Checklist (pp. 164–166), providing support for criterion-related validity.

Clinical Utility

High. The CTS2 is useful in quantifying the frequency of a variety of conflict tactics used by the respondent and his/her partner. Additionally, the time frame for responses may be modified, making the CTS2 useful as an outcome measure.

Research Applicability

High. The CTS2 is time efficient and may be modified in various ways to measure relevant time frames or situations. For example, the CTS2 may be modified to assess violence between parents of adolescents by asking adolescents to respond about the behavior of their parents toward each other. The CTS2 has also been used to code categories to analyze documents such as data from police records, orders of protection, and psychiatric intake interviews. If a shortened scale is needed, the CTS2 may be shortened to include the most crucial scales, such as the three original scales of the CTS.

Original Citation

Straus, M. A., Hamby, S. L., Boney-McCoy, S., & Sugarman, D. B. (1996). The revised Conflict Tactics Scales (CTS2). *Journal of Family Issues, 17*, 283–316.

Source

Murray A. Straus, Professor of Sociology and Co-Director Family Research Laboratory, University of New Hampshire, Durham, NH 03824. The CTS2 is available from Western Psychological Services, 2031 Wilshire Blvd, Los Angeles, CA 90025-1251, 1-800-648-8857, Fax: (310) 478-7838, http://portal.wpspublish.com/portal/page?_pageid=53,70488&_dad=portal&_schema=PORTAL

Cost

A kit that includes a handbook, 10 CTS2 autoscore forms, and 10 CTS PC autoscore forms (the parent–child version of the CTS) can be purchased from Western Psychological Services for $82.50.

Alternative Forms

The original CTS has three forms: Form A, Form N, and Form R. The three forms are very similar and differ only in the number of items for each scale and the number of response categories respondents can choose from. Form A was the first form of the scale and was a written questionnaire that had six response categories (Bulcroft & Straus, 1975, as cited in Straus, 1979). In contrast, Form N was part of a telephone interview and Form R was an in person interview. Both Forms N and R had seven response categories. Form N had more violence items than Form A and fewer reasoning items. Form R is very similar to Form N and differs only in that it has an additional parent–child item and an additional spouse item.

Parent–Child Conflict Tactics Scales (CTS PC) were developed to assess the psychological and physical abuse of children by their parents. There are two versions of the scale; one version is completed by the parent whereas the other version is completed by the child. The Parent–Child Conflict Tactics Scales were found to measure child maltreatment better than the original CTS (Straus, Hamby, Finkelhor, Moore, & Runyan, 1998).

References

Bulcroft, R., & Straus, M. A. (1975). *Validity of husband, wife, and child reports of intrafamily violence and power*. Unpublished manuscript, Family Violence Research Program, University of New Hampshire.

Lucente, S. W., Fals-Stewart, W., Richards, H. J., & Goscha, J. (2001). Factor structure and reliability of the revised Conflict Tactics Scales for incarcerated female substance abusers. *Journal of Family Violence, 16*, 437–450.

Straus, M. A. (1979). Measuring intrafamily conflict and violence: The Conflict Tactics (CT) Scales. *Journal of Marriage and Family, 41*, 75.

Straus, M. A., Hamby, S. L., Finkelhor, D., Moore, D. W., & Runyan, D. (1998). Identification of child maltreatment with the Parent-Child Conflict Tactics Scales: Development and psychometric data for a national sample of American parents. *Child Abuse and Neglect, 22*, 249–270.

Criminal Sentiments Scale-Modified (CSS-M)

Purpose

To quantify the attitudes of convicted criminals.

Population

All ages.

Background and Description

The Criminal Sentiments Scale-Modified (CSS-M) is a modified version of the Criminal Sentiments Scale. Whereas the Criminal Sentiments Scale employed a 5-point scale, the modified version uses a 3-point scale. The wording of the CSS was also clarified and the scoring of a subscale changed to allow a higher score to indicate a more pro-criminal attitude. The 41-item CSS-M measures attitudes, values, and beliefs related to law breaking. The three subscales assess attitudes toward law–court–police (LCP), tolerance for law violations (TLV), and identification with criminal others (ICO). Responses are recorded on a 3-point scale ranging from 0 (acceptance of prosocial statements or rejection of antisocial statements) to 2 (acceptance of antisocial statements or rejection of prosocial statements). Sample items follow:

- Almost any jury can be fixed.
- The police are honest.
- A hungry man has the right to steal.

Administration

The CSS-M is estimated to take 8–12 min to complete.

Scoring

The CSS-M yields three subscale scores (LCP, TLV, and ICO) and a total score. Endorsing antisocial statements (or rejecting prosocial statements) adds 2 points to the cumulative total score. Endorsing an undecided response to antisocial statements (or prosocial statements) receives a score of 1.

Interpretation

Higher scores are indicative of more pro-criminal attitudes.

Psychometric Properties

Reliability. Internal consistency, assessed by Cronbach's alpha, was .73 for the total score, .73 for the LPC Scale, .70 for the TLV Scale, and .73 for the ICO Scale. Additional total scale coefficients were .75 for a sample of violent and nonviolent offenders, .73 for violent offenders, and .75 for nonviolent offenders. Item–total correlations ranged from .54 to .91.

Validity. Scores on the CSS-M correlated with scores on the Pride in Delinquency Scale (pp. 210–213) in samples of violent and nonviolent offenders. Total scores and scores on the subscales correlated with scores on the Level of Service Inventory-Revised (pp. 200–201) and Factor-2 of the Psychopathy Checklist (pp. 220–223). TLV, ICO, and total scores correlated with scores on the Statistical Information on Recidivism scale (pp. 247–249). These correlations provide support for the convergent validity of the CSS-M.

Data support the criterion-related validity of the CSS-M. A modest correlation was found between the CSS-M and both incarceration and misconduct criteria. Scores covaried with rearrest and reincarceration criteria for a sample of violent and nonviolent offenders. Additionally, the total and LCP scores correlated with recidivism in a sample of violent offenders. Total scores on the CSS-M and scores on the LCP and ICO subscales correlated with the total number of institutional conducts, but none of the scales on the CSS-M correlated with total number of convictions, number of different offenses, previous violent offense, and previous property offense (Simourd & Van de Ven, 1999).

Clinical Utility

Moderate. The scale may be useful in predicting relapse. It is important to note that the scale did not predict recidivism in violent criminals (Mills & Kroner, 1997). Recidivism was, however, predictable in sexual offenders. If research continues to consistently find this measure to be reliable and valid, it could be very useful in studies that relate to sexual offenses.

Research Applicability

Moderate. The measure could be useful for researchers interested in evaluating the relationship between pro-criminal attitudes and subsequent criminal behavior.

Original Citation

Simourd, D. J. (1997). The Criminal Sentiments Scale-Modified and Pride in Delinquency scale: Psychometric properties and construct validity of two measures of criminal attitudes. *Criminal Justice and Behavior, 24,* 52–70.

Source

Dr. David Simourd, Algonquin Correctional Evaluation Services, 86 Braemar Road, Kingston, Ontario K7M 4B6 Canada, (613) 384-6637, Fax: (613) 384-6637, dave@acesink.com

Cost

Please contact the source (above) for permission to use the CSS-M.

References

Mills, J. F., & Kroner, D. G. (1997). The Criminal Sentiments Scale: Predictive validity in a sample of violent and sex offenders. *Journal of Clinical Psychology, 53,* 399–404.

Simourd, D. J., & Van de Ven, J. (1999). Assessment of criminal attitudes: Criterion-related validity of the Criminal Sentiments Scale-Modified and Pride in Delinquency Scale. *Criminal Justice and Behavior, 26,* 90–106.

Danger Assessment Instrument (DA)

Purpose

To help battered women assess their risk of homicide.

Population

Adult women.

Background and Description

The Danger Assessment Inventory (DA) is a means of quantifying the risk of serious injury resulting from domestic abuse. Items were developed to tap four risk factors obtained from retrospective studies of cases where women were killed or seriously injured by their abusers (e.g., Berk, Berk, Loseke, & Rauma, 1983). It is based on the assumption that the woman is the victim and the man is the perpetrator, although it may be used in reverse situations (i.e., male victim, woman perpetrator) with slight modification in directions and language. The measure consists of 15 yes–no items. Estimating the frequency of violence requires the use of a calendar to identify each episode of battering and the subsequent noting of how long each incident lasted (in hours) as well as the type of incident (e.g., beaten up, threat of weapon use, and weapon use). Several sample items are listed below.

- Has the physical violence increased in frequency during the past year?
- Does he ever try to choke you?
- Is there a gun in the house?

Administration

The measure was initially intended to allow nurses to assess the danger of severe injury, but may be administered by anyone who is in contact with battered women. The DA can be completed by either the interviewer or the victim and takes approximately 10 min to complete.

Scoring

A total score is obtained by summing the affirmative answers. Scores can range from 0 to 15. On the initial pilot sample, the mean score was 7 with a standard deviation of 3.

Interpretation

A higher score indicates the presence of more risk factors for homicide. Currently there are no cutoff scores or weighting of the items.

Psychometric Properties

Reliability. Measures of internal consistency from different samples have ranged from .60 to .86 (Campbell, 1995). Campbell (1995) reported temporal stability from several studies ranged from .89 to .94.

Validity. Content validity of the DA was assessed through discussions with battered women, shelter workers, law enforcement officials, and other experts on battering (Campbell, 1986). Additionally, the DA was piloted with battered women in shelters who reported that the DA, combined with discussions with the author about the measure, increased their awareness of danger and provided information useful for making future decisions.

Construct validity was assessed by examining correlations with both prevalence and severity of abuse measured by the Conflict Tactics Scale (pp. 177–180) and severity of injuries (Campbell, 1986). Stuart and Campbell (1989) also found moderate correlations between the DA and severity and type of abuse. McFarlane, Willson, Malecha, & Lemmey (2000) obtained a correlation of .75 between the DA with the Index of Spouse Abuse (pp. 196–198), providing further support for the validity of the measure.

Clinical Utility

Moderate. The DA might be useful in clinical settings because it provides a means for caregivers to warn battered women about possible outcomes of their situation and to give them information (through discussion of risk factors) that will increase their ability for self-care (e.g., McFarlane, Soeken, Campbell, Parker, Reel, & Silva, 1998). Stuart and Campbell (1989) reported that after completing the DA, many women verbally expressed feeling less isolation and increased knowledge that other women had similar experiences. Follow-up discussion with the interviewer required, on average, an additional five minutes. A lack of normative and predictive validity data limits the clinical utility.

Research Applicability

Moderate. The DA possesses acceptable levels of reliability and could prove useful for researchers seeking an instrument to quantify potential risk of severe family violence.

Original Citation

Campbell, J. C. (1986). Nursing assessment for risk of homicide with battered women. *Advances in Nursing Science, 8*, 36–51.

Source

Jacquelyn C. Campbell, Johns Hopkins University School of Nursing 525 N. Wolfe Street Baltimore, MD 21205, (410) 955-2778, jcampbel@son.jhmi.edu.

Cost

The DA may be obtained from the Nursing Network on Violence Against Women, International website NNVAWI.ORG.

References

Berk, R. A., Berk, S. F., Loseke, D. R., & Rauma, D. (1983). Mutual combat and other family violence myths. In D. Finkelhor, R. J. Gelles, & G. T. Hotaling (Eds.), *The dark side of families* (pp. 197–212). Beverly Hills: Sage.

Campbell, J. C. (1995). Prediction of homicide of and by battered women. In J. C. Campbell (Ed.), *Assessing dangerousness: Violence by sexual offenders, batterers, and child abusers* (pp. 96–113). Thousand Oaks, CA: Sage Publications.

Hudson, W., & McIntosh, S. (1981). The assessment of spouse abuse: Two quantifiable dimensions. *Journal of Marriage and the Family, 43*, 873–888.

McFarlane, J., Soeken, K., Campbell, J., Parker, B., Reel, S., & Silva, C. (1998). Severity of abuse to pregnant women and associated gun access of the perpetrator. *Public Health Nursing, 15*, 201–206.

McFarlane, J., Willson, P., Malecha, A., & Lemmey, D. (2000). Intimate partner violence: A gender comparison. *Journal of Interpersonal Violence, 15*, 158–169.

Stuart, E. P., & Campbell, J. C. (1989). Assessment of patterns of dangerousness with battered women. *Issues in Mental Health Nursing, 10*, 245–260.

Date Rape Decision-Latency Measure (DRDLM)

Purpose

To measure the ability of college males to determine when a man should terminate unwanted sexual advances toward a woman.

Population

College-age males.

Background and Description

The Date Rape Decision-Latency Measure (DRDLM) is based on the decision latency method. This methodology represents a series of procedures that can be adapted for use in a variety of experimental situations. The paradigm was applied to the study of date rape by Marx and Gross (1995) and involved allowing men to listen to an audiotaped depiction of a couple engaging in sexual foreplay, ostensibly leading toward sexual intercourse. Physical intimacy was portrayed through dialogue and audible breathing and kissing sounds. During the course of the audiotape, the man's use of persuasion to obtain sex gradually increases from verbal persuasion to the use of physical force. The woman's responses escalate from ambiguous verbal responses to clear verbal refusals and resistance, and finally to pleading and crying. The total running time of the audiotape is 390 s.

Response latency is defined as the length of time needed by subjects to determine whether the man in the audiotape should refrain from making further sexual advances. Subjects press a button that activates a buzzer when they think the man in the audiotape should stop his advances. The time between the beginning of the audiotape and the activation of the buzzer is the decision latency (measured in seconds). This basic paradigm has been utilized in related studies (e.g., Bernat, Stolp, Calhoun, & Adams, 1997; Bernat, Wilson, & Calhoun, 1999).

Administration

The DRDLM is administered individually and the audiotape lasts 6 min and 30 s.

Scoring

Scoring of the DRDLM requires timing the interval between the start of the analogue audiotape and the sound of the buzzer. As the interval is typically measured in seconds, a simple stopwatch is sufficient, although more elaborate devices can be used.

Interpretation

Longer intervals between beginning and termination of the analogue situation suggest decreased responsivity to a female's resistance toward engaging in sexual intercourse.

Psychometric Properties

Reliability. Test–retest reliability was assessed over a 2-week period in a subset of the original sample that was asked to return and take the DRDLM a second time. The Pearson product–moment correlation between decision latencies from these two measurements was .87.

Validity. Convergent validity was indicated by significant intercorrelations between the DRDLM and a number of self-report predictors of sexual aggression. Significant correlations ranged from .20 between the DRDLM and the Acceptance of Interpersonal Violence Scale (pp. 166–168) to .39 between the DRDLM and

self-report measures for sexual aggression and calloused sexual beliefs. Discriminant validity was indicated by the lack of significant correlations between the DRDLM and social desirability, weekly alcohol consumption, and current drug use.

Clinical Utility

Limited. The DRDLM is essentially an adjunctive laboratory-based methodology requiring specialized equipment, facilities, and training.

Research Applicability

High. The DRDLM has a flexible format and acceptable psychometric properties. The DRDLM appears to be an excellent laboratory-based experimental paradigm for the investigation of the phenomenon of date rape.

Original Citation

Marx, B. P., & Gross, A. M. (1995). Date rape: An analysis of two contextual variables. *Behavior Modification, 19*, 451–463.

Source

Brian P. Marx, Ph.D., Behavioral Science Division, National Center for PTSD, VA Boston Healthcare System, Boston, MA 02130, brian.marx@va.gov or

Alan M. Gross, Ph.D., Department of Psychology, University of Mississippi, Mississippi, 38677, (662) 915-5186, Fax: (662) 915-5398, pygross@olemiss.edu.

Cost

Please contact the source (above) for permission to use the DRDLM.

References

Bernat, J. A., Stolp, S., Calhoun, K. S., & Adams, H. E. (1997). Construct validity and test-retest reliability of a date rape decision-latency measure. *Journal of Psychopathology and Behavioral Assessment, 19*, 315–330.

Bernat, J. A., Wilson, A. E., & Calhoun, K. S. (1999). Sexual coercion history, calloused sexual beliefs and judgments of sexual coercion in a date rape analogue. *Violence and Victims, 14*, 147–160.

Deviant Peers (DP)

Purpose

To determine the level of exposure a child or adolescent has to deviant peers.

Population

Children and adolescents.

Background and Description

The scale was developed to investigate correlates and implications of Agnew's General Strain Theory (GST, 1992). According to GST, the likelihood of deviant responses increases as a function of the interaction among exposure to strain, level of prior experience with deviance, moral constraints against deviance, and exposure to deviant peers. The 12 items were taken from the Moral Beliefs Scale, also develop by Mazerolle and Piquero (1997). Respondents are asked to list the number of friends they have who engage in deviant acts. These acts range from trivial behaviors (e.g., cheating on exams) to serious acts of violence. Responses are rated on a 10-point scale, ranging from 0 ("no friends at all") to 5 ("some friends have") to 10 ("a lot of friends have"). Sample items follow.
• Stolen something worth more than $50.
• Hit or threatened to hit someone without any reason.

Administration

The scale is estimated to take 3–5 min to complete.

Scoring

Item responses are summed to create a total score.

Interpretation

Higher scores are indicative of higher levels of deviant peer exposure.

Psychometric Properties

Factor analysis. The results of a factor analysis support the scale's unidimensionality.

Reliability. Internal consistency, measured by Cronbach's alpha was .88.

Validity. Research has shown that scores on the scale were positively associated with measures of intention to assault. The effects of strain on delinquency were weakened when exposure to delinquent peers, moral beliefs, and total risks were lessened. Additionally, when these latter variables had strong influences on the individual, the effects of strain on delinquency were strengthened.

Clinical Utility

Limited. The scale may be useful as a brief assessment of the type of interpersonal relationships a client maintains. Lack of normative and predictive validity data set limits on the clinical utility.

Research Applicability

Moderate. The scale could serve as a unidimensional measure of affiliation with deviant peers.

Original Citation

Mazerolle, P., & Piquero, A. (1997). Violent responses to strain: An examination of conditioning influences. *Violence and Victims, 12*, 323–343.

Source

Paul Mazerolle, Mt Gravatt campus, Griffith University, 176 Messines Ridge Rd, Mt Gravatt, Queensland 4122, phone (07) 373 55710, p.mazerolle@griffith.edu.au

Cost

Please contact the source (above) for permission to use the DP.

Alternate Form

A 9-item scale measuring the same concept has also been created (Mazerolle & Maahs, 2000). It was found to have adequate internal consistency with Cronbach's alpha .80.

References

Agnew, R. (1992). Foundation for a general strain theory of crime and delinquency. *Criminology, 30*, 47–88.

Mazerolle, P., & Maahs, J. (2000). General strain and delinquency: An alternative examination of conditioning influences. *Justice Quarterly, 17*, 753–778.

Domestic Violence Inventory (DVI)

Purpose

To assess the risks and needs of perpetrators of physical, emotional, or verbal abuse.

Population

Adults.

Background and Description

The Domestic Violence Inventory (DVI) was developed as a means for early identification of domestic violence perpetrators and to collect information pertinent to decisions concerning levels of probation supervision, counseling, treatment, and incarceration. Items were generated by doctoral level psychologists at domestic violence treatment agencies, shelters, and batterers programs. The 155 items contained in the DVI were selected through a procedure that identified items that were statistically related to known domestic violence offender groups.

The DVI consists of six scales: Violence (use of force to injure, damage, or destroy), Alcohol (alcohol use and abuse), Drugs (drug use and abuse), Control (attempts to control others), Stress and Coping Ability (coping effectiveness), and Truthfulness (a lie scale measuring denial, guardedness, problem minimization, and faking). Depending on the content, items are presented in a true–false or a multiple-choice format.

Administration

The DVI requires approximately 30–40 min to complete. It may be administered as a pencil-and-paper measure or via computer. A human voice audio version presents items through a headset and responses are typed into a computer.

Scoring

The DVI is computer scored. Space is provided to record subjective observations.

Interpretation

Scores should be considered in conjunction with evaluator judgments, as well as available court and adjustment records. "Truth-corrected" scores are provided as a means of controlling for socially desirable responding. Scores for each of the six scales are given as percentiles and classified in one of the following ranges: low risk (0–39 %), medium risk (40–69 %), problem risk (70–89 %), or severe problem risk (90–100%). For the Truthfulness Scale, scores at or above the 90th percentile reflect a respondent who was uncooperative, concerned with self-presentation, deceptive, or who misunderstood the test items. According to the publishers, higher scores on the Violence Scale, coupled with high scores on the Alcohol or Drugs Scales, are indicative of the worst prognosis. In general, elevated scores on the Alcohol Scale or Drugs Scale magnify the severity of the other scale scores. The computer scoring program provides a three page narrative summarizing the respondent's self-report history, the meaning of attained scale scores, and specific score-related recommendations. The report also highlights critical items and provides answers to a built-in interview.

Psychometric Properties

Norms. The DVI was standardized on over 45,000 male and female domestic violence offenders. Gender-specific norms and separate norms for ethnicity (Caucasian, African American, and Hispanic) are available. Risk range percentiles were derived from this same sample.

Reliability. Based on 7,941 domestic violence abusers screened in the year 2000, Cronbach's alpha coefficients ranged from .88 to .93 for the six scales. The publishers reported that further analyses have demonstrated high reliability coefficients with minimum interscale correlations.

Validity. Each scale is treated separately in validity studies. DVI scales have been related to MMPI validity scales (L-Scale and F-Scale), the 16 PF, the MMPI MacAndrews Scale, the MMPI Psychopathic Deviate scale, the Taylor-Manifest Anxiety Scale, the MMPI Depression Scale, the Treatment Intervention Inventory, the SAQ-Adult Probation scales ($r=.34$–.76), and professional staff ratings and screening interviews ($r=.03$–.54).

Clinical Utility

High. Reviewers of the DVI described it as a satisfactory and useful measure for assessing the level and risk of offending (Collins, 2001; Kaplan & Vanduser, 2001). The inventory is easy to take, provides for immediate scoring, and contains objective and subjective components, allowing the evaluator to conduct a thorough assessment. The DVI has been used in clinics, court settings, and service provider offices. The risk ranges allow one to use the instrument as a screening tool to identify cases requiring referral for a more comprehensive evaluation and/or treatment.

Research Applicability

High. Filled diskettes are returned to the publisher (names are eliminated to ensure confidentiality before being returned) and the data on the diskettes are compiled into a national database. Currently, the database consists of over 45,000 entries and the publishers use these data as a source for continual analyses of the scale (e.g., summary reports and further analyses of reliability and validity). Additionally, the DVI requires only a fifth-to sixth-grade reading level and is available in four formats, allowing a broader range of people to be assessed (e.g., those with reading impairments may use the human voice audio format, and the optimal scanning format can be given to large groups).

Although the publishers reported user satisfaction when using the DVI for prediction, screening in research, and in clinical and criminal justice settings, some concerns have been expressed about the lack of document organization, the need to be computer literate, and the danger of taking scores at face value (Collins, 2001; Kaplan & Vanduser, 2001).

Original Citation

Domestic Violence Inventory. Risk & Needs Assessment, Inc., P.O. Box 44828, Phoenix, AZ 85064-4828

Source

Domestic Violence Inventory. Risk & Needs Assessment, Inc. P.O. Box 44828, Phoenix, AZ 85064-4828, (800)231-2401, http://www.riskan-dneeds.com/TestsA_DVI.asp

Cost

Prices range from $7.00 to $8.00 per test, depending upon the number of tests administered during the course of a year and the organization requesting the tests.

Alternate Forms

The DVI has four versions: the DVI-J (a juvenile form for ages 12–18), an adult form (ages 18 and older), the DVI-short form which contains 76 items, and a pre–post-form for outcome comparison. The DVI-J has similar properties to the adult version but contains one additional item, making it a 156-item measure. The pre–post-form consists of 142 items, which are variations of the standard DVI scales, and requires approximately 30 min to complete. The DVIs are available in both English and Spanish.

References

Collins, C. (2001). Review of the Domestic Violence Inventory. In O. K. Buros (Ed.), *Mental measurements yearbook*. Highland Park, NJ: Gryphon Press.

Kaplan, D. M., & Vanduser, M. L. (2001). Review of the Domestic Violence Inventory. In O. K. Buros (Ed.), *Mental measurements yearbook*. Highland Park, NJ: Gryphon Press.

Domestic Violence Myth Acceptance Scale (DVMAS)

Purpose

To assess the degree to which an individual believes myths about domestic violence to be true.

Population

Adults.

Background and Description

The Domestic Violence Myth Acceptance Scale (DVMAS) was created to provide a measure of domestic violence myths. Domestic violence myths were defined as "stereotypical beliefs about domestic violence that are generally false but widely and persistently held, and which serve to minimize, deny, or justify physical aggression against intimate partners" (Peters, 2008, p. 5). The DVMAS is an 18-item, multi-dimensional scale with items assessing myths related to character blame of victim, behavior blame of victim, minimization of seriousness and extent of abuse, and exoneration of the perpetrator. It uses a 7-point, Likert style scale with responses ranging from 1 (strongly disagree) to 7 (strongly agree). Samples items follow.
- When a man is violent it is because he lost control of his temper.
- If a woman continues living with a man who beats her then it's her own fault if she is beaten again.
- Women who flirt are asking for it.

Administration

The DVMAS requires approximately 10–15 min to complete.

Scoring

Scores are summed and then divided by 18 to calculate the mean score.

Interpretation

Higher mean scores indicate greater acceptance of domestic violence myths.

Psychometric Properties

Factor analysis. Factor analyses were conducted separately for males and females in a sample of 345 students, staff, and faculty members at a New England college. Using varimax rotation, factor analysis of female responses resulted in five interpretable factors: character blame, behavior blame, exoneration of perpetrator, women's unconscious desire to be battered, and minimization. Factor analysis of male responses resulted in four interpretable factors: character blame, behavior blame, exoneration of perpetrator, and minimization.

Factor analyses were conducted on a separate sample of 290 students, staff, and faculty at the same New England college. Factor analysis of female responses resulted in four factors. Four of the factors were replicated from the original factor analysis, however, the factor "women's unconscious desire to be battered" was not found. Factor analysis of male responses resulted in five factors. Four of the factors were replicated from the original factor analysis, whereas the fifth factor was deemed uninterpretable.

Reliability. Internal consistency, as measured by Cronbach's alpha, was .81 for a sample of 345 students, staff, and faculty at a New England college. Cronbach's alpha was .88 in a similar sample of 290 students, staff, and faculty from the same New England college. Internal consistency reliability of the DVMAS factors ranged from .64 to .88.

Validity. Men's scores on the DVMAS were significantly higher than women's scores, which is consistent with previous studies of the closely related construct of rape myth endorsement. Evidence of convergent validity was found; the DVMAS was significantly related to Burt's Rape Myth Acceptance Scale ($r=.65$, pp. 224–226), the Attitudes Toward Women scale ($r=.47$, Spence, Helmreich, & Stapp, 1974), sex role stereotypes ($r=.51$), and attitudes toward wife abuse ($r=.37$). Evidence of divergent validity is not as clear. The DVMAS was found to weakly, but sig-

nificantly, correlate with social desirability. The DVMAS was unexpectedly related to attitudes toward violence in war and violence toward criminals.

Clinical Utility

Moderate. The DVMAS may be a useful tool in identifying domestic violence myths held by men and women. It may be used to assess treatment related changes in domestic violence myth acceptance.

Research Applicability

Moderate. The DVMAS may be a useful tool for investigating possible correlates of domestic violence myth acceptance such as negative, stereotypical views of women. It may also be useful to determine if the acceptance of domestic violence myths is related to, or predicts domestic violence, and if acceptance of these myths can be changed.

Original Citation

Peters, J. (2008). Measuring myths about domestic violence: Development and initial validation of the Domestic Violence Myth Acceptance Scale. *Journal of Aggression, Maltreatment, and Trauma, 16,* 1–21.

Source

Jay Peters, University of Maine, School of Social Work, Orono, ME, 04469, (207) 581-2355, jpeters@maine.edu

Cost

The DVMAS is free to use for research and evaluation purposes. Please contact the source (above) for additional information.

Reference

Spence, J. T., Helmreich, R. L., & Stapp, J. (1974). A short
  version of the Attitudes Toward Women Scale (ATW).
  Bulletin of the Psychonomic Society, 2, 219–220.

Dominance Scale (DS)

Purpose

To assess three forms of dominance perceived as
risk factors for intimate partner violence.

Population

Adults.

Background and Description

The three forms of dominance (authority, restrictiveness, and disparagement) assessed by the
Dominance Scale (DS) are conceptualized as deviations from an egalitarian relationship. Authority
involves an imbalance in decision-making power.
Restrictiveness entails restricting the behavior of
another, even when the restricted behavior does not
directly affect the person who is doing the restricting. Disparagement results from one person failing
to equally value the other or one person holding a
negative view of another's worth. Each of the
above forms of dominance is viewed as a contrib-
uting cause of partner aggression and violence.

The DS contains 32 items that are worded in
the present tense to elicit current ways of relating
to or thinking about one's partner. Twelve items
refer to the amount of authority held, nine items
refer to how restrictive one partner is toward the
other, and 11 items refer to how disparaging one
partner is toward the other. Items are rated using a
4-point Likert-type format (1 = strongly disagree,
4 = strongly agree). Sample items are listed below.
• I hate losing arguments with my partner.
• I have a right to know everything my partner
  does.
• My partner makes a lot of mistakes.

Administration

The DS requires about 10 min to complete and
can be administered individually or in a group
format.

Scoring

There are 10 reverse-scored items. Items from
each subscale are summed to produce a total
score for each form of dominance.

Interpretation

Higher scores on a subscale indicate more dominant behavior. Comparing subscale scores after
controlling for the different number of items provides an indication of the pattern of dominance
manifested.

Psychometric Properties

Factor analyses. Factor analysis of data collected
from a sample of 131 male and female undergraduates provided support for the three-factor model.

Reliability. Alpha coefficients for the Authority,
Restrictiveness, and Disparagement subscales
were .80, .73, and .82, respectively. Among
the subscales, the Authority and Disparagement
subscales correlated significantly ($r = .58$) and
the Authority and Restrictiveness subscales
were moderately correlated ($r = .38$). The
Restrictiveness and Disparagement subscales
were not correlated.

Validity. Each subscale of the dominance con-
struct was compared with four measures: the
Decision-Making in Intimate Relationships Scale
(Hamby, 1992), the Jourard Self-Disclosure
Questionnaire (Jourard, 1971; Raphael &
Dohrenwend, 1987), the Conflict Tactics Scale,
Revised (pp. 177–180), and the Marlowe-Crowne
Social Desirability Scale (Crowne & Marlowe,
1960). As predicted, the Decision Making in

Intimate Relationships Scale not only achieved the highest correlation with the Authority subscale ($r=.39$) but also correlated with the Disparagement subscale ($r=.27$). It was expected that the Jourard Self-Disclosure Questionnaire would have a high correlation with the Restrictiveness subscale, a hypothesis that was confirmed ($r=.26$). The Marlowe-Crowne Social Desirability Scale was inversely related to the Authority ($r=-.35$) and the Disparagement subscales ($r=-.18$). The three DS subscales correlated with the Conflict Tactics Scale, supporting the idea of dominance as a risk factor for physical violence against an intimate partner. When rating one's own behavior, the Authority subscale correlated inversely with Negotiation and positively with Psychological Aggression; the Restrictiveness subscale correlated with Psychological Aggression, Physical Assault, and Injury; and the Disparagement subscale correlated inversely with Negotiation and positively with Psychological Aggression. When rating the partner's behavior, the Authority subscale was inversely related to Negotiation and positively related to Psychological Aggression and Physical Assault; the Restrictiveness subscale correlated with Psychological Aggression, Physical Assault, and Injury; and the Disparagement subscale was inversely related to Negotiation and positively related to Psychological Aggression and Physical Assault.

Clinical Utility

Moderate. The DS shows promise for clinical use. The DS is easily administered, brief, and requires a only a seventh-grade reading level. Preliminary evidence suggests the DS may be useful in assessing the distribution of power within a relationship and may predict partner abuse. However, research with clinical samples is needed prior to routine clinical application.

Research Applicability

Moderate. The DS correlates in the expected directions with relevant measures. Hamby (1996)

noted that more research on the construct of dominance is needed, and additional research is needed on the DS.

Original Citation

Hamby, S. L. (1996). The Dominance Scale: Preliminary psychometric properties. *Violence and Victims, 11,* 199–212

Source

Sherry L. Hamby, Ph.D., Sewanee: The University of the South, 735 University Ave, Sewanee, TN 37383, (931) 598-1000, slhamby@sewanee.edu

Cost

Please contact the source (above) for permission to use the DS.

References

Crowne, D. P., & Marlowe, D. (1960). A new scale of social desirability independent of psychopathology. *Journal of Consulting Psychology, 24,* 349–354.

Hamby, S. L. (1992). Women's attitudes towards the use of force in intimate relationships. *Dissertation Abstracts International, 53,* 5976B (Order No. AAC9309886).

Jourard, S. M. (1971). *Self-disclosure: An experimental analysis of the transparent self.* New York: Wiley.

Raphael, K. G., & Dohrenwend, B. P. (1987). Self-disclosure and mental health: A problem of confounded measurement. *Journal of Abnormal Psychology, 96,* 214–217.

Feelings and Acts of Violence Scale-Short Form (PFAV)

Purpose

To measure the risk of violence.

Population

Adults.

Background and Description

The Feelings and Acts of Violence Scale-Short Form (PFAV) was developed from the 36-item Feelings and Acts of Violence Scale (FAV) by examining item response frequencies and item–total correlations. Items with the highest correlations and most normal distributions were selected. The PFAV contains 12 items that focus on feelings of anger in various forms, as opposed to overt behavior or past history. Respondents choose the frequency with which they experience or engage in the acts described for the first nine questions. The response options are as follows: "never," "sometimes," "often," or "very often." Two questions have the following response options: "never," "once," "twice," or "more than twice." One question is answered yes/no.

Administration

The PFAV is estimated to take 3–5 min to complete.

Scoring

Responses to items 1–9 are weighted and summed. A response of "never" is scored 0, "sometimes" is scored 1, "often" is scored 2, and "very often" is scored 3.

Interpretation

Higher scores indicate a greater likelihood that the individual will become violent. Plutchik and van Praag (1990) considered respondents violent if they answered "sometimes," "often," or "very often" to items 6 and 7, or if they answered "sometimes," "often," or "very often" to items 8 and 11.

Psychometric Properties

Reliability. Internal consistency, measured by Cronbach's alpha, was .77 in a sample of 100 psychiatric patients.

Validity. Sensitivity and specificity scores for a PFAV score of 4 was approximately 75 % in a normal college sample. In a sample of 157 psychiatric inpatients, a history of violence obtained from hospital records was associated with violence defined by PFAV scores in 66 % of cases. All items of the PFAV were found to discriminate between violent and nonviolent individuals.

Clinical Utility

Limited. Although the brevity of the PFAV is advantageous, more research needs to be conducted to establish its psychometric properties.

Research Applicability

Moderate. The PFAV allows for a brief evaluation of an individual's overt behavior and feelings in regards to anger and violence.

Original Citation

Plutchik, R., & van Praag, H. M. (1990). A self-report measure of violence risk, II. *Comprehensive Psychiatry, 31*, 450–456.

Source

Plutchik, R., & van Praag, H. M. (1990). A self-report measure of violence risk, II. *Comprehensive Psychiatry, 31*, 450–456.

Cost

Unavailable.

Alternative Forms

The original 36-item scale demonstrated a coefficient alpha of .83. The FAV scale has been correlated with a history of family violence, presence of episodic dyscontrol, total life problems, and scores on several Minnesota Multiphasic Personality Inventory (MMPI) and Emotion Profile Index Scales (Plutchik, Climent, & Ervin, 1976).

Reference

Plutchik, R., Climent, C., & Ervin, F. (1976). Research strategies for the study of human violence. In W. L. Smith, A. Kling (Eds.), *Issues in Brain/Behavior Control* (pp. 69–94). New York, NY: Spectrum.

Firestone Assessment of Violent Thoughts (FAVT)

Purpose

To assess negative thoughts about self and others.

Population

Ages 17 and older.

Background and Description

The theory behind the development of the Firestone Assessment of Violent Thoughts (FAVT) derives from Robert Firestone's concept of the "inner voice"—an integrated system of negative, cynical, and hostile thoughts and attitudes toward the self and others. Derived from the Firestone Assessment of Self-Destructive Thoughts, the FAVT specifically assesses negative thoughts about self and the self in relationship to others. The 56 items contained in the FAVT require a reading level at or below the sixth grade and are organized into four subscales: social mistrust, perceived disrespect/disregard, negative-critical thoughts, and expression of overt anger. Respondents indicate the frequency with which they experience each thought using a 5-point Likert-type scale.

Administration

The FAVT is estimated to take 10–20 min to complete.

Scoring

A total score and four subscale scores are derived from summing relevant items.

Interpretation

Higher scores indicate greater levels of negative thoughts about the self and others.

Psychometric Properties

Factor analysis. Analysis using item response theory reduced the pool of original items to 56. The 56 items were then subjected to a factor analysis with a varimax rotation. A four-factor solution (social mistrust, perceived disrespect/disregard, negative-critical thoughts, and expression of overt anger) was determined to best represent the results. Items loading on more than one scale were reviewed for content by three raters and consensus reached for factor assignment.

Reliability. Internal consistency was assessed using Cronbach's alpha. Coefficients for the social mistrust, perceived disrespect/disregard, negative critical thoughts, and expression of overt anger scales were .89, .89, .90 and .88, respectively. Alpha for the total scale was .96.

Validity. Subscale correlations ranged from .61 (expression of overt anger subscale with perceived disrespect subscale) to .78 (social mistrust subscale with perceived disrespect subscale). Content validity was assessed by having two therapists with experience in treating violent and aggressive populations review the items for relevance. The resulting FAVT scores were higher for violent individuals across incarcerated and parolee subsamples, providing initial support for criterion validity.

Clinical Utility

Limited. The FAVT is currently being developed and more research in construct validity and normative data are needed prior to widespread clinical use.

Research Applicability

Moderate. The FAVT is easily understood by most adults. The measure assesses negative thoughts about the self and others; therefore, it might prove to be useful for modeling psychological antecedents to aggressive and violent behavior.

Original Citation

Doucette-Gates, A., Firestone, L.A., & Firestone, R.W. (1999) Assessing violent thoughts: The relationship between thought processes and violent behavior. *Psychologica Belgica, 39*(2/3), 13–134.

Source

The FAVT may be purchased from Psychological Assessment Resources, 16204 N. Florida Ave, Lutz, FL 33549, 1-800-331-8378, Fax: 1-800-727-9329, http://www3.parinc.com/products/product.aspx?Productid=FAVT

Cost

The Introductory kit, which includes a manual, 25 rating forms and 25 score summary/profile forms, costs $125 from Psychological Assessment Resources (PAR).

Historical–Clinical–Risk Assessment (HCR-20)

Purpose

To assess the risk of future violence in mentally ill, personality disordered, and/or forensic populations.

Population

Adults with a history of violence and a likelihood of mental illness and/or a personality disorder.

Background and Description

The original version of the Historical–Clinical–Risk Assessment (HCR-20) was published in 1995. It was designed to provide clinicians with a more structured means for assessing and quantifying the risk of future violent behavior in forensic inpatients and outpatients. The revised HCR-20 was published in 1997. The primary purpose of the revision was to clarify administration and coding procedures for clinicians who were using it as an assessment tool. The 20 Historical, Clinical, and Risk items from the original version were retained.

The current version of the HCR-20 is a semistructured interview that assesses the risk for future violence. The interview scale consists of 20 items that are divided into three categories (Historical-10 items, Clinical-5 items, Risk-5 items) that have been found to have predictive validity for future violent behavior. The Historical category concerns past information related to an individual's previous violence, age at first violent incident, relationship instability, employment problems, substance use, mental illness, psychopathy, early maladjustment, personality functioning, and prior supervision failure. The Clinical category involves present information related to an individual's insight, attitudes, symptoms of mental illness, impulsivity, and responsiveness to treatment. The Risk category assesses destabilizers, future plans, personal support, compliance with remediation attempts, and stress. Items are rated using a three-point, ordinal scale that ranges from 0 to 2 (0 = The item definitely is absent or does not apply, 1 = The item possibly is present, or is present only to a limited extent, 2 = The item definitely is present).

Administration

The HCR-20 structured interview requires approximately 90 min to administer, though the amount of time will vary according to the depth and breadth of the person's past history. Additional time must be allotted for the review of collateral information (e.g., review of criminal history material, collateral contacts with family members, etc.). The total amount of time required to complete the HCR-20 is estimated to be 2 1/2–3 h.

Scoring

Items from the three scales (Historical, Clinical, and Risk) are summed to provide a total score that quantifies the risk for future violence. The higher an individual's full scale score, the greater their risk for future violent behavior. The total score can range from 0 to 40. Items may be omitted if the information required to code them is insufficient to permit a decision concerning the presence or absence of the item. The HCR-20 provides some flexibility to the interviewer in that four items (two historical, one clinical, one risk management) can be omitted without invalidating total scores.

Interpretation

The HCR-20 provides a dimensional score for factors related to recidivism, rather than a categorical diagnosis of future risk for violent behavior. Coding for one of the items (e.g., current major mental illness) may place an individual at a great risk for future violent behavior, even if other coding items are not present. Conversely, an individual may code on a high number of historical, clinical, and risk factors, but be at a low risk for future violent behavior because of a current physical condition (e.g., paralysis). Contextual factors also play a role. For example, if an individual will be residing in a forensic setting, then the HCR-20 assessment should refer to that individual's potential for future violent behavior within that setting. If the individual will be residing in the community, then the HCR-20 assessment should refer to their risk for future violent behavior within that community. Risk is assessed on a case-by-case basis, after a careful

review of all pertinent information. There is no specific cutoff point for risk assessment.

Psychometric Properties

Reliability. The Historical scale of the HCR-20 is reported to have a Cronbach's alpha of .73. In a sample of 74 Canadian incarcerated inmates, the interrater reliability of the Historical and Clinical scales of the HCR-20 was found to be .80. The total score on the HCR-20 correlated .44 with previous violent behavior (Douglas & Webster, 1999). Interrater reliability has been found in the range of .80 to .99 in several studies for the Historical scale, .49 to .95 for the Clinical scale, and .56 to .94 for the Risk scale (Douglas, 2004).

Validity. The HCR-20 correlated .54 with the Violence Risk Appraisal Guide (VRAG; pp. 258–260). The Historical scale correlated .61 with the VRAG and .54 with the Hare Psychopathy Checklist-Revised (PCL-R; pp. 220–222). The Clinical scale correlated .28 with the VRAG and .47 with the PCL-R.

In a retrospective study, the predictive validity of the HCR-20 and PCL-R was assessed using a sample of 80 forensic psychiatric patients who had been released in 1986 from a psychiatric hospital. The HCR-20 and PCL-R correlated at approximately .30 with several measures of later community violence. Readmission to a forensic hospital was predicted by the HCR-20 at .38 and the PCL-R at .25. Later psychiatric hospitalizations were predicted by the HCR-20 at .45 and the PCL-R at .36.

In a sample of 887 male forensic psychiatric patients, the HCR-20 was a good predictor of violent offenses (AUCs = .70–.76; Gray, Taylor, & Snowden, 2008). It was also found that the predictive ability of the HCR-20 declined slightly over longer follow-up periods.

Clinical Utility

Moderate. The semistructured interview is fairly easy to administer. The review of collateral material and the final assessment of risk requires professional skill and judgment. The HCR-20 has been used successfully in forensic populations but is still in the process of development. As normative data and additional reliability and validity studies are made available, clinical utility should increase.

Research Applicability

Moderate. The HCR-20 correlates strongly with the VRAG and the PCL-R, which are two instruments found to have high research utility. Like the VRAG and the PCL-R, the HCR-20 is designed for use by qualified professionals.

Original Citation

Webster, C. D., Douglas, K. S., Eaves, D., & Hart, S. D. (1997). HCR-20: Assessing risk for violence. Version 2. Burnaby, BC, Canada: Simon Fraser University and Forensic Psychiatric Services Commission of British Columbia.

Source

Information regarding the use of the HCR-20 may be obtained from Mental Health, Law, and Policy Institute, Simon Fraser University, Burnaby, British Columbia, Canada V5A 1S6 (604) 291-5868.

The HCR-20 can also be obtained from Psychological Assessment Resources, 16204 N. Florida Ave, Lutz, FL 33549, 1-800-727-9329, Fax: 1-800-899-8378, http://www3.parinc.com/products/product.aspx?Productid=HCR-20

Cost

The HCR-20 Manual costs $30 (Canadian). It includes one sample scoring form that may be photocopied. The HCR-20 may also be purchased from PAR. An introductory kit that includes the manual, 50 coding sheets, and the

HCR-20 Violence Risk Management Companion Guide costs $130.

References

Douglas, K. S. (2004). Making structured clinical decisions about violence risk: Reliability and validity of the HCR-20 violence risk assessment scheme. *Dissertation Abstracts International: Section B: The Sciences and Engineering, 64,* 4032.

Douglas, K. S., & Webster, C. D. (1999). The HCR-20 violence risk assessment scheme: Concurrent validity in a sample of incarcerated offenders. *Criminal Justice and Behavior, 26,* 3–19.

Gray, N. S., Taylor, J., & Snowden, R. J. (2008). Predicting violent reconvictions using the HCR-20. *The British Journal of Psychiatry, 192,* 384–387.

Index of Spouse Abuse (ISA)

Purpose

To measure frequency and severity of intimate partner violence.

Population

Women who are suspected of experiencing intimate partner violence.

Background and Description

The Index of Spouse Abuse (ISA) was developed to provide a means of assessing the degree or intensity of domestic violence perpetrated by a male against a female in an intimate relationship. It was designed to be completed by the abused female and can be used on a regular basis to monitor abuse in treatment settings. The ISA contains 30 items that relate to behaviors or interactions that are considered to be abusive. The ISA has two scales that measure physical abuse (ISA-P) and nonphysical abuse (ISA-NP). The items are weighted based on the severity of abuse represented by the item. Respondents rate each statement using a scale that ranges from 1 (never) to 5 (very frequently).

Administration

The ISA takes approximately 5 min to complete.

Scoring

There is a four-step procedure to scoring the ISA that should be followed for each of the scales separately. A global score can also be calculated. The first step involves examining the items to ensure that they were answered correctly. Any incorrectly answered items (e.g., score outside the range 1–5) should be given a 0. The second step involves calculating weighted item scores. Items (I) are weighted based on the severity of abuse represented by the item, with more severe items assigned greater weight (W). Each item response is multiplied by the item weight to obtain the product score (P; $P = I*W$). The third step involves calculating the lowest sum–score possible by summing the item weights ($MIN = \Sigma W$). The fourth step involves calculating the ISA scale score (S) by using the following equation: $S = (\Sigma P - MIN)*100/((MIN*4)*3)$. This results in a scale score that ranges from 0 to 100. If all of the items are responded to correctly, simpler equations may be used. For the ISA-P scale the following equation may be used: ISA-P = $(\Sigma P/(682-1))*25)$. The following equation may be used for the ISA-NP scale: ISA-NP = $(\Sigma P/(387-1))*25)$.

Interpretation

Higher scores indicate a greater amount or severity of abuse.

Psychometric Properties

Factor analysis. A principal components analysis with varimax rotation was conducted on data from 398 graduate and undergraduate female students from the University of Hawaii who were involved in a serious intimate relationship with a male partner. This analysis included all of the ISA items and items from the Index of Marital Satisfaction (IMS; Hudson & Glisson, 1976) in order to evaluate whether the ISA contained two scales (as hypothesized) and was distinct from the IMS. The results suggested the presence of three factors: Factor-1 contained items from the IMS, Factor-2 contained items related to physical abuse, and Factor-3 contained items related to nonphysical abuse. The factor structure of the ISA has not been consistently replicated using diverse populations (Campbell, Campbell, King, Parker, & Ryan, 1994; Cook, Conrad, Bender, & Kaslow, 2003; Torres et al., 2010).

Reliability. Internal consistency, as measured by Cronbach's alpha, was calculated for a sample of graduate and undergraduate students and for a sample of women from clinical settings. The alpha coefficient for the ISA-P scale was .90 for the university sample and .94 for the clinical sample. The alpha coefficient for the ISA-NP scale was .91 for the university sample and .97 for the clinical sample.

Validity. Discriminant validity of the ISA was examined in a clinical sample of 107 women, 64 who had been identified as experiencing partner abuse and 43 who had been identified as not experiencing partner abuse. The ISA was able to discriminate between the criterion groups, with discriminant validity coefficients of .73 and .80 for the ISA-P and ISA-NP scales, respectively. The ISA scales were found to significantly correlate with measures of self-esteem problems (as measured by the Index of Self-Esteem; Hudson & Proctor, 1976), marital problems (as measured by the IMS), and sexual relationship problems (as measured by the Index of Sexual Satisfaction; Hudson, Harrison, & Crosscup, 1981) with $r = .12$ to .56. The ISA scales were also found to correlate highly with abuse status, $r = .73$ and .80, with ISA-P and ISA-NP, respectively.

Cut-scores were developed for use in clinical settings using frequency distributions from a clinical sample. A cut-score of 10 on the ISA-P resulted in correct classification of 90.7 % of the sample. A cut-score of 25 on the ISA-NP also resulted in a correct classification of 90.7 % of the sample. Separate cut-scores have been developed for use with diverse populations. For instance, in a Spanish sample a cut-score of 7 for ISA-P and 14 for ISA-NP were shown to most effectively classify women as abused or non-abused (Torres et al., 2010).

Clinical Utility

High. The ISA has been used in a variety of clinical settings to identify women experiencing intimate partner violence. It has good psychometric properties and has been validated in diverse populations. The factor structure has not been consistent in use with diverse samples, so attention to scale structure may be warranted.

Research Applicability

High. The ISA has good psychometric properties and has been used in several research studies to validate other measures of spousal abuse. It provides a quick and effective means of assessing intimate partner violence, which makes it convenient for research contexts where time constraints are present.

Original Citation

Hudson, W. W., & McIntosh, S. R. (1981). The assessment of spouse abuse: Two quantifiable dimensions. *Journal of Marriage and the Family, 43*, 873–888.

Source

Copyright Sally R. McIntosh and Walter W. Hudson, 1978.

Cost

Unavailable.

Alternative Forms

The ISA has been adapted for use in Chinese populations and Spanish populations (So-Kum Tang, 1998; Torres, Garcia-Esteve, Torres, Navarro, Ascaso, Imaz, et al., 2010). The Chinese ISA contains 19 items and two scales, physical and nonphysical abuse. The Chinese ISA has good internal consistency, $\alpha = .91$ and .79 for ISA-NP and ISA-P, respectively, and has been shown to effectively discriminate between women who have and have not experienced spousal abuse. The Spanish ISA contains 30 items and has two scales, physical and nonphysical abuse. However, the item loadings on the scales differ slightly from the original version of the ISA. The Spanish ISA has good internal consistency, $\alpha = .98$ and .88 for ISA-NP and ISA-P, respectively, and has been shown to be valid for differentiating between abused and non-abused women.

References

Campbell, D. W., Campbell, J., King, C., Parker, B., & Ryan, J. (1994). The reliability and factor structure of the Index of Spouse Abuse with African-American women. *Violence and Victims. Special Issue: Violence Against Women of Color, 9*, 259–274.

Cook, S. L., Conrad, L., Bender, M., & Kaslow, N. J. (2003). The internal validity of the Index of Spouse Abuse in African American women. *Violence and Victims, 18*, 641–657.

Hudson, W. W., & Glisson, D. H. (1976). Assessment of marital discord in social work practice. *Social Service Review, 50*, 293–311.

Hudson, W. W., Harrison, D. F., & Crosscup, P. C. (1981). A short-form scale to measure sexual discord in dyadic relationships. *Journal of Sex Research, 17*, 157–174.

Hudson, W. W., & Proctor, E. K. (1976). *A short-form scale for measuring self-esteem.* Honolulu, HI: University of Hawaii School of Social Work.

So-Kum Tang, C. (1998). Psychological abuse of Chinese wives. *Journal of Family Violence, 13*, 299–314.

Torres, A., Garcia-Esteve, L., Torres, A., Navarro, P., Ascaso, C., Imaz, M. L., et al. (2010). Detecting domestic violence: Spanish external validation of the Index of Spouse Abuse. *Journal of Family Violence, 25*, 275–286.

Interview Schedule for Violent Events

Purpose

To qualitatively and quantitatively assess physical attacks and the situations in which they occurred.

Population

Adult women.

Background and Description

Interviews with 109 battered women living in a shelter were used to gather information about the situations in which violent acts occurred. This information was used to generate questions that are administered in an in-depth interview. Using a series of identical questions, respondents are asked about three specific physical attacks: the worst violent episode, the violent episode that resulted in their leaving the relationship, and the most typical or usual violent episode. Each series of questions begins with a question similar to, "Can you tell me exactly what happened during the first assault?" Respondents are asked to discuss the event from beginning to end, including the argument, physical attack, injuries, and contact. Respondents are encouraged to provide responses in sequence, relating the event as it was experienced in an elaborate and detailed fashion. Following each series of questions, respondents are prompted for additional information using both open and close-ended questions.

Administration

The administration time varies depending on the amount of information provided by interviewees.

Scoring

The interview provides qualitative and quantitative data about two processes: the progression of a particular violent event from beginning to end and changes in violent events over time from the first to the last attack.

Interpretation

Qualitative and quantitative approaches to interpretation are used. The details about violent events are qualitatively analyzed whereas the overall patterns of violent events are analyzed quantitatively.

Psychometric Properties

Reliability. Reliability data have not been published for the Interview Schedule for Violent Events.

Validity. Data collected from the interviews have corroborated general findings obtained from other settings and individuals about the behavioral sequencing of violent events. The violent events experienced by women at the hands of their significant others followed similar patterns as violent events between males. Specifically, there are three major stages of a violent incident that have been found in male–male conflicts that were identified in the interviews about male–female conflicts: verbal argument, threats and attempts to leave by the victim that might involve the help of others, and physical attack (Felson & Steadman, 1983).

Clinical Utility

Limited. The interview provides a means of gathering detailed information about the nature and sequence of violent events experienced by women in abusive relationships.

Research Applicability

Moderate. The interview has the benefit of providing detailed information about violence toward women by their partners, as well as details about the shaping and progression of violent events. However, it is a lengthy interview making it difficult to collect data in situations where there are time constraints.

Original Citation

Dobash, R. E., & Dobash, R. P. (1984). The nature and antecedents of violent events. *British Journal of Criminology, 24*(3), 269–288.

Source

R. Emerson Dobash, University of Manchester, Social Policy and Social Work, 13 Oxford Road, Manchester, UNI M13 9PL, United Kingdom, Phone: 0161-275-4490, Fax: 0161-275-4724

Cost

Please contact the source (above) for additional information.

Reference

Felson, R. B., & Steadman, J. (1983). Situational factors in disputes leading to criminal violence. *Criminology, 21,* 59–74.

Level of Service Inventory-Revised (LSI-R)

Purpose

To assess offenders for criminal risk and need for treatment.

Population

Ages 16 and older.

Background and Description

The Level of Service Inventory-Revised (LSI-R) was developed within a social learning perspective using primarily probationers and offenders with sentences less than 2 years. The measure was designed to reflect both dynamic and static risk factors from four areas conceptualized as responsible for criminal behavior: antisocial cognitions, antisocial associates, history of antisocial behavior, and antisocial personality.

The LSI-R contains 54 items that assess personal history and interpersonal interactions. Items are divided into 10 subscales: Criminal History, Education/Employment, Finances, Family/Marital, Accommodations, Leisure/Recreation, Companions, Alcohol/Drug, Emotional/Personal, and Attitude/Orientation. The measure is administered using a semistructured interview, with additional information gathered from individuals' files and collateral contacts. Items are scored as 0 or 1 to indicate the absence or presence of an item, or using a 0–3 rating scale, dependent upon item content.

Administration

The LSI-R is estimated to take 30–45 min to complete.

Scoring

Item scores are summed to produce subscale scores and subscale scores are summed to produce a total score.

Interpretation

Higher scores indicate an increased chance of antisocial behavior and a need for treatment.

Scores are compared to normative data. Cutoff scores are provided to guide decisions regarding placement in probation, halfway house, or institutional setting.

Psychometric Properties

Norms. The scale has been normed using two distinct populations. It was normed using a sample of 956 males and 1,414 females from detention centers in Ontario, Canada. It was also normed using two different US populations, inmates and community offenders. The inmate sample was comprised of 19,481 males and females from various correctional institutions in the USA. The community offender sample was comprised of 4,240 males and females on parole or probation.

Factor analysis. A principal components analysis using total LSI-R scores from sex offenders resulted in a two-factor solution the authors labeled Criminal Lifestyle and Emotional/ Personal Problems, respectively. The Criminal Lifestyle reflects attitude, peer, and antisocial behavior domains. The Emotional/Personal factor reflects personal distress. Together, the two factors accounted for 47 % of the explained variance in LSI-R total scores (Simourd & Malcolm, 1998).

Reliability. Interrater reliabilities range from .80 to .96. In a sex offender population, Cronbach's alphas for internal consistency ranged from .29 for the Family/Marital subscale to .89 for the total score, with all coefficients, except Family/ Marital and Attitude/Orientation subscales, above .50. Test–retest reliabilities ranged from .80 to .99 (Simourd & Malcolm, 1998). In a sample of 334 African American male offenders, Cronbach's alphas ranged from .11 (Accommodations subscale) to .81 (Alcohol/ Drug subscale), with a total score alpha .55 (Schlager & Simourd, 2007). Cronbach's alphas ranged from -.08 (Accommodations subscale) to .83 (Alcohol/Drug subscale) with a total score alpha .56 in a sample of 112 Hispanic male offenders (Schlager & Simourd, 2007).

Validity. LSI-R scores were correlated with the number of parole violations and re-incarceration, recidivism, and number of institutional misconducts (Barnoski, 2006; Kroner & Mills, 2001). Convergent validity was demonstrated in a sex offender population by correlating LSI-R scores with the Psychopathy Checklist-Revised (pp. 220–222) and the General Statistical Inventory on Recidivism (pp. 247–249). Discriminant validity was examined in three groups of sex offenders (Simourd & Malcolm, 1998). The adult-victim sex aggressor groups had higher total scores and subscale scores measuring criminal history, accommodation, companions, and attitude/orientations in comparison to a child molestation group. The extrafamilial child molester group scored higher than the familial child molester group on the total score and criminal history, education/employment, financial, accommodation, companions, and attitude/orientation subscales. The adult offenders had higher scores than the extrafamilial child molesters on the attitude/orientation subscale and lower scores on the financial subscale. The LSI-R was found to have much lower predictive validity in a sample of African American and Hispanic male offenders. The LSI-R was weakly related to rearrest ($r=.06$, nonsignificant) and reconviction ($r=.09$, nonsignificant) (Schalger & Simourd, 2007).

Clinical Utility

High. Although training in the LSI-R is required, the resulting profile of static and dynamic risk factors can aid prediction. The authors report potential uses such as classifying offenders, allocating treatment and security resources, monitoring offender risk, making halfway house placement decisions, deciding appropriate security level classification, making probation supervision decisions, and assessing likelihood of recidivism. Additionally, researchers have reported that the measure is valid for both male and female offenders and that scores are not significantly impacted by the presence of childhood abuse (Lowenkamp, Holsinger, & Latessa, 2001). Additional normative data would be helpful to determine the applicability of the measure for varied populations.

Research Applicability

High. The LSI-R has been used to predict the total number of convictions and the total number of violent convictions among offenders and has performed statistically comparable to the Psychopathy Checklist-Revised (pp. 220–222), the HCR-20 (pp. 194–196), and the Violence Risk Appraisal Guide (pp. 258–260). Additionally, the LSI-R allows researchers to investigate both dynamic and static factors related to criminal risk.

Original Citation

Andrews, D. A., & Bonta, J. L., (1995). *The Level of Service Inventory-Revised*. Toronto, Ontario, Canada: Multi-Health Systems.

Source

Multi-Health Systems, 3770 Victoria Park Avenue, Toronto, ON M2H 3M6 (phone: 1-800-268-6011) or P.O. Box 950, North Tonawanda, NY 14120-0950 (US address; phone: 1-800-456-3003). https://ecom.mhs.com/(rh2abwqqg4aj0h-vfwbab5ban)/inventory.aspx

Cost

The LSI-R complete kit, which includes a manual, 25 interview guides, 25 quikscore forms, and 25 colorplot profiles costs $130.

Alternative Forms

The LSI-R is available in English, French-Canadian, and Spanish. It can be given in a paper-and-pencil format or on a computer. A shorter version (8 items) is also available called the Level of Service Inventory-Revised: Screening Version (LSI-R: SV). The measure has also been adapted for use with adolescents ages 12–17 and is called the Youth Level of Service/Case Management Inventory (YLS/CMI).

References

Barnoski, R. (2006). *Sex offender sentencing in Washington state*: *Predicting recidivism based on the LSI-R* (Document No. 06-02-1201). Olympia: Washington State Institute for Public Policy.

Kroner, D. G., & Mills, J. F. (2001). The accuracy of five risk appraisal instruments in predicting institutional misconduct and new convictions. *Criminal Justice and Behavior, 28*(4), 471–489.

Lowenkamp, C. T., Holsinger, A. M., & Latessa, E. J. (2001). Risk/need assessment, offender classification, and the role of childhood abuse. *Criminal Justice and Behavior, 28*(5), 543–563.

Schlager, M. D., & Simourd, D. J. (2007). Validity of the Level of Service Inventory – Revised (LSI-R) among African American and Hispanic male offenders. *Criminal Justice and Behavior, 34*, 545–554.

Simourd, D. J., & Malcolm, P. B. (1998). Reliability and validity of the Level of Service Inventory-Revised among federally incarcerated sex offenders. *Journal of Interpersonal Violence, 13*(2), 261–274.

Levenson Self-Report Psychopathy Scale (LSRP)

Purpose

To assess primary and secondary psychopathic traits in noninstitutionalized individuals.

Population

Noninstitutionalized samples.

Background and Description

The most widely used measures of psychopathy are generally used in forensic settings and rely on a combination of psychopathic traits and antisocial behavior to calculate total scores. The Levenson Self-Report Psychopathy Scale (LSRP) is a 26-item, paper-and-pen measure that assesses psychopathic traits in noninstitutionalized populations. Rather than assessing criminal behavior, the LSRP elicits information regarding personality and interpersonal traits related to the construct of psychopathy.

Test items on the LSRP are subdivided into two scales: primary and secondary psychopathic traits.

Items on the primary psychopathy scale assess traits such as selfishness, manipulativeness, callousness, and tendency to lie. Items on the secondary psychopathy scale assess traits such as impulsivity and self-destructive lifestyle choices. Items are rated on a 4-point Likert-type scale, with some items reverse-scored to control for response bias. Response options include "disagree strongly," "disagree somewhat," "agree somewhat," and "agree strongly." Sample items follow.

Primary Scale

• Success is based on survival of the fittest; I am not concerned about the losers.
• For me, what's right is whatever I can get away with.

Secondary Scale

• I find myself in the same kinds of trouble, time after time.
• I am often bored.

Administration

The LSRP takes approximately 15–20 min to complete.

Scoring

Scores are summed to obtain a total psychopathy score based on 26 items (with some items reverse scored to minimize response bias). Primary and secondary psychopathy scales are also summed, with the primary scale consisting of items 1–16 and the secondary scale consisting of items 17–26.

Interpretation

A high total score indicates a higher general level of psychopathy. High scale scores indicate greater propensities for primary and/or secondary traits related to the construct of psychopathy.

Psychometric Properties

Norms. The LSRP was normed on 487 undergraduates. Of the 481 subjects who endorsed their gender on testing materials, 346 were female and 135 were male. Subjects ranged from 17 to 49 years of age, with a mean age of 20.82 ($SD = 3.25$).

Factor analysis. A principal components analysis of the test items yielded two factors: Factor-1 Primary Psychopathy and Factor-2 Secondary Psychopathy. The two-factor structure was not found in a sample of female inmates, instead a three-factor structure was a better fit. The three factors were: Egocentric, Antisocial, and Callous (Brinkley, Diamond, Magaletta, & Heigel, 2008).

Reliability. Cronbach's coefficient alpha was .85, .82, and .63 for the LSRP total score, the primary scale, and the secondary scale, respectively. Results indicate moderate to high internal consistency. Cronbach's alphas for the factors Egocentric, Antisocial, and Callous identified in a sample of female inmates were .82, .69 and .63, respectively.

Validity. The LSRP total scores correlate significantly with Hare's Psychopathy Checklist-Revised (PCL-R, pp. 220–222) scores, indicating good construct validity. Factor scores for the LSRP were found to correlate significantly with corresponding factor scores of the PCL-R, also indicating good construct validity (Brinkley, Schmitt, Smith, & Newman, 2001). Factor-1 of the LSRP was related to low agreeableness and narcissistic personality disorder in a sample of undergraduates (Miller, Gaughan, & Pryor, 2008). In the same sample, Factor-2 was related to neuroticism and low conscientiousness.

Clinical Utility

Moderate. The LSRP is a psychopathy measure designed for self-report use with noninstitutionalized populations. It is relatively easy and brief to administer, and the initial psychometric properties appear promising.

Research Applicability

High. Though designed for noninstitutionalized populations, the LSRP measures constructs of psychopathy that are uniform among both forensic and non-forensic populations. The measure has promise for further research due to its brevity, ease of administration, reliability, construct validity, and significant correlation with the PCL-R.

Original Citation

Levenson, M. R., Kiehl, A. K., & Fitzpatrick, C. M. (1995). Assessing psychopathic attributes in a noninstitutionalized population. *Journal of Personality and Social Psychology, 68*(1), 151–158.

Source

Dr. Michael R. Levenson, Department of Human Development and Family Sciences, Oregon State University, 203 Bates Hall, Corvallis, OR 97331, (541) 737-9241, Fax: (541) 737-5549, rick.levenson@oregonstate.edu

Cost

Contact the source (above) for permission to use the LSRP.

References

Brinkley, C. A., Diamond, P. M., Magaletta, P. R., & Heigel, C. P. (2008). Cross-validation of Levenson's Psychopathy Scale in a sample of federal female inmates. *Assessment, 15*, 464–482.

Brinkley, C. A., Schmitt, W. A., Smith, S. S., & Newman, J. P. (2001). Construct validation of a self-report psychopathy scale: Does Levenson's Self-Report Psychopathy Scale measure the same constructs as Hare's Psychopathy Checklist-Revised? *Journal of Personality and Individual Differences, 31*, 1021–1038.

Miller, J. D., Gaughan, E. T., & Pryor, L. R. (2008). The Levenson Self-Report Psychopathy Scale: An examination of the personality traits and disorders associated with LSRP factors. *Assessment, 15*, 450–463.

Maudsley Violence Questionnaire (MVQ)

Purpose

To assess thoughts related to violent behavior.

Population

Ages 16 and older.

Background and Description

The Maudsley Violence Questionnaire (MVQ) is a violence-specific measure designed to assess thoughts held by individuals about violence, violent acts, and what is acceptable, justifiable and reasonable in specific contexts. Items were created to reflect Gilligan's (1996) theory of aggression which postulates that several factors are needed for aggression: low self-esteem, anger, perceived humiliation, and lack of nonviolent alternatives to "saving face". As such, items were included that assessed hiding self-esteem through aggression and using violence in response to threats against self-esteem. The MVQ contains 56 items and two subscales, Machismo and Acceptance of Violence, which assess beliefs and rules that provide support, or justification, for violence. The items were created through conversations with violence researchers and reviewing common beliefs reported by violent offenders in treatment. A true/false response format is used. Sample items follow.

- Being violent shows you are a man.
- I am totally against violence.
- People who irritate you deserve to be hit.

Administration

The MVQ is estimated to require 10–15 min to complete.

Scoring

Items are scored in the keyed direction and summed to produce subscale scores and a total score.

Interpretation

Higher scores indicate greater endorsement of violence-related thoughts. Higher scores on the Machismo subscale indicate endorsement of beliefs related to embarrassment resulting from backing down from a conflict, violence as justified in response to a threat or attack, violence as a male characteristic, and fear and nonviolence associated with weakness. Higher scores on the Acceptance of Violence subscale indicate endorsement of beliefs related to acceptance and enjoyment of violence in the media or in sports.

Psychometric Properties

Norms. Normative data were obtained for 785 high school students (480 males, 305 females). Normative data are provided separately for males and females.

Factor analysis. A principal components analysis was conducted on data for male and female high school students. The results were analyzed separately for the genders, and the same two factors were found: Machismo and Acceptance of Violence. There were slightly different loadings of items on the two factors for males and females; the authors chose to use only the male factor structure because the sample was larger than the female sample and most individuals that will complete the measure in clinical and forensic settings will be male.

Reliability. Internal consistency, as measured by Cronbach's alpha, ranged from .73 to .91 for the MVQ subscales in male and female high school students.

Validity. Scores on the MVQ were correlated with self-reported violence and delinquency in a high school student sample. The MVQ was significantly related to self-reported violence for males and females, with the Machismo subscale for males having the highest correlation with self-reported violence ($r = .50$). The MVQ Acceptance of Violence subscale was related to nonviolent delinquency in males and females. The MVQ Machismo subscale was related to nonviolent delinquency in males but not in females (Walker & Gudjonsson, 2006).

In a separate high school sample, scores on the Machismo subscale for males were significantly related to psychoticism ($r = .34$) and violent and nonviolent delinquency ($r = .33$ to .50). In contrast, scores on the Machismo subscale for females were most strongly related to violent delinquency ($r = .26$). Acceptance of Violence was related to psychoticism and delinquency for males and females. Acceptance of Violence was also related to self-esteem, extraversion, and neuroticism in males. A high Machismo score was the most predictive factor (compared to Acceptance subscale, self esteem, Lie Scale, extraversion, and psychoticism) for violent offending behavior in males. In contrast, a high Acceptance of Violence score was the most predictive factor of violent offending behavior in females (Walker & Bright, 2009).

The validity of the MVQ was also assessed in an adult male, forensic population. Scores on the Machismo subscale were significantly related to criminal convictions ($r = .25$) and institutional violent incidents ($r = .36$). Scores on the Acceptance of Violence scale were significantly related to institutional violent incidents ($r = .29$), but the correlation with criminal convictions was nonsignificant ($r = .07$) (Warnock-Parkes, Gudjonsson, & Walker, 2008).

Clinical Utility

Moderate. The MVQ can be used with offender and non-offender populations to evaluate dysfunctional assumptions or rules related to the use, justification, and acceptability of violence. The MVQ may be a useful measure for assessing treatment-related changes in cognitive styles that promote the use of violence. Additional normative, reliability, and validity data for adult, female, and forensic populations would improve the clinical utility of the measure.

Research Applicability

High. The MVQ may be a useful measure for examining the relationship between violent thoughts, anger, and aggressive behavior. It has also been used in several studies to examine the relationship between self-esteem and aggression.

Original Citation

Walker, J. S. (2005). The Maudsley violence questionnaire: Initial validation and reliability. *Personality and Individual Differences, 38*, 187–201.

Source

Dr. Julian Walker, Fromeside Clinic, Blackberry Hill, Stapleton, Bristol BS16 1EG, UK, Phone: 0117 378 4123, Fax: 0117 958 5477, Julian.walker@awp.nhs.uk

Cost

Please contact the source (above) for permission to use the MVQ.

References

Walker, J. S., & Gudjonsson, G. H. (2006). The Maudsley Violence Questionnaire: Relationship to personality and self-reported offending. *Personality and Individual Differences, 40*, 795–806.
Walker, J. S., & Bright, J. A. (2009). False inflated self-esteem and violence: A systematic review and cognitive model. *The Journal of Forensic Psychiatry & Psychology, 20*, 1–32.

Warnock-Parkes, E., Gudjonsson, G. H., & Walker, J. (2008). The relationship between the Maudsley Violence Questionnaire and official recordings of violence in mentally disordered offenders. *Personality and Individual Differences, 44*, 833–841.

Multidimensional Measure of Emotional Abuse (MMEA)

Purpose

To assess emotional abuse that occurs in the context of dating relationships.

Population

Adults in dating relationships.

Background and Description

The Multidimensional Measure of Emotional Abuse (MMEA) was created to assess emotional abuse that occurs in dating relationships. Emotional abuse was conceptualized as "coercive or aversive acts intended to produce emotional harm or threat of harm" (Murphy & Hoover, 1999, p. 40). The MMEA contains 54 items that were created to reflect four forms of emotional abuse: Restrictive Engulfment, Hostile Withdrawal, Denigration, and Dominance/Isolation. Restrictive Engulfment items reflected behaviors intended to isolate the partner and control the partner's activities and also included acts of jealously and possessiveness. Hostile Withdrawal items reflected the tendency to withhold emotional contact and withdraw from the partner in an attempt to punish the partner and increase their anxiety about the relationship. Items in the Denigration subscale were comprised of behaviors intended to humiliate or degrade the partner. Dominance/Intimidation items included threats, property violence, and intense verbal aggression carried out to cause fear or submission in the partner. Respondents report the frequency with which they or their partner committed each behavior during the previous 4 months using a 7-point scale (0 = never, 6 = more than 20 times).

Administration

The MMEA is estimated to require 10–15 min to complete.

Scoring

Two scoring schemes are possible; for both, items for self and partner are calculated separately. The items can be scored as 0 if the behavior never occurred or 1 if the behavior occurred regardless of the frequency. Alternatively, scores can be calculated using the 7-point scale and taking frequency into account. In both scoring schemes, the items are summed to calculate subscale scores and a total score.

Interpretation

Higher scores are indicative of greater levels of emotionally abusive behaviors committed by the respondent, the respondent's partner, or both.

Psychometric Properties

Factor analysis. A principal components analysis with varimax rotation was conducted on responses of 157 undergraduate females about reports of abuse by their relationship partners. This analysis revealed four factors: Hostile Withdrawal, Domination/Intimidation, Denigration, and Restrictive Engulfment.

Reliability. The internal consistency, as measured by Cronbach's alpha, for the MMEA subscales

for reports of abusive behaviors by female respondents ranged from .83 (Domination/ Intimidation) to .89 (Denigration). Alphas for the MMEA subscales for reports of abusive behaviors by the respondents' partners ranged from .85 (Restrictive Engulfment) to .92 (Denigration).

Validity. The subscales of the MMEA were correlated with related constructs including physical aggression and interpersonal problems. All of the MMEA subscales were significantly related to physical aggression as measured by the Conflict Tactics Scale (CTS; pp. 177–180). Denigration and Dominance/Intimidation had the highest correlations with physical aggression for reported abuse by partner ($r = .72$ and .74, respectively) and abuse by self ($r = .56$ and .67, respectively). The MMEA subscales were significantly related to interpersonal problems associated with dominance, coercion and aggression as measured by the Inventory of Interpersonal Problems (Horowitz, Rosenberg, Baer, Ureno, & Villasenor, 1988). The MMEA was also correlated with the Reciprocal Attachment Questionnaire (West & Sheldon-Keller, 1992) to investigate problematic attachment styles and their relationship to emotional abuse. High scores on the Restrictive Engulfment subscale were related to anxious/ insecure attachment qualities ($r = .34$ to .52). Restrictive Engulfment, Hostile Withdrawal, and Denigration were all significantly correlated with compulsive care seeking, suggesting that emotional abuse is related to attachment concerns.

The MMEA subscales were correlated with a measure of social desirability (Balanced Inventory of Desirable Responding-Version 6, Paulhus, 1991) to determine the extent of social desirable responding on the MMEA. For reports of abuse by self, all of the MMEA subscales were significantly related to impression management. The Hostile Withdrawal subscale was the only MMEA subscale to be significantly related to social desirability for reports of abuse by partner. This suggests the MMEA is impacted by socially desirable responding, especially for reports of abuse by self.

Clinical Utility

Moderate. The MMEA has good psychometric properties and can be adapted to measure abuse that occurred during varying time periods. The MMEA may be helpful in identifying individuals and couples that are not only emotionally abusive but are also more likely to be physically abusive that could benefit from treatment. It can also be used to identify specific patterns of emotionally abusive behaviors committed by couples to be targeted in treatment. Additional information on the psychometric properties of the MMEA would increase the clinical utility of the measure.

Research Applicability

Moderate. The MMEA may be a useful tool in investigating developmental processes associated with interpersonal violence. The MMEA may also be used to study the relationship between physical abuse and emotional abuse and to better clarify our understanding of the consequences of emotional abuse in dating relationships.

Original Citation

Murphy, C. M., & Hoover, S. A. (1999). Measuring emotional abuse in dating relationships as a multifactorial construct. *Violence and Victims, 14*, 39–53.

Source

Dr. Christopher Murphy, Department of Psychology, University of Maryland, Baltimore County, 1000 Hilltop Circle, Baltimore, MD, 21250, (410) 455-2367, Fax: (410) 455-1055, chmurphy@umbc.edu

Cost

Please contact the source (above) for permission to use the MMEA.

Alternative Forms

A 56-item (28 self abuse items and 28 partner abuse items) version of the MMEA exists that consists of the same four subscales and response format. It has been found to have adequate to good reliability with alphas ranging from .77 to .91 for the total score and .52 to .92 for the subscales. It was found to significantly correlate with other measures of psychological aggression including the Test of Negative Social Exchange (pp. 81–83) and the CTS (pp. 177–180) (Ro & Lawrence, 2007).

References

Horowitz, L. M., Rosenberg, S. E., Baer, B. A., Ureno, G., & Villasenor, V. S. (1988). Inventory of Interpersonal Problems: Psychometric properties and clinical applications. *Journal of Consulting and Clinical Psychology, 56*, 885–892.

Paulhus, D. L. (1991). Measurement and control of response bias. In J.P. Robinson, P.R. Shaver, & L.S. Wrightsman (Eds.), *Measures of personality and social psychological attitudes* (pp.17–59). New York: Academic Press.

Ro, E., & Lawrence, E. (2007). Comparing three measures of psychological aggression: Psychometric properties and differentiation from negative communication. *Journal of Family Violence, 22*, 575–586.

West, M., & Sheldon-Keller, A. (1992). The assessment of dimensions relevant to adult reciprocal attachment. *Canadian Journal of Psychiatry, 37*, 600–606.

My Exposure to Violence (My ETV)

Purpose

To assess child and youth exposure to violence.

Population

Children to young adults.

Background and Description

The My Exposure to Violence measure (My ETV) was developed in response to the methodological problems with previous measures. A wide range of violent events are sampled and items about sexual violence are included. Moreover, respondents indicate whether the event was observed or personally experienced. The My ETV is administered as a structured interview that covers 18 different events. The format was designed in a similar format to diagnostic interviews. Frequency of exposure, both during the past year and lifetime, is measured on a 6-point scale (never, once, 2 or 3 times, 4–10 times, 11–50 times, more than 50 times).

Administration

The measure is estimated to require 30–45 min to complete.

Scoring

Items are summed to produce three subscales for lifetime exposure and three subscales for exposure during the past year. The subscales are: Witnessing Violent Events, Experiencing Violent Events, and Total Violence Exposure.

Interpretation

Higher scores indicate greater exposure to violence.

Psychometric Properties

Norms. Initial data were obtained from 80 participants that were distributed at 3-year intervals across age cohorts (9, 12, 15, 18, 21, and 24). Based upon the neighborhood-level crime statistics, 50 % of the sample resided in low crime areas, 17 % in moderate crime areas, and 33 % in high crime neighborhoods.

Reliability. Internal consistency estimates for the six scales ranged from .68 to .93. Internal consistency was lowest for the experiencing subscales. Subscale test–retest reliability estimates, based on 23 participants who were sampled

between 2 and 4 weeks following the initial interview, ranged from .75 to .94.

Validity. Evidence of construct validity was obtained using item analysis, which revealed a theoretically sensible ordering of item extremity. The My ETV was meaningfully linked to demographic characteristics in theoretically predicted ways. For instance, age was inversely related to total exposure to violence, males reported more exposure than females, violent offenders reported more exposure than did non-offenders, and those living in high crime areas reported more exposure than those residing in low crime areas (Selner-O'Hagan, Kindlon, & Buka, 1998).

Clinical Utility

Limited. Preliminary psychometric data are promising. Few studies have used the measure in a clinical setting. Additional validity and normative data are needed prior to recommending widespread clinical use.

Research Applicability

Moderate. The measure is relatively easy to administer. The My ETV could help with providing additional data on experiencing versus witnessing violence, and research in this area may be useful in guiding the development of models for understanding the initiation and maintenance of violent behavior.

Original Citation

Buka, S., Slener-O'Hagan, M., Kindlon, D., & Earls, F. (1996). *My exposure to violence and my child's exposure to violence.* Unpublished manual.

Source

Mary Beth Selner-O'Hagan, Harvard School of Public Health, Department of Maternal and Child Health, Huntington Avenue, Boston, MA 02115.

Cost

Please contact source (above) for permission to use the My ETV.

Reference

Selner-O'Hagan, M. B., Kindlon, D. J., & Buka, S. L. (1998). Assessing exposure to violence in urban youth. *Journal of Child Psychology and Psychiatry,* *39*(2), 215–224.

Pride in Delinquency Scale (PID)

Purpose

To assess the degree of shame and pride associated with participation in specific criminal behaviors.

Population

Adults and adolescents.

Background and Description

Past research has supported the link between criminal attitudes and criminal behavior. The Pride in Delinquency scale (PID) was developed to complement the Criminal Sentiments Scale (pp. 180–181) by measuring the degree of pride associated with participation in criminal activities. Respondents are asked to rate their likely reaction to engaging in 10 criminal behaviors using a 21-point scale that ranges from –10 (high degree of shame) to +10 (high degree of pride). A rating of 0 reflects that the subject is undecided. A sample item is listed below:
• Beating up a child molester.

Administration

The PID takes approximately 15 min to complete.

Scoring

Scores from each item are summed and added to a constant value of 100, so that all total scores are a positive value.

Interpretation

Higher scores reflect a greater degree of pro-criminal attitudes.

Psychometric Properties

Norms. The PID has been used with probationers, provincial prisoners, federal and forensic inmates, young offenders, college students, and community volunteers. No easily accessible normative data have been published.

Factor analysis. A principal components analysis using varimax rotation and the Kaiser criterion resulted in two factors: Attitude Toward Offenses, which accounted for 42 % of the variance and reflected attitudes regarding specific types of criminal behavior, and Criminal Subculture, which accounted for 13 % of the variance and reflected attitudes regarding specific criminal morals.

Reliability. Cronbach's coefficient alpha was .75, .78, and .79 for the PID total scale, the Attitude Toward Offenses factor, and the Criminal Subculture factor, respectively. Results indicate moderate levels of internal consistency.

Validity. The PID significantly correlated with the Criminal Sentiments Scale-Modified (pp. 180–181). Convergent validity was obtained by comparing the PID to alternative measures of criminal behavior/risk, specifically the Level of Service Inventory-Revised (pp. 202–204), the Statistical Information on Recidivism (pp. 247–249), and the Psychopathy Checklist-Revised (pp. 220–222). Correlations were .42, .36, and .24, respectively.

Clinical Utility

Moderate. The PID is a relatively new measure of criminal attitudes. Initial results appear promising. Easily accessible normative data would enhance the clinical utility.

Research Applicability

Moderate. The measure has promise due to its brevity, ease of administration, acceptable reliability, and acceptable construct validity. Further research is needed to further ascertain its applicability for use with varied populations and settings.

Original Citations

Simourd, D. J. (1997). The Criminal Sentiments Scale-Modified and Pride in Delinquency Scale: Psychometric properties and construct validity of two measures of criminal attitudes. *Criminal Justice and Behavior,* 24, 52–70.

Source

Dr. David Simourd, Algonquin Correctional Evaluation Services, 86 Braemar Road, Kingston, Ontario K7M 4B6 Canada, (613) 384-6637, Fax: (613) 384-6637, dave@acesink.com

Cost

Please contact the source (above) for additional information.

Alternative Forms

Both paper-and-pencil and interview formats are available.

Reference

Simourd, D. J., & Van de Ven, J. (1999). Assessment of criminal attitudes: Criterion-related validity of the Criminal Sentiments Scale-Modified and Pride in Delinquency Scale. *Criminal Justice and Behavior,* 26, 90–106.

Propensity for Abusiveness Scale (PAS)

Purpose

To measure males' propensity to abuse female partners.

Population

Adults.

Background and Description

The Propensity for Abusiveness Scale (PAS) was created to serve as a measure of abuse potential in males that would be less susceptible to biased self-report styles. The items were derived from scales that measured constructs strongly associated with emotional and physical abusiveness that were less susceptible to reactivity bias. As such, the items do not directly reference abuse, but instead measure personality traits, anger expression, experiences of trauma symptoms, and recollections of treatment by the father. Respondents rate items 1–12 using a 5-point, Likert style scale, ranging from 1 (completely undescriptive) to 5 (completely descriptive). Items 13–22 are frequency ratings in which respondents rate how often the specified event occurred during their childhood using a 4-point Likert-type scale ranging from 1 (never occurred) to 4 (always occurred). The final items (numbers 23–29) are frequency ratings of how often the specified event occurred in the previous 2 months using a 4-point, Likert style scale ranging from 0 (never) to 3 (very often). Sample items follow.

• I can make myself angry about something in the past just by thinking about it.
• If I let people see the way I feel, I'd be considered a hard person to get along with.
• My parent punished me even for small offenses.

Administration

The PAS is estimated to require 15–20 min to complete.

Scoring

The scoring for items is detailed above. The item scores are summed to produce a total score.

Interpretation

Higher scores indicate a greater propensity for abusiveness.

Psychometric Properties

Factor analysis. A principal components analysis revealed three factors that accounted for 54 % of the variance. These factors were labeled: Recalled Negative Parental Treatment, Affective Instability, and Trauma Symptoms.

Reliability. Internal consistency, as measured by Cronbach's alpha, was .92 in the original test construction sample. In a separate sample of 100 men and 76 women, Cronbach's alpha was .88. The 2 year, test–retest reliability of the PAS was found to be adequate in a sample of 64 college men ($n = 27$) and women ($n = 37$) with PAS total score test–retest reliability .63 for men and .85 for women. Test–retest reliability of the PAS scales ranged from .53 to .67 for men and .62 to .79 for women (Clift, Thomas, & Dutton, 2005).

Validity. The PAS was significantly related to abusiveness as measured by the Psychological Maltreatment of Women Inventory (PMWI, pp. 215–216). The PAS total score correlated with the dominance/isolation subscale of the PMWI ($r = .51$) and with the emotional abuse subscale ($r = .47$). The PAS was able to correctly classify 80 % of men on the dominance/isolation factor of the PMWI, and 84.4 % of the men on the emotional abuse factor of the PMWI using cutoff criteria of one standard deviation away from the mean for each factor.

In a separate sample using the same cutoff criteria, the PAS correctly classified 82.2 % of men on the dominance/isolation factor and 81.3 % of men on the emotional abuse factor. The PAS total score was significantly related to the dominance/isolation factor ($r = .52$) and the emotional abuse factor ($r = .45$) of the PMWI.

The PAS has been found to significantly predict use of intimidation, emotional abuse, and use of male privilege by assaultive men. The PAS was cross-validated on diverse samples of men including a nonviolent clinical outpatient population, male college students, gay men in committed relationships, and men in spousal assaultive treatment groups. The PAS was significantly related to reports of physical and emotional abuse by the partners of assaultive men. PAS scores were significantly related to partners' reports of emotional abuse in the college and gay samples (Dutton, Landolt, Starzomski, Bodnarchuk, 2001).

The PAS has been found to not only predict potential abuse but also predict general arousal levels prior to an interpersonal conflict and following an interpersonal conflict. The PAS was significantly related to anger, anxiety, sub-anger, and general arousal levels experienced in anticipation of an interpersonal conflict (Thomas & Dutton, 2004).

Clinical Utility

High. The PAS has adequate psychometric properties and appears to be minimally affected by reactive and social desirability bias. It has been shown to be effective in predicting abuse in diverse populations of men. As such, the

PAS may be a useful instrument to use with court-referred men to predict potential for abusiveness. The PAS may also be utilized in high schools or prevention programs to identify individuals likely to become abusive.

Research Applicability

Moderate. The PAS may be a useful measure for assessing correlates of abusiveness in men including emotional priming that may occur in anticipation of an interpersonal conflict. The PAS could also be utilized to investigate possible similarities and differences in abusiveness potential in men and women.

Original Citation

Dutton, D. G. (1995). A scale for measuring propensity for abusiveness. *Journal of Family Violence, 10,* 203–221.

Source

Dr. Donald Dutton, University of British Columbia, Department of Psychology, 2136 West Mall, Vancouver, B.C., V6T 1Z4, (604) 822-4592, dondutton@shaw.ca

Cost

Please contact the source (above) for permission to use the PAS.

References

Clift, R. J. W., Thomas, L. A., & Dutton, D. G. (2005). Two-year reliability of the Propensity for Abusiveness Scale. *Journal of Family Violence, 20,* 231–234.

Dutton, D. G., Landolt, M. A., Starzomski, A., & Bodnarchuk, M. (2001). Validation of the propensity for abusiveness scale in diverse male populations. *Journal of Family Violence, 16,* 59–73.

Thomas, L. A., & Dutton, D. G. (2004). The propensity for abusiveness scale (PAS) as a predictor of affective priming to anticipated intimate conflict. *Journal of Applied Social Psychology, 34,* 2166–2178.

Proximal Antecedents to Violent Episodes Scale (PAVE)

Purpose

To identify events that are likely to elicit partner violence committed by males.

Population

Adult males.

Background and Description

The Proximal Antecedents to Violent Episodes Scale (PAVE) was developed to differentiate among types of partner related violence, as well as to identify triggering events likely to elicit male-to-female aggression. The typology developed by Holtzworth-Munroe and Stuart (1994), which classifies violent males as family only violence, borderline/dysphoric, or generally violent/antisocial guided item development. Items were selected to tap instrumental and expressive acts of violence. The resulting self-report measure consists of 20 hypothetical situations. Respondents use a 6-point scale (1=not at all likely, 6=extremely likely) to indicate the likelihood that they would employ physical aggression in each of the given situations. The following are sample items.

- My partner threatens to leave me.
- My partner does not include me in important decisions.

Administration

The PAVE is estimated to take 10 min to complete.

Scoring

Responses are summed to create a total score. Three factor scores can also be computed: Violence to Control, Violence out of Jealousy, and Verbal Abuse.

Interpretation

Higher scores indicate that the individual is more likely to respond with physical aggression.

Psychometric Properties

Factor analysis. Preliminary analyses were conducted using a clinical sample whose positively skewed distribution was normalized using a log linear transformation. A principal components analysis of the transformed scores resulted in a 3-factor solution. The factors were labeled violence to control (14 situations), violence out of jealousy (4 situations), and violence following verbal abuse (11 situations). A factor analysis using responses from a general community was used to refine the measure to 20 items. A confirmatory factor analysis revealed an adequate fit for the previously identified 3-factor model.

Reliability. Internal consistency was assessed in a community sample of men and found to be adequate. Cronbach's alphas for the factor scores ranged from .73 to .93, and the total scale alpha was .94.

Validity. Using a clinical sample of aggressive males, the total score on the PAVE correlated with scores on the Conflict Tactics Scale ($r = .24$, pp. 177–180). A cluster analysis of standardized scores from the Conflict Tactics Scale (frequency of marital violence), breadth of general violence, and the MCMI-III (antisocial personality and borderline personality; Millon, 1994) resulted in four clusters (family only violence, intermediate, borderline/dysphoric, and generally violent). Males classified as generally violent scored highest on the violence to control and violence following verbal abuse factors and were more likely than males classified as family only violence to obtain higher scores when their partners exerted autonomy or were verbally threatening or critical. Males classified as borderline scored highest on the violence out of jealousy factor and reported more violence than antisocial batterers in situations involving jealousy or infidelity.

In a community sample, a cluster analysis (conducted as described above) produced a 3-cluster solution (family only, borderline, and generally violent/antisocial). Males categorized as borderline and generally violent/antisocial reported more violence than males categorized as family only on the violence as a means of control factor. Males categorized as generally violent/antisocial were more likely than males categorized as family only violence to obtain high scores on the violence following verbal abuse factor.

Clinical Utility

Moderate. The PAVE is a short and easy measure to administer and score. The measure is potentially useful for identifying antecedents to partner violence, and identification of such situations can help to guide treatment. Additional normative data would enhance the clinical utility, as well as to better establish the reliability and validity using clinical samples.

Research Applicability

Moderate. The measure appears useful for developing models of male violence that acknowledge the interaction between individual differences and contextual influences. Situations could be selected or added to explore the role of specific contextual factors.

Original Citation

Babcock, J. C., Costa, D. M., Green, C. E., & Eckhardt, C. I. (2004). What situations induce intimate partner violence?: A reliability and validity study of the Proximal Antecedents to Violent Episodes Scale (PAVE). *Journal of Family Psychology, 18,* 433–442.

Source

Julia C. Babcock, Department of Psychology, The University of Houston, 126 Heyne Building, Houston, TX 77204, (713) 743-8500, jbabcock@uh.edu

Cost

Contact the source (above) for permission to use the PAVE.

References

Holtzworth-Munroe, A., & Stuart, G. L. (1994). Typologies of male batterers: Three subtypes and the differences among them. *Psychological Bulletin, 116,* 476–497.

Millon, T. (1994). *Manual for the Millon Clinical Multiaxial Inventory—III.* Minneapolis, MN: National Computer Systems.

Psychological Maltreatment Inventory (PMI)

Purpose

To retrospectively rate an individual's negative experiences with their parents.

Population

Adults.

Background and Description

The Psychological Maltreatment Inventory (PMI) was constructed to reflect five major categories of psychological maltreatment: reject, terrorize, isolate, corrupt, and denial of emotional responsiveness. A review of the psychological maltreatment literature resulted in an initial pool of 74 items. Clinicians then sorted the items into five categories. The 47 items that achieved 100 % interrater reliability were kept and statistical analyses were conducted. On the basis of a principal component analysis, 25 of these items were used to develop the final self-report measured designed to assess negative parent–child experiences. Respondents use a 6-point scale to indicate how negatively they were affected by each of the 25 parent–child experiences ranging from 0 (this didn't happen) to 5 (extremely negative effect on me).

Administration

The PMI is estimated to take 5–10 min to complete.

Scoring

Responses to items are summed to produce a total score and subscale scores. Subscale scores assess perceived emotional neglect, hostile rejection, and being isolated.

Interpretation

Higher scores indicate that the individual perceived a greater degree of emotional abuse or neglect during childhood.

Psychometric Properties

Reliability. The alpha coefficients for the entire scale range from .81 to .94. Subscale test–retest reliability for intervals between 18 months and 2 years ranged from .75 to .78.

Validity. Emotional neglect correlated with the Neglect/Indifference scale of the Parental Acceptance and Rejection Questionnaire (PARQ, Rohner, 1991), and Hostile rejection correlated with the PARQ Aggression/Hostility scale. Scores on the modified PMI mother scale and father scale were significantly related to scores on the Codependency Assessment Tool Hughes-Hammer, Martsolf, & Zeller, 1998 (Reyome & Ward, 2007).

Clinical Utility

Limited. The PMI may provide insight into childhood experiences but provides little information about current functioning. The retrospective nature of the measure has the added risk of being susceptible to inaccurate responding due to current biases.

Research Applicability

Moderate. The PMI requires little time to administer and may be used to investigate the influence of perceived emotional abuse and neglect during childhood.

Original Citation

Engels, M. L., & Moisan, D. (1994). The Psychological Maltreatment Inventory: Development of a measure of psychological maltreatment in childhood for use in adult clinical settings. *Psychological Reports, 74,* 595–604.

Source

Engels, M. L., & Moisan, D. (1994). The Psychological Maltreatment Inventory: Development of a measure of psychological maltreatment in childhood for use in adult clinical settings. *Psychological Reports, 74,* 595–604.

Cost

Unavailable.

Alternative Forms

A modified version of the PMI exists that allows for the evaluation of maternal and paternal psychological maltreatment separately. The modified PMI has good split-half reliability ($r = .88$).

References

Hughes-Hammer, C., Martsolf, D., & Zeller, R. (1998). Development and testing of the codependency assessment tool. *Archives of Psychiatric Nursing, 12,* 264–272.

Reyome, N. D., & Ward, K. S. (2007). Self-reported history of childhood maltreatment and codependency in undergraduate nursing students. *Journal of Emotional Abuse, 7,* 37-50.

Rohner, R. P. (1991). *Handbook for the study of parental acceptance and rejection.* Storrs, CT: University of Connecticut.

Psychological Maltreatment of Women Inventory (PMWI)

Purpose

To quantify the psychological maltreatment experienced by women in intimate relationships.

Population

Adults.

Background and Description

The Psychological Maltreatment of Women Inventory (PMWI) was developed to assess the function and consequence of nonphysical abuse. The goal was to create a measure of psychological abuse that could be administered with the Conflict Tactics Scale (pp. 177–180) and the Index of Spouse Abuse (pp. 196–198) to provide a more robust understanding of intimate partner abuse. Twenty-one items were modified from either the Conflict Tactics Scale or the nonphysical abuse scale of the Index of Spouse Abuse. Other items were developed from scanning the literature and clinical observations. The 58 items contained in the PMWI are organized into a dominance-isolation subscale and an emotional–verbal abuse subscale. Items on the dominance-isolation subscale depict behaviors such as isolation from resources, demands for subservience, and rigid observance of traditional sex roles. Items on the emotional–verbal abuse subscale depict behaviors such as verbal attacks, behavior that demeans women, and withholding emotional resources. Respondents are asked to rate how often each of the behaviors occurred during the past 6 months on a 5-point scale (1 = never occurs, 5 = always occurs). Both female and male versions are available; differences exist in the pronouns and the direction of abuse. Several sample items from the female version are listed below:

- My partner called me names.
- My partner demanded obedience to his whims.
- My partner used our money or made important financial decisions without talking to me about it.

Administration

The PMWI is estimated to take 10–15 min to complete.

Scoring

Responses are summed to produce dominance-isolation and emotional–verbal abuse subscale scores.

Interpretation

Higher scores on the dominance-isolation subscale are indicative of higher occurrences of psychological maltreatment using behaviors involving dominance and isolation. Higher scores on the emotional–verbal subscale indicate a higher occurrence of psychological maltreatment using emotional and verbal behaviors.

Psychometric Properties

Factor analysis. A principal component analysis was conducted separately for male and female versions and the results supported the two-factor model. A confirmatory factor analysis, using the multiple-group method, revealed that the factor structure for men was similar to the factor structure for women. (Hudson & McIntosh, 1981).

Reliability. Intra-couple reliability was examined using 28 couples. Spearman's Rho coefficients revealed low agreement between men and women's reports, a finding confirmed by Wilcoxon tests for each item pair. Items with high social acceptability revealed the largest correlations. Total scores on the dominance-isolation subscale were significantly correlated between men and women, but total scores on the emotional–verbal subscale were not. Cronbach's alpha coefficients for the subscales were similar for men and women and ranged from .91 to .95.

Validity. Face and content validity of the PMWI were established by obtaining feedback from individuals working with victims and perpetrators of spousal assault. The subscales of the PMWI were highly correlated with the physical abuse scale of the Conflict Tactics Scale and the nonphysical and physical abuse subscales of the Index of Spouse Abuse. The correlation between the PMWI and the nonphysical subscale of the Index of Spouse Abuse was higher than the latter two correlations. Additionally, subscales of the PMWI had moderate to high correlations with marital satisfaction and the General Symptom Index of the Brief Symptom Inventory (Derogatis, 1975).

The PMWI was able to differentiate between battered women, maritally distressed but not battered women, and nonbatterred women who were satisfied with their relationship. In a different sample, the PMWI differentiated between service-seeking battered women, battered women recruited from the community, maritally distressed nonbattered women, and nonbattered and nondistressed women from a community sample. The inventory, however, failed to differentiate between battered women from the community and maritally distressed nonbattered women (Tolman, 1999).

Clinical Utility

Moderate. The PMWI can help to identify and quantify psychological abuse. The time frame can make the measure suitable for assessing treatment gains following a course of couple's therapy. A drawback of the use of the PMWI in clinical settings is that it may not yield agreements between males and females and normative data are not readily available.

Research Applicability

Moderate. This measure could prove useful for assessing how perceptions of psychological abuse impact overall relationship satisfaction.

Original Citation

Tolman, R. M. (1989). The development of a measure of psychological maltreatment of women by their male partners. *Violence and Victims, 4*(3), 159–177.

Source

Dr. Richard M. Tolman, University of Michigan, School of Social Work, 1080 S. University, Ann Arbor, MI 48109, (734) 764-5333, Fax: (734) 763-3372, rtolman@umich.edu.

Cost

Please contact the source (above) for permission to use the PMWI.

Alternative Forms

A short version of the PMWI was constructed forming two, 7-item subscales from the original items representing psychological maltreatment that were most distinct from general relationship distress. On the short form, Cronbach's alpha was .88 for the dominance-isolation subscale and .92 for the verbal–emotional subscale. A factor analysis revealed identical factors as the long form, a dominance-isolation factor and a verbal–emotional factor. The short form was able to differentiate between battered women, nonbattered and

nondistressed women, and maritally distressed nonbattered women. In a different sample, the short version differentiated between service-seeking battered women, battered women recruited from community, maritally distressed nonbattered women, and nonbattered and nondistressed community sample. Battered women from the community, however, were not differentiated from maritally distressed nonbattered women.

References

Derogatis, L. R. (1975). *Brief Symptom Inventory.* Baltimore, MD: Clinical Psychometric Research.
Hudson, W., & McIntosh, S. (1981). The assessment of spouse abuse: Two quantifiable dimensions. *Journal of Marriage and the Family, 43*, 873–885.
Tolman, R. M. (1999). The validation of the Psychological Maltreatment of Women Inventory. *Violence and Victims, 14*, 25–37.

Psychological Maltreatment Rating Scales (PMRS)

Purpose

To code dimensions of psychological abuse and neglect in parent–child interactions.

Population

Parents interacting with their 5–9 year old children.

Background and Description

The National Center on Child Abuse and Neglect funded the research to create the Psychological Maltreatment Rating Scales (PMRS). Categories of psychological abuse and neglect were combined. The PMRS is a global assessment of psychological maltreatment used to code parent–child interactions. The PMRS consists of 15 scales: four scales assess psychological abuse and neglect (e.g., spurning, terrorizing, and corrupting/exploiting); nine scales assess prosocial parenting (e.g., maternal support, emotionality, and touching); and two scales measure aspects of the interaction between the parent and the child (e.g., experience of mutual pleasure such as laughing together).

Administration

The described procedure used 15-min tapes of a parent–child interaction. Mothers are instructed to teach the child and help him/her perform the task correctly. For preschool children, the task is a board game. For school-age children, the task is a paper construction project.

Scoring

Raters score 15 min of video taped from the mother–child interaction. Behaviors are coded using the 15 PMRS scales.

Interpretation

A qualitative analysis is used to evaluate the types of behaviors displayed during the parent–child interaction.

Psychometric Properties

Factor analysis. The authors interpreted a 3-factor solution: Facilitation of Social and Cognitive Development, Psychological Abuse, and Quality of Emotional Support.

Reliability. Interrater reliabilities for the scales ranged from .72 to .94. Test–retest rating agreements for a 2-week interval were as follows: spurning 60 %, terrorizing 100 %, corrupting/exploiting 87 %, and denying emotional responsiveness 46 %.

Validity. The PMRS accurately identified 82 % of mothers who were confirmed perpetrators of physical and emotional abuse or neglect. The scale correctly identified 92 % of psychologically maltreating mothers, but misclassified 29 % of mothers in the non-abusive comparison group as psychologically maltreating (Brassard, Hart, & Hardy, 1993).

Clinical Utility

Limited. The PMRS shows promise as a useful means for coding abusive parent–child interactions, but more research is needed to establish norms for community samples. Moreover, the time required for coding tapes might limit the usefulness in routine clinical practice.

Research Applicability

Moderate. The extensiveness and thoroughness of the PMRS is impressive. Interrater agreements and the stability of the scores are also promising. The PMRS is likely to prove useful in research settings where accurate depiction of the frequency, intensity and duration of abusive parenting is important.

Original Citations

Hart, S. N., & Brassard, M. R. (1990). Final report addendum: *Developing and validating operationally defined measures of emotional maltreatment.* NCCAN Research Grant final Report, HHS Grant ID# 90CA1216HART.

Hart, S. N., & Brassard, M. R. (1990). Psychological maltreatment of children. In R. T. Ammerman, & M. Hersen (Eds.), *Treatment of family violence: A sourcebook* (pp. 77–112). New York: Wiley.

Source

Marla R. Brassard, Ph.D., Department of Health and Behavior Studies, Teachers College, Columbia University, 525 W 120th St, New York, NY 10027, (212) 678-3368, mrb29@columbia. edu

Cost

Contact the source (above) for permission to use the PMRS.

Reference

Brassard, M. R., Hart, S. N., & Hardy, D. B. (1993). The Psychological Maltreatment Rating Scales. *Child Abuse and Neglect, 17*, 715–729.

Psychopathy Checklist-Revised (PCL-R)

Purpose

To assess antisocial and psychopathic behaviors and traits.

Population

Adults.

Background and Description

The original Hare Psychopathy Checklist was a semistructured interview that contained 22 items. Two items from the Hare Psychopathy Checklist were deleted, descriptions on several items were modified, and more detailed scoring instructions were included in the Hare Psychopathy Checklist-Revised (PCL-R). Construction, standardization, and validation involved 1,192 adult male prisoners and 440 adult male forensic psychiatric inpatients (Hart, Cox, & Hare, 1995). The PCL-R has subsequently been used with a variety of other populations (females, juveniles, and ethnic minority offenders), though no normative data have been reported for these specific populations.

The PCL-R is a semistructured interview designed to quantify the extent to which an individual meets prototypical criteria for the diagnosis as a psychopathic individual. Items are divided into three factors and coded after considering information gleaned from both clinical observations and collateral documentation (i.e., review of past records, collateral contacts with family members, etc.). Factor one contains eight items that code interpersonal-affective traits on narcissistic and exploitative dimensions. The author described these traits as capturing selfishness, callousness, and remorseless use of others. Factor-2 contains nine items that relate to unstable, impulsive, and antisocial behaviors. The author described these items as reflecting a chronically unstable, antisocial, and socially deviant lifestyle. Items on factor-1 and -2 are rated using a 3-point ordinal scale: (0) Item does not apply; (1) Item may apply or applies somewhat; or (2) Item definitely applies. Factor-3 scores are derived from combining factors-1 and -2 scores, as well as scores from three additional items. Factor-3 yields a total dimensional score that reflects the severity of psychopathic traits.

Administration

The semistructured interview component of the PCL-R requires up to 90 min to complete. An additional 60 min is allotted for the review of collateral information. The total amount of time required to complete the PCL-R is estimated to range from 2½ to 3 h. The PCL-R provides some flexibility to the examiner and 5 items can often be omitted without invalidating total scores.

Scoring

Items are summed to provide a final dimensional score on the construct of psychopathy that ranges from 0 to 40. Raw scores can be converted to percentile ranks and compared with normative data from prison and forensic populations. In addition, the PCL-R yields two factor scores that reflect two specific dimensions of psychopathy: interpersonal-affective traits (Factor-1) and criminal/impulsive/antisocial behavioral characteristics (Factor-2).

Interpretation

The PCL-R provides a dimensional score for traits related to psychopathy, rather than a categorical diagnosis of psychopathy. The manual acknowledges that diagnoses may be required and a cutoff score of 30 or higher on the PCL-R has been found to have an overall hit rate of .85, a specificity of .93, a sensitivity of .72, and a kappa of .67.

Psychometric Properties

Norms. Norms and psychometric properties were based on factor scores and total scores for seven samples of adult male prisoners ($N = 1,192$) and four samples of adult male forensic psychiatric patients ($N = 440$). The means and standard deviations for these samples are provided by Hart, Hare, and Harpur (1992).

Reliability. Coefficient alpha estimate for the 11 samples was .87, with a mean inter-item correlation of .25. A 1-month test–retest reliability study conducted with a sample of 88 adult males attending a methadone treatment program yielded a total score test–retest reliability coefficient of .89. Interrater agreements across various studies have yielded a kappa coefficient from .50 to .80. According to Hare (1991), the PCL and PCL-R may be viewed as parallel forms. Total scores on both measures have been found to correlate at .88 without attenuation for unreliable scales and .95–1.0 with attenuation for unreliable scales.

Validity. The PCL-R has good content validity, though the base rate of psychopathic symptoms for noncriminal populations may differ from the forensic populations on which the measure was normed. Accordingly, the reliability and validity of the items may be diminished somewhat with noncriminal populations. Hare indicates that preliminary data show that the PCL-R is still a useful tool for evaluating psychopathic symptoms in noncriminal populations, though the utility of the measure may be slightly diminished. The PCL-R is highly correlated with Cleckley's criteria for psychopathy, global clinical ratings for psychopathy, and antisocial personality disorder diagnoses. Numerous studies conducted in the USA and Canada indicate that the PCL-R performs better than other measures of psychopathology (Minnesota Multiphasic Personality Inventory and Antisocial Personality Disorder) in assessing future criminal behavior and risk for recidivism. Analyses of the two factor scales in the PCL-R indicate that the items have acceptable convergent and discriminant validity, as well as specificity for DSM-IV Axis I and Axis II Cluster B disorders. Evidence of construct validity is obtained from years of research by various investigators indicating the presence of abnormal physiological, behavioral, and emotional responsiveness to affective stimuli in persons categorized as psychopathic.

Clinical Utility

Moderate. The PCL-R is best suited to the assessment and description of psychopathic symptoms in the forensic populations on which it was developed. The PCL-R requires a considerable amount of time to administer and should be administered by professionals who received specific training in the use of the PCL-R. The PCL-R is not appropriate for the routine screening of non-forensic samples.

Research Applicability

High. The PCL-R is one of the most widely used instruments for evaluating psychopathy and predicting future criminal behavior. Research with the instrument suggests that the PCL-R provides an accurate assessment of the psychopathy construct.

Original Citations

Hare, R. D. (1985). A comparison of procedures for the assessment of psychopathy. *Journal of Consulting and Clinical Psychology, 53*, 7–16.

Hare, R. D. (1991). *Manual for the Hare Psychopathy Checklist-Revised*. Toronto: Multi-Health Systems.

Source

Information regarding the use of the PCL-R may be obtained from Multi-Health Systems, Incorporated, PO Box 950, North Tonawanda, NY 14120-0950, 1-800-456-3003.

Cost

A complete Hardcover Kit (includes PCL-R Manual, 1 Rating Booklet, 25 Quikscore Forms, and 25 Interview Guides) costs $250.00 US dollars. A Softcover Kit (contents similar to Hardcover Kit) costs $215.00 US dollars. Manuals and Rating Booklets may be purchased separately for $100 and $40, respectively. Quikscore Forms may be purchased separately in packages of 25 ($50) or 100 ($100). Interview Guides may be purchased separately in packages of 25 ($170) or 100 ($340).

Alternative Forms

The PCL-R is available in English, French, Spanish, Dutch, and Danish languages.

A shortened version of the PCL-R, the Hare Psychopathy Checklist-Screening Version (PCL-SV) exists to be used in research and applied settings because it requires less time to administer and score. Six items from Part I were derived from the PCL-R and assess the interpersonal and affective symptoms of psychopathy. Part II contains six new items that tap symptoms related to social deviance. Internal consistency is adequate, with Cronbach's alpha for the total score .84, and alphas of .81 and .75 for Parts I and II, respectively. A Spearman–Brown estimate of test–retest reliability for a 1-month interval yielded a correlation coefficient of .90. Interrater agreements between raters of seven validation studies yielded a mean weighted reliability coefficient of .84 for total scores, .77 for Part I, and .82 for Part II. Total scores on the PCL-SV and PCL-R yielded a mean weighted correlation of .80 (range=.55 to .84). Part I of the PCL-SV correlated higher with Factor-1 of the PCL-R (.68)

than it did with Factor-2 (.40) or PCL-R total scores (.61). Part II of the PCL-SV correlated higher with Factor-2 of the PCL-R (.81) than it did with Factor-1 (.48) or PCL-R total scores (.78). The PCL-SV is available in English, German, and Swedish (Hart, Cox, & Hare, 1995).

References

Hart, S. D., Cox, D. N., & Hare, R. D. (1995). *Manual for the Psychopathy Checklist: Screening Version (PCL:SV)*. Toronto, Canada: Multi-Health Systems.

Hart, S. D., Hare, R. D., & Harpur, T. J. (1992). The psychopathy checklist: Overview for researchers and clinicians. In J. Rosen & P. McReynolds (Eds.), *Advances in psychological Assessment*, Vol. 8 (pp. 103–130). New York, NY: Plenum Press.

Rape Conformity Assessment (RCA)

Purpose

To assess potential to commit rape.

Population

Adult males.

Background and Description

The Rape Conformity Assessment (RCA) was revised from a similar version presented by Schewe and O'Donohue (1993). It was designed as an outcome measure of rape prevention programs, and the authors sought to make the RCA less susceptible to social desirability response bias and more criterion-relevant. The RCA places a single participant in a room with two experimental confederates. A facilitated small-group discussion is held with participants publicly responding to 19 multiple-choice questions. Confederates always respond first with identical answers. Responses to the first two questions, which are non-rape related, reflect high base-rate content, and establish a history of agreement between the confederates and the participant. The remaining questions address sexual interactions and confederates' answers are biased toward justifying victimization. This procedure serves to create a norm of conformity that argues for victimization. The following are sample items.

- Once a couple has had sexual intercourse, then that issue is resolved and it is no longer possible for that man to rape that woman.
  (a) Yes   (b) No
- In World War II Russians raped German women. Given how the Russians suffered under the Germans, was this justified?
  (a) Yes   (b) No
- If I forced a woman to have sexual intercourse with me, she would probably begin to enjoy it.
  (a) Yes   (b) No

Administration

The RCA is estimated to take 35–45 min to complete. Following the procedures carefully is crucial in order to create a realistic atmosphere of conformity.

Scoring

The score consists of the number of times the respondent did not conform to the confederate response (i.e., the number of times the subject indicated that rape is not justified).

Interpretation

Higher scores indicate less potential to engage in rape.

Psychometric Properties

Reliability. In a sample of 19 undergraduate males, 2-week test–retest reliability was .78.

Cronbach's alpha was .84 and .83 for samples of 86 and 21 undergraduate men, respectively.

Validity. In a sample of 86 undergraduate men, scores on the RCA correlated positively with scores on the Acceptance of Interpersonal Violence (pp. 166–168), Adversarial Sexual Beliefs (Burt, 1980), and Rape Myth Acceptance (pp. 222–224) scales, but did not correlate significantly with Attraction to Sexual Aggression (Malamuth, 1989) or the Marlowe-Crowne Social Desirability Scale (Reynolds, 1982).

Clinical Utility

Limited. The RCA requires considerable time to administer and requires two confederates and one experimenter; therefore, the procedure is cumbersome to employ in a typical clinical setting. Additional research is needed to further establish age-based norms for both clinical and nonclinical samples.

Research Applicability

Moderate. The RCA disguises the purpose of the procedure and appears to diminish socially desirable responding. It may prove useful as a measure of sexually coercive thinking. However, additional psychometric data are needed.

Original Citation

Schewe, P. A., & O'Donohue, W. (1998). Psychometrics of the Rape Conformity Assessment and other measures: Implications for rape prevention. *Sexual Abuse: A Journal of Research and Treatment, 10*(2), 97–112.

Source

Paul A. Schewe, Ph.D., University of Illinois at Chicago, Department of Psychology, 1007

W. Harrison St., Chicago, IL 60607, (312) 413-2626, schewepa@uic.edu.

Cost

Contact the source (above) for additional information on the RCA.

Reference

Burt, M. (1980). Cultural myths and supports for rape. *Journal of Personality and Social Psychology, 38,* 217–230.

Malamuth, N. M. (1989). The Attraction to Sexual Aggression scale: Part one. *Journal of Sex Research, 26,* 26–49.

Reynolds, W. M. (1982). Development of reliable and valid short forms of the Marlowe-Crowne Social Desirability Scale. *Journal of Clinical Psychology, 38,* 119–124.

Schewe, P. A., & O'Donohue, W. T. (1993). Rape prevention: Methodological problems and new directions. *Clinical Psychology Review, 13,* 667–682.

Rape Myth Acceptance Scale (RMAS)

Purpose

To assess the degree to which an individual believes false information about rape, rapists, and rape victims.

Population

Adults.

Background and Description

The Rape Myth Acceptance Scale (RMAS) was designed to explore correlates of rape myth acceptance. The RMAS uses 19 items to measure beliefs about rape, rape victims, and rapists. Items are rated using a 7-point scale ranging from strongly agree to strongly disagree. Select items use a different rating scale. Two items are rated as almost all, about 3/4, about half, about 1/4, or almost none. One item uses the rating scale: always, frequently, sometimes, rarely, or never. Sample items follow.

• A woman who goes to the home or apartment of a man on their first date implies that she is willing to have sex.
• Any healthy woman can successfully resist a rapist if she really wants to.

Administration

The RMAS is estimated to take 4–7 min to complete.

Scoring

Several items are reverse scored, responses are then summed. Scores can range from 19 to 133.

Interpretation

Higher scores are indicative of greater adherence to rape myths.

Psychometric Properties

Reliability. Internal consistency, reported by Burt (1980), was estimated at .88. Subsequent studies using undergraduate students found alpha coefficients ranging from .82 to .87. Item–total correlations ranged from .27 to .62. Two-week test–retest coefficients using undergraduates ranged from .70 to .88.

Validity. Burt (1980) found RMAS scores correlated with sex role stereotyping, feelings about sexuality, adversarial sexual beliefs, and acceptance of interpersonal violence. The RMAS was related to measures of loneliness ($r = .39$), intimacy ($r = .68$), and hostility toward women ($r = .82$) in a sample of rapists (Marshall & Hambley, 1996).

Other research demonstrated the RMAS differentiated between male and female respondents and between non-rapists and convicted rapists. The RMAS was not correlated with the Marlowe-Crowne Social Desirability Scale (Reynolds, 1982; Schewe & O'Donohue, 1998; Spohn, 1993).

Clinical Utility

Moderate. Although normative data for relevant subsamples are not readily available, the RMAS can be used to assess treatment related changes in rape myth acceptance.

Research Applicability

Moderate. The RMAS is an efficient means to investigate the correlates of rape myth acceptance.

Original Citation

Burt, M. R. (1980). Cultural myths and supports for rape. *Journal of Personality and Social Psychology, 38*(2), 217–230.

Source

Martha R. Burt, Urban Institute, 2100 M ST NW, Washington, DC 20037-1264, (202) 261-5709, mburt@urban.org

Cost

Contact the source (above) for additional information regarding the RMAS.

Alternative Forms

The Illinois Rape Myth Acceptance Scale (IRMAS) was created to address some of the shortcomings of the original RMAS such as awk-ward wording and the inclusion of outdated rape myths (Payne, Lonsway, & Fitzgerald, 1999). The 45-item IRMAS has adequate reliability with Cronbach's alpha .93. A 20-item short version of the IRMAS (IRMAS-SF) was also developed that has adequate reliability, $\alpha = .87$ and is significantly related to the IRMAS ($r = .97$). The IRMAS and IMRAS-SF were related to the Acceptance of Interpersonal Violence scale (pp. 166–168) and other measures of violence.

The RMAS has been adapted for use in Korea. A translated and slightly modified version of the RMAS was used with professionals in Korea; it was found that rape myth acceptance was related to holding rigid sex role stereotypes, viewing violence against women as acceptable, and endorsing a double-bind sexual ethic Kim, 1989 as cited in Oh & Neville, 2004.

The Korean Rape Myth Acceptance Scale (KRMAS) was created to overcome some of the shortcomings of the RMAS such as awkward wording of items. The KRMAS contains 28 items and was found to have acceptable psychometric properties with 2-week test–retest reliability .87 and was related to correlates of violence against women such as sex role attitudes (Oh & Neville, 2004).

References

Kim, S. (1989). *Kangkan-e taehan tongny_om-ui suyong-e kwanhan y_on'gu* [Study of rape myth acceptance in Korea]. Unpublished master's thesis, Ewha Women's University, Seoul, Korea.

Marshall, W. L., & Hambley, L. S. (1996). Intimacy and loneliness, and their relationship to rape myth acceptance and hostility toward women among rapists. *Journal of Interpersonal Violence, 11*, 586–592.

Oh, E., & Neville, H. (2004). Development and validation of the Korean Rape Myth Acceptance Scale. *The Counseling Psychologist, 32*, 301–331.

Payne, D. L., Lonsway, K. A., & Fitzgerald, L. F. (1999). Rape myth acceptance: Exploration of its structure and its measurement using the Illinois Rape Myth Acceptance Scale. *Journal of Research in Personality, 33*, 27–68.

Reynolds, W. M. (1982). Development of reliable and valid short forms of the Marlowe-Crowne Social Desirability Scale. *Journal of Clinical Psychology, 38*, 119–124.

Schewe, P. A., & O'Donohue, W. (1998). Psychometrics of the Rape Conformity Assessment and other measures:

Implications for rape prevention. *Sexual Abuse: A Journal of Research and Treatment, 10*(2), 97–112.

Spohn, R. B. (1993). Social desirability correlates for acceptance of rape myth. *Psychological Reports, 73*, 1218.

Relationship Conflict Inventory (RCI)

Purpose

To assess the process and content of conflict in relationships.

Population

Adults.

Background and Description

The Relationship Conflict Inventory (RCI) was developed by the Task Force on Family Diagnosis of the Family Psychology Division of the American Psychological Association. The goals were to target areas of greatest conflict, to accumulate normative data on verbal and physical conflict, to create a hierarchical scale assessing the severity of verbal and physical conflict, to assess process as well as content of conflict, to assess frequency and distress level of conflict, and to create a concise, broad, and sensitive inventory for measuring changes in relationships. Forms of dysfunctional communication were reviewed to develop items.

The RCI is a 114-item self-report measure of verbal and physical conflict among couples. Items are written to focus on the occurrence and nature of the conflict and to avoid assignment of blame. The measure contains process (verbal and physical) and content scales. Process scales are written at less than an eighth-grade level and content items are written at a fifth-grade level. Items on the verbal and physical scales are ordered in an approximate hierarchy of seriousness. The 23 verbal conflict items are categorized into six areas: Communication Difficulties (6 items), Arguments (6 items), Painful/Deteriorating Relationship

(6 items), Distancing (2 items), Intimidation (2 items), and Separation (1 item). The 12 physical conflict items are grouped into six levels. (each with 2 items): Physical Coercion/Intimidation; Indirect Aggression; Physical Abuse (level I); Physical Abuse (level II); Physical Abuse (level III); and Use of Weapons (beyond the prior levels). The content items are clustered in nine categories: Activities, Change, Characteristics, Communication, Habits, Preferences, Relationships, Responsibilities, and Values.

Respondents indicate whether the conflict has occurred, rate the frequency of occurrence using a scale ranging from 0 to 20+ occurrences, and rate the degree of distress that was generated ranging from 0 ("no distress") to 6 ("extreme distress").

Administration

The RCI is estimated to take up to 40 min to complete.

Scoring

Scoring is based on weights and the number of items endorsed. A scoring form is provided with the instrument.

Interpretation

If scores are obtained from a couple, the degree of agreement may be ascertained between partners. Quantitative and qualitative assessment of individual data can indicate patterns in individual actions or interactions.

Psychometric Properties

Reliability. Reliability data for the RCI has not been published (Aldarondo & Straus, 1994).

Validity. Validity data were provided for the true/false version. The verbal conflict scores correlated positively with the verbal and physical scales of the Conflict Tactics Scale (pp. 177–180), the Global Distress and Problem Solving Communication Scales of the Marital Satisfaction Inventory (Snyder, 1979) and correlated negatively with the Cohesion and Adaptability Scales of the FACES II (Olson, Portner, & Bell, 1982). For females, the physical conflict scores correlated with physical conflict on the Conflict Tactics Scale, the Marital Satisfaction Inventory Global Distress and Problem Solving Communication scales, and FACES II Cohesion and Adaptability scales. For males, only the physical scale of the Conflict Tactics Scale correlated with the physical scale of the RCI. The relationship between conflict and dissatisfaction was found to be .74 in a sample of 21 men and women.

Clinical Utility

Moderate. The RCI is a comprehensive instrument that identifies processes and content of conflict that can be targeted by interventions. More research is needed to establish the psychometric properties of the instrument.

Research Applicability

Moderate. The RCI takes a considerable amount of time to complete and score, and therefore may not be well suited to research investigations with time constraints. However, the RCI may be useful in investigating the nature of intimate conflicts and their relationship to intimate partner violence.

Original Citation

Bodin, A. M. (1992). Relationship conflict inventory. Palo Alto, CA: Mental Research Institute.

Source

Arthur M. Bodin, Ph.D., 555 Middlefield Road, Palo Alto, CA 94301-2124. Phone: (650) 328-3000. The RCI may also be obtained online at http://www.familyandmarriage.com/rciusage.html

Cost

There is a usage fee of $50 for the RCI.

Alternative Forms

A sibling form, a truncated version of the RCI with dual Likert scales, was developed by the author for research on programs to reduce sibling conflict. A shortened version of the RCI exists that contains 35 items (Fernandez & Veshini, 2004).

References

Aldarondo, E., & Straus, M. A. (1994). Screening for physical violence in couple therapy: Methodological, practical, and ethical considerations. *Family Process, 33*, 425–439.

Fernandez, M. S., & Veshini, S. E. (2004). Child custody and divorce assessment: Strategies and inventories. In L. Sperry (Ed.), *Assessment of couples and families: Contemporary and cutting-edge strategies*. New York, NY: Brunner-Routledge.

Olson, D. H., Portner, J., & Bell, R. Q. (1982). *FACES II: Family Adaptability and Cohesion Evaluation Scales.* St. Paul, MN: Family Social Science, University of Minnesota.

Snyder, D. K. (1979). *Marital Satisfaction Inventory (MSI) administration booklet.* Los Angeles, CA: Western Psychological Services.

Risk of Eruptive Violence Scale (REV)

Purpose

To measure the general tendency to act violently and/or erupt into "sudden and unexpected episodes of violence."

Population

Ages 15 and older.

Background and Description

The rationale underlying the Risk of Eruptive Violence Scale (REV) is that outward appearances of quiet, withdrawn, and restraint behavior may mask seething anger and frustration. These pent-up emotions may subsequently "erupt" into violent action. The REV is a 35-item self-report measure assessing frustrated and pent-up urges toward violence. Items deal primarily with various persistent fantasies, including wishes to harm, injure, or destroy others. Respondents rate their level of agreement with each item using a 9-point scale. Sample items are as follows:

- People who know me well would not describe me as an angry person.
- If I had the ability, there are some people I definitely would hurt physically.

Administration

The REV is estimated to take 8 min to complete.

Scoring and Interpretation

Responses may be hand-scored or computer scored. Hand-scored responses are used to calculate a total-scale score. Computer scoring also provides percentile and z-scores. The REV manual provides detailed information on scoring and interpretation.

Psychometric Properties

Factor analysis. A principal components analysis of the 35 items in an undergraduate sample was conducted. A one-factor solution was interpreted, suggesting the REV is unidimensional.

Reliability. Internal consistency, as measured by Cronbach's alpha, was reported as .95.

Validity. Convergent, concurrent, and discriminant validity were assessed by comparing scores on the REV with violent history scores,

and scores on measures of aggression and empathy. REV scores correlated .71 with violent history scores and correlated positively with scores on the Brief Anger–Aggression Scale (pp. 101–103) and the Violence Risk Scale (Plutchik & van Pragg, 1990). REV scores correlated negatively with scores on the Balanced Emotional Empathy (Mehrabian, 1996) and Emotional Empathic Tendency scales (Mehrabian, 1997; Mehrabian & Epstein, 1972).

Original Citation

Mehrabian, A. (1996). *Manual for the risk of Eruptive Violence Scale.* (Available from Albert Mehrabian, 1130 Alta Mesa Road, Monterey, CA, 93940.)

Source

Albert Mehrabian, Department of Psychology, UCLA, 1130 Alta Mesa Rd, Monterey, CA 93940, (888) 363-1732, am@kaaj.com. Additional information may be found on the following website: http://kaaj.com/psych/scales/vio.html

Cost

Contact the source (above) for information on obtaining the REV.

References

Mehrabian, A. (1996). *Manual for the balanced emotional empathy scale (BEES).* (Available from Albert Mehrabian, 1130 Alta Mesa Road, Monterey, CA, USA 93940.)

Mehrabian, A. (1997). Relations among personality scales of aggression, violence, and empathy: Validational evidence bearing on the Risk of Eruptive Violence Scale. *Aggressive Behavior, 23,* 433–445.

Mehrabian, A., & Epstein, N. (1972). A measure of emotional empathy. *Journal of Personality 40,* 525–543.

Plutchik, R., & van Pragg, H. M. (1990). A self-report measure of violence risk, II. *Comprehensive Psychiatry, 31*, 450–456.

Sensational Interests Questionnaire (SIQ)

Purpose

To assess sensational interests in forensic and non-forensic populations.

Population

Adults.

Background and Description

Sensational interests have been described in case studies and anecdotal stories of seriously disturbed offenders and others bordering or meeting criteria for a mental illness. There is, however, a lack of systematic and rigorous research to explore this domain. The Sensational Interests Questionnaire (SIQ) was created to address this gap in the literature by providing a means of measuring sensational interests. Sensational interests were defined as interests that are vivid, exciting, savage, or violent. The original 60 pilot items for the SIQ were developed from clinical consensus by forensic clinical psychologists and from a paper presented by Brittain (1970). Additional items reflected normal activities and pastimes (e.g., reading).

The SIQ is a 29-item measure of sensational interests, consisting of five subscales: militarism, violent-occultism, intellectual activities, credulousness, and wholesome interests. The two primary scales are militarism and violent-occultism, which both share an interest in weaponry and a value of power over others. The remaining three scales were derived from the filler items. Respondents choose one of five responses (ranging from "great dislike" to "great interest") to describe their interest in the activity.

Administration

The SIQ is estimated to take 5–10 min to complete.

Scoring

Responses to each item are weighted from –2 ("great dislike") to +2 ("great interest"). Six scores can be calculated, one for each subscale and a total score. A total score is obtained by summing scores to 19 items (3–5, 7–10, 13, 14, 16–19, 22–25, 27, and 28). Scores for each of the five subscales are obtained by summing scores on each of the items forming the subscale. All total scores are then transformed into T-scores.

Interpretation

Higher scores on each of the subscales reflect a greater interest in activities represented by the subscale. Scores are compared to norms to facilitate interpretation.

Psychometric Properties

Norms. Normative data are available and can be obtained from Dr. Vincent Egan, East Midlands Centre for Forensic Mental Health, Arnold Lodge, Cordelia Close, Leicester LE5 OLE.

Factor analysis. Using a sample size of 301, and the original pool of 60 items, an exploratory factor analysis was conducted. Five factors were extracted, with 29 items loading substantially on the factors. Using these 29 items, a principal components factor analysis with varimax rotation was conducted and produced a single factor on which 20 items loaded significantly. The five factors were labeled: militarism, violent-occultism, intellectual recreation, credulousness, and wholesome activities.

Reliability. Reliability was assessed using 301 participants from outpatient referrals, inpatient referrals, and nonclinical individuals (i.e., fishermen, security guards, domestic assistants, teachers, nursing and clerical staff, and students). Additionally, a control group consisting of community people, ancillary workers, and support staff at university halls of residence, were utilized. Cronbach's coefficient alpha was used to assess internal consistency of each of the following subscales: militarism ($\alpha = .84$), violent-occultism ($\alpha = .77$), intellectual recreation ($\alpha = .75$), credulousness ($\alpha = .75$), and wholesome activities ($\alpha = .68$). The factor consisting of 20 items had an alpha coefficient of .84.

Validity. Subscales on the SIQ were correlated with measures of personality (i.e., the five factors of the NEO-Five Factor Inventory: neuroticism, agreeableness, conscientiousness, openness, and extraversion; Costa & McCrae, 1985), verbal IQ, and social desirability. Small to moderate, but statistically significant, correlations emerged. The total SIQ score correlated positively with neuroticism and negatively with agreeableness, conscientiousness, verbal IQ, and age. The militarism subscale correlated negatively with openness, agreeableness, verbal IQ, and age. The violent-occultism subscale covaried positively with neuroticism and negatively with agreeableness, conscientiousness, social desirability, verbal IQ, and age. The intellectual recreation scale correlated positively with extraversion, openness, agreeableness, and verbal IQ and negatively with neuroticism. The credulousness subscale correlated positively with openness and negatively with conscientiousness and age. The wholesome activities subscale covaried positively with age and negatively with neuroticism and verbal IQ.

A stepwise multiple regression analysis was employed to predict interest patterns, using the five personality traits on the NEO-FFI, verbal IQ, social desirability, and age. Higher scores on the violent-occultism subscale were predicted by low agreeableness, low conscientiousness, and younger age. High extraversion, low verbal IQ, and younger age predicted higher scores on the militarism subscale. High extraversion, lower agreeableness, low verbal IQ, and younger age predicted higher total SIQ scores. The authors of the SIQ noted that more individual factors were essential in predicting scores on the SIQ, as the

variance accounted for by the predictors for each of the listed subscales ranged from 13 % to 20 %. The SIQ, particularly the militarism and violent-occultism subscales, have also been associated with higher scores on sensation seeking; data have suggested that sensation seeking is a mediator between scores on the SIQ and measures of antisocial and borderline personality (Weiss, Egan, & Figueredo, 2004).

Clinical Utility

Moderate. The SIQ has been found to differentiate between normals and forensic populations. For example, normals are less interested in sensational topics in general (i.e., they have lower total scores on the SIQ) and less interest in activities represented by the militaristic and violent-occultism subscales.

It was suggested by the authors that property of an individual be examined and the SIQ scored based on such observations to crosscheck self-reported information and to monitor an individual's progress in eliminating deviant interests. The rationale behind this suggestion is that individuals surround themselves with property reflective of their interests.

Research Applicability

Moderate. The SIQ requires little time to complete and has potential for examining the prevalence and magnitude of sensational interests. The developers of the SIQ criticized the scoring system, suggesting that negative responses to some interests may cancel out positive response to others, thus creating artificially low scores. Additionally, the authors suggested the possibility that the SIQ is a measure of offense types, not psychopathology.

Original Citation

Egan, V., Auty, J., Miller, R., Ahmadi, S., Richardson, C., & Gargan, I. (1999). Sensational interests and general personality traits. *The Journal of Forensic Psychiatry, 10*(3), 567–582.

Source

Dr. Vincent Egan, Forensic Section School of Psychology, University of Leicester, 106 New Walk, Leicester, LE1 7EA, Phone: +44 (0)116 252 3658, Fax: +44 (0)116 252 3994, ve2@le.ac.uk.

Cost

Contact the source (above) for permission to use the SIQ.

Alternative Forms

The SIQ has been updated to include indicators of how important an interest is to an individual by asking about interest, knowledge, and importance for each item. The revised SIQ (SIQ-R) does not contain any filler items, and contains additional sensational interests (e.g., Green Berets, bomb making). The SIQ-R was found to contain three subscales: militarism, paranormal interests, and criminal identity. The subscales have good internal consistency, ranging from .78 to .92 and were found to significantly correlate with each other, suggesting the presence of an underlying sensational interests factor. Males have been found to have higher scores on the SIQ-R subscales militarism and criminal identity, and scores on the SIQ-R have been related to mating effort.

References

Brittain, R. P. (1970). The Sadistic Murderer. *Medicine, Science, and the Law, 10,* 198–207.

Costa, P.T., Jr., & McCrae, R.R. (1985). *The NEO Personality Inventory Manual.* Odessa, FL: Psychological Assessment Resources.

Egan, V., Charlesworth, P., Richardson, C., Blair, M., & McMurran, M. (2001). Sensational interests and sensation seeking in mentally disordered offenders. *Personality and Individual Differences, 30,* 995–1007.

Weiss, A., Egan, V., & Figueredo, A. J. (2004). Sensational interests as a form of intrasexual competition. *Personality and Individual Differences, 36,* 563–573.

Seventh Grade Inventory of Knowledge and Attitudes

Purpose

To measure adolescents' knowledge and attitudes about relational abuse.

Population

Adolescents.

Background and Description

The Seventh Grade Inventory of Knowledge and Attitudes was designed to evaluate an educational program (*Skills for Violence-Free Relationships; SVFR*) that teaches children definitions related to abuse and domestic violence, disseminates facts and dispels myths about battered women, and presents causes of battering. The program attempts to teach children skills to reduce the likelihood of them becoming an abuser or being a victim of abuse. The inventory was designed to reflect the goals of the SVFR program. Middle school was identified as a time to address the issue of relational abuse, as early- and pre-adolescents are beginning to develop their own intimate relationships.

The Seventh Grade Inventory of Knowledge and Attitudes is a 44-item self-report measure consisting of four sections: demographics, knowledge, attitudes, and safety plans. The demographics section consists of 6 items in which respondents circle a response or fill in answers. The knowledge section consists of 18 items in which respondents circle "True" or "False." The attitudes section consists of 12 items in which respondents rate their agreement, from "strongly agree" to "strongly disagree." The safety plans section consists of 8 free-response items. The measure was written at a seventh-grade reading level.

Administration

The Seventh Grade Inventory of Knowledge and Attitudes is estimated to take 35–45 min to complete.

Scoring

Knowledge items are scored by identifying the number of correct and incorrect responses, as identified by the authors. Attitude items are scored by comparing responses with the provided expected directions of each response.

Interpretation

Scores on the Seventh Grade Inventory of Knowledge and Attitudes provide an indication of current knowledge and attitudes about relational abuse.

Psychometric Properties

Reliability. Test–retest reliability was evaluated on a sample of 99 (57 male, 42 female), 12–14-year olds. The inventory was given 2 weeks apart. Spearman's rho was used to calculate correlations between the two administrations. The test–retest correlation for the knowledge scale was .57, and .67 for the attitude scale. Internal consistency of the knowledge and attitude scales was evaluated using Cronbach's alpha. For the knowledge scale, $\alpha = .32$. For the attitude scale, $\alpha = .72$.

Validity. Content validity was established by having 19 national experts, known for their work in the areas of domestic violence, child abuse, or child development, rate the acceptability of each item on a 5-point Likert-type scale (1 = not acceptable, 5 = indispensable). Ratings assessed the degree to which items revealed knowledge or attitudes toward battering. Ratings were averaged across judges. Comments from judges were

examined, and items revised, moved to a different scale, or eliminated before administering the inventory to respondents. All items on the inventory, with the exception of one, had mean ratings of 4 or higher.

Clinical Utility

Limited. The Seventh Grade Inventory of Knowledge and Attitudes has potential to be useful in evaluating programs designed to increase knowledge and change attitudes concerning abusive relationships. Further research needs to be done, however, to improve the psychometric properties.

Research Applicability

Limited. The Seventh Grade Inventory of Knowledge and Attitudes is still in its initial phases of development. Additionally, to increase the potential of generalization, the inventory should be administered to more diversified samples. Research could be done to improve the psychometric properties of the inventory, as well as to investigate the knowledge and attitudes held by adolescents regarding abusive relationships.

Original Citation

Rybarik, M. F., Dosch, M. F., Gilmore, G. D., & Krajewski, S. S. (1995). Violence in relationships: A seventh grade inventory of knowledge and attitudes. *Journal of Family Violence, 10*(2), 223–251.

Source

Rybarik, M. F., Dosch, M. F., Gilmore, G. D., & Krajewski, S. S. (1995). Violence in relationships: A seventh grade inventory of knowledge and attitudes. *Journal of Family Violence, 10*(2), 223–251.

Cost

Unavailable.

Severity of Violence Against Men Scales (SVAMS)

Purpose

To measure how serious, aggressive, abusive, violent, and threatening an act is when a woman does the act to a man.

Population

Adult men.

Background and Description

The Severity of Violence Against Men Scales (SVAMS) were developed to address the lack of measures assessing threatened, attempted, and completed behaviors likely to result in physical or emotional harm to a male. An additional concern was the need to develop an instrument that takes into account how sex based differences affect the physical and emotional implications of the violence. The SVAMS was designed as a counterpart to the Severity of Violence Against Women Scales (SVAWS. pp. 235–237) to assess female violence against males. Items on the SVAMS were developed by having men rate their perceptions (i.e., likelihood of physical and emotional harm) of the behaviors described on the SVAWS, except the behaviors were performed by a woman against a man.

Forty-nine behaviors cited in the violence literature were given to 587 male college students. Behaviors were representative of symbolic violence, threats of physical violence, actual violence, and sexual violence. Three items were dropped due to feedback indicating that they were not indicative of violence and may have had different connotations to males and females. The

46 remaining behaviors are identical to those used on the SVAWS.

The resulting SVAMS consists of 46 items that describe behaviors or acts with a component of physical threat done by a woman to a man. The described acts represent symbolic violence, threats of physical violence, actual violence, and sexual violence. Male respondents rate the frequency with which each act is committed by their female partners. The SVAMS can also be completed by females to rate how often they commit each act against their male partners. Two rating scales have been used depending on the assessment question. One format uses a 6-point scale ranging from 0 (never) to 5 (a great many times). A 10-point scale has also been used that elicits greater detail in the frequency of acts, with responses ranging from 0 (never) to 9 (almost daily). The SVAMS assesses three levels of threats (mild, moderate, serious), four levels of physical violence (minor, mild, moderate, severe), and sexual violence.

Samples of items are printed below.
- Hit or kick a wall, door, or furniture.
- Hold you down pinning you in place.
- Demand sex whether you wanted it or not.

Administration

The SVAMS is estimated to take 10–15 min to complete.

Scoring

SVAMS scores are calculated by assigning weights (mean severity score for aggressiveness, abusiveness, threat, and violence) to each of the items endorsed. Weights are obtained from the normative samples (student or community) cited in the original article (Marshall, 1992). Weights are multiplied by the frequency given for the item and summed to yield a score for each dimension. Additionally, values can be added to produce single scores for each of the two broad factors.

Interpretation

Higher scores are reflective of greater levels of severity in violent acts committed by a woman against a man.

Psychometric Properties

Norms. Impact weightings for college and community men are provided. These were derived from having males rate on 10-point scales how serious, aggressive, abusive, threatening, and violent the behavior was perceived. Males also rated the amount of physical harm and emotional/psychological harm they perceived the behavior to cause.

Factor analysis. Using scores from the five severity scales, exploratory factor analyses were conducted using maximum likelihood procedures with oblique rotation revealed an eight-factor solution accounted for 78 % of variance in severity rating scores. The factors were labeled as minor violence, threats of mild violence, sexual violence, moderate violence, threats of moderate violence, threats of serious violence, and serious violence. To support the eight-factor solution, alpha coefficients were calculated for each factor, mean scores on each factor were compared, and between and within-factor correlations were calculated. Results were consistent in supporting the eight-factor solution.

These results were replicated on a second sample consisting of 115 men, ranging in age from 18 to 82 years. A second order factor analysis, using maximum likelihood procedures, was conducted. From the eight dimensions, two higher order factors emerged: physical violence and threats of physical violence and sexual violence.

Reliability. Cronbach's alpha coefficients for the eight factors ranged from .93 to .95, indicating the factors had excellent internal consistency.

Validity. Results indicated that community men perceived acts more extremely than male students.

Clinical Utility

Moderate. Scores on the SVAMS do not allow actual effects, feelings, or injury to the victim to be determined. Nor do scores provide insight into the intent of the perpetrator. However, scores on the SVAMS can be used to help men track the increase or decrease of violence committed against them. Furthermore, the use of weighted scores has been shown to be effective in increasing men's acceptance of the impact of the behavior they sustained.

Research Applicability

Moderate. The author reported that the SVAMS has several uses in research: assessment of one violent incident or the comparison of violent incidents, the determination of escalating or decreasing violence, and a means of tracking violence received. Additionally, the SVAMS may be used in conjunction with the SVAWS to assess the impact of violence done to and done by the responder.

Original Citation

Marshall, L. L. (1992). The severity of violence against men scales. *Journal of Family Violence, 7*(3), 189–203.

Source

Linda L. Marshall, University of North Texas, Department of Psychology, 1155 Union Circle #311280, Denton, TX 76203, (940) 565-2339, linda.marshall@unt.edu.

Cost

Please contact the source (above) for permission to use the SVAMS.

Alternative Forms

A student version exists (SVAMS-S) which uses identical items but different weights. Additionally, community and student versions exist using the same items to assess perceptions of violence of men against women (SVAWS-S and SVAWS).

Severity of Violence Against Women Scales (SVAWS)

Purpose

To measure how serious, aggressive, abusive, violent, and threatening an act is when a man does the act to a woman.

Population

Adult women.

Background and Description

The Severity of Violence Against Women Scales (SVAWS) were developed to address the lack of measures assessing threatened, attempted, and completed behaviors likely to result in physical harm or to limit a woman's well-being. An additional concern was the need to develop an instrument that takes into account intent, and perceived intent, of the violent acts. The instrument originally consisted of 49 physical abuse-related behaviors which were frequently cited in the family violence literature. Items were worded in the third person to facilitate the development of a normative scale. Three items were dropped due to lack of agreement of whether the act was physically abusive or because of discrepancies concerning whether the act was positive or harmful.

The SVAWS consists of 46 items that describe behaviors or acts with a component of physical threat done by a man to a woman. The

described acts represent symbolic violence, threats of physical violence, actual violence, and sexual violence. Female respondents rate the frequency with which their male partners committed each act. The SVAWS can also be completed by males to rate how often they commit each act against their female partners. Two rating scales have been used depending on the assessment question. One format uses a 6-point scale ranging from 0 (never) to 5 (a great many times). A 10-point scale has also been used that elicits greater detail in the frequency of acts, with responses ranging from 0 (never) to 9 (almost daily). The SVAWS assesses four levels of actual physical violence (minor, mild, moderate, and severe), three levels of threats of physical violence (mild, moderate, and serious), and sexual violence. Samples of items are printed below:

- Threaten to destroy property
- Pull your hair
- Physically force you to have sex

Administration

The SVAWS is estimated to take 10–15 min to complete.

Scoring

SVAWS scores are calculated by assigning weights (mean severity score for aggressiveness, abusiveness, threat, and violence) to each of the items endorsed. Weights are obtained from the normative samples (student or community) cited in the original article (Marshall, 1992). Weights are multiplied by the frequency given for the item and summed to yield a score for each dimension. Additionally, values can be added to produce single scores for each of the two broad factors.

Higher scores are reflective of greater levels of severity of violence in acts carried out by a man against a woman.

Psychometric Properties

Norms. Impact weightings for college and community women are provided.

Factor analysis. The instrument was given to 707 female students. Using scores from the five severity scales, exploratory factor analyses were conducted using Maximum Likelihood procedures with oblique rotation. A nine-factor solution accounted for 80.6 % of variance in severity ratings. The factors were labeled as follows: minor violence, serious violence, threats of serious violence, sexually violent acts, symbolic violence, threats of moderate violence, threats of mild violence, moderate violence, and mild violence. To support the nine-factor solution, alpha coefficients were calculated for each factor, mean severity scores on each factor were compared, and between and within-factor correlations were calculated. Results were consistent in supporting the nine-factor solution.

These results were replicated on a second sample consisting of 208 women from the community, ranging in age from 19 to 75 years. Using the second sample, a second order factor analysis, using Maximum Likelihood procedures, was conducted. From the nine dimensions, two higher order factors emerged: physical violence and threats of violence. The physical violence factor consisted of minor, moderate, serious, mild, and sexual violence. The threats of violence factor consisted of serious and moderate threats, symbolic violence, and mild threats.

Reliability. Cronbach's alpha coefficients for the nine factors ranged from .92 (symbolic violence) to .96 (moderate threats, and mild, moderate, and serious violence), indicating the factors had excellent internal consistency. In a second sample of 208 women from the community, alpha coefficients for the nine factors ranged from .89 (symbolic violence) to .96 (mild and serious violence), indicating that the factors again had good to excellent internal consistency.

Validity. Results indicated that community women perceived acts more extremely than female students.

Clinical Utility

Moderate. Scores on the SVAWS do not allow actual effects, feelings, or injury to the victim to be determined. Nor do scores provide insight into the intent of the perpetrator. However, scores on the SVAWS can be used to help women track the increase or decrease of violence committed against them. The SVAWS weighted scores have also been used in clinical settings to emphasize the impact these behaviors have on an individual.

Research Applicability

Moderate. The SVAWS is useful for discriminating between nine dimensions of violence committed by men against women, as well as distinguishing between the effects of receiving physical violence, threats of physical violence, and sexual violence. The author reported that the SVAWS has several uses in research: assessment of one violent incident or the comparison of violent incidents, the determination of escalating or decreasing violence, and a means of tracking violence received. Additionally, the SVAWS may be used in conjunction with the SVAMS to assess the impact of violence done to and done by the responder.

Original Citation

Marshall, L. L. (1992). Development of the severity of violence against women scales. *Journal of Family Violence, 7*(2), 103–121.

Source

Linda L. Marshall, University of North Texas, Department of Psychology, 1155 Union Circle

#311280, Denton, TX 76203, (940) 565-2339, linda.marshall@unt.edu.

Cost

Please contact the source (above) for permission to use the SVAWS.

Alternative Forms

A student version exists (SVAWS-S) which uses identical items but weights obtained from college students. Additionally, community and student versions exist using the same items to assess perceptions of violence of women against men (SVAMS-S and SVAMS).

Sex Inventory (SI)

Purpose

To assess various aspects of sexuality, including sex interests, drives, attitudes, adjustment, conflict, cathexes, controls, and sociopathic tendencies.

Population

Adults.

Background and Description

The Sex Inventory (SI) was designed to aid in gathering information about actual or potential sex offenders. The inventory was developed from an atheoretical stance; items do not reflect one particular theory of sexuality. Sexuality was conceptualized as a non-static aspect of personality. Items on the SI were developed empirically using interview methods, personality inventory questions, and projective items. Initial items were used in pilot studies, allowing the author to clarify wording, semantic meaningfulness, and clinical significance of the items.

The SI is a 200-item, self-report measure of sexual deviancy. The inventory consists of nine scales, or factors: Sex Drive and Interest (Factor A), Sexual Maladjustment and Frustration (Factor B), Neurotic Conflict Associated with Sex (Factor C), Sexual Fixations and Cathexes (Factor D), Repression of Sexuality (Factor E), Loss of Sex Controls (Factor F), Homosexuality (Factor G), Sex Role Confidence (Factor H), and Promiscuity and Sociopathy (Factor I).

The SI consists of 40 subtle-indirect items and 160 obvious-direct items. Items were written at an eighth-grade reading level. Respondents are instructed to answer "true" or "false" to each item and are told that there is no penalty for omission of items. Many of the questions are worded such that a response of "true" is indicative of affirmation of a symptom of sexual deviance, whereas the remaining questions are worded such that a response of "false" is indicative of affirmation of a symptom of sexual deviance. After the initial administration, examiners should follow-up with a clinical interview, as the SI is used primarily for the purpose of gathering information.

Administration

The SI is estimated to take 45–60 min to complete.

Scoring

All items should be reviewed by the examiner to assess deviant or atypical responses, most notably on the Sexual Cathexes and Loss of Sex Control clusters. "Stop" items (i.e., items indicative of pathognomonic or antisocial deviances if answered positively) should be examined. Any noteworthy item should be followed by further inquiry.

Most factor scores are obtained by summing items that are marked in the direction indicated by the answer guide. The Sexual Fixations and Cathexes scale is not unidimensional and, therefore, should be interpreted qualitatively. The Repression of Sexuality Scale may be scored by splitting the scale items into their two clusters: repression of sexuality and conservative attitudes. The Homosexuality scale may be scored by splitting its items into two clusters: admission and denial of homosexual tendencies.

Interpretation

A qualitative appraisal of all items provides the following information: general level of sexuality, radicalism or conservatism of sexual attitudes, patterns of sexual cathexes, incidence of sexual sociopathies, and marker items suggestive of dangerous trends. Items endorsed on the Sexual Fixations and Cathexes scale are reflective of individual patterns of sexual expression. Endorsement of items on the Loss of Sex Controls scale is indicative of possibly socially dangerous symptoms in need of further investigation. Higher scores on the remaining scales reflect greater deviance from respective aspects of sexuality.

Psychometric Properties

Factor analysis. An original factor analysis produced the nine factors outlined in the description of the SI. In a second factor analysis using varimax rotation of 545 males, the same nine factors were obtained.

Reliability. The magnitude of interrcorrelations among subscales ranged from .01 to .67 for males and .00 to .63 for females. In a sample of 84 participants, test–retest reliabilities for a period of 3 months were reported for each factor: (A) .83, (B) .79, (C) .67, (D) .75, (E) .79, (F) .76, (G) .80, (H) .79, and (I) .75. Test–retest reliabilities over a 3 month period of individual items ranged from .00 to 1.00; 156 items had coefficients of .40 or higher, 124 items had coefficients of .50 or higher, and 14 items had coefficients of zero or nearly zero due to the lack of inter-subject variability (Thorne, 1966).

Validity. Scores on the Sex Drive and Interest and Promiscuity and Sociopathy scales of the SI correlated negatively with scores on the Sex-guilt

subscale of the Mosher Forced-Choice Guilt Inventory (Mosher, 1966). Scores on the Repression of Sexuality scale of the SI correlated positively with scores on the Sex-guilt subscale. The Sexual Maladjustment and Frustration, Loss of Sex Controls, and Homosexuality scales were found to differentiate between sexually deviant inmates and randomly chosen inmates. Additionally, the Sexual Maladjustment and Frustration and Loss of Sex Controls scales differentiated between sex offenders considered deviant and sex offenders not considered deviant.

Clinical Utility

Moderate. The SI appears to be a thorough inventory for collecting information about potential or known sex offenders. The format allows for easy follow-up questions about specific items in the context of a clinical interview.

Research Applicability

Moderate. The SI is rather lengthy to administer. Additionally, the breadth of topics it covers may make it less feasible to use if investigating a particular aspect of sexuality.

Original Citation

Thorne, F. C. (1966). The sex inventory. *Journal of Clinical Psychology, 22*(4), 367–374

Source

A full listing of the items can be found in Thorne, F. C. (1966). A factorial study of sexuality in adult males. *Journal of Clinical Psychology, 22,* 378–386.

Cost

Unavailable.

Alternate Forms

The SI has separate forms for male and female respondents.

References

Allen, R. M., & Haupt, T. D. (1966). The sex inventory: Test-retest reliabilities of scale scores and items. *Journal of Clinical Psychology, 22*, 375–378.

Cowden, J. E., & Pacht, A. R. (1969). The sex inventory as a classification instrument for sex offenders. *Journal of Clinical Psychology, 25*, 53–57.

Mosher, D. L. (1966). The development and multitrait-multi-method matrix analysis of three measures of three aspects of guilt. *Journal of Consulting and Clinical Psychology, 30*, 25–29

Thorne, F. C. (1966). A factorial study of sexuality in adult males. *Journal of Clinical Psychology, 22*, 378–386.

Sexual Adjustment Inventory (SAI)

Purpose

To assess attitudes and behaviors of accused or convicted sexual offenders.

Population

Accused or convicted adult sexual offenders.

Background and Description

The Sexual Adjustment Inventory (SAI) was developed to help fulfill the need for screening and assessment in criminal justice settings. The SAI is a 214-item, self-report measure of sexually deviant behaviors, and commonly associated problematic behaviors and attitudes (e.g., substance abuse). The SAI consists of 13 scales: 2 truth scales (Test Item Truthfulness, Sex Item Truthfulness), 5 sex-related scales (Sexual Adjustment, Child Molest, Sexual Assault, Exhibitionism, Incest), and 6 non-sex-related scales (Alcohol, Drugs, Violence, Antisocial, Distress, Judgment). Item format consists of true/false and multiple choice.

Administration

The SAI is estimated to take one hour to complete. It may be given as a paper-and-pencil measure or on the computer screen using optical scanners and human voice audio.

Scoring

Scores are computed on-site with a computer program and a printed report is provided. Reports summarize self-reported history, explain the scores, and offer specific score related recommendations. Scores reported as truth corrected are more accurate than raw scores.

Interpretation

Using truth-corrected scores, scores at or above the 90th percentile on the Sex Item Truthfulness and Test Item Truthfulness scales are inaccurate and indicate that the respondent may be minimizing problems or attempting to fake good. The higher score of these two scales is indicative of the greatest area of concern for the client.

For the remaining 11 scales, scores in the 70th percentile or higher indicate a problem in that area, with scores in the 90th percentile or higher indicative of severe problems. Risk classifications are as follows:

Low risk (0–39 %)

Medium risk (40–69 %)

Problem risk (70–89 %)

Severe problem (90–100 %)

It is suggested that a configural interpretation be utilized, examining the problems indicated by a particular scale as well as interactions between scale scores.

Psychometric Properties

Norms. The SAI has been standardized on thousands of sex offenders.

Reliability. Internal consistency was measured using Cronbach's coefficient alpha. The following are coefficients for each scale obtained from initial research and in a sample of sex offenders, respectively: Test Item Truthfulness Scale ($\alpha=.88$, $\alpha=.88$), Sex Item Truthfulness Scale ($\alpha=.85$, $\alpha=.85$), Sexual Adjustment Scale ($\alpha=.84$, $\alpha=.88$), Child (Pedophile) Molest Scale ($\alpha=.85$, $\alpha=.85$), Sexual (Rape) Assault Scale ($\alpha=.87$, $\alpha=.84$), Exhibitionism Scale ($\alpha=.84$, $\alpha=.89$), Incest Scale ($\alpha=.84$, $\alpha=.91$), Violence Scale ($\alpha=.89$, $\alpha=.85$), Alcohol Scale ($\alpha=.94$, $\alpha=.93$), Drugs Scale ($\alpha=.92$, $\alpha=.92$), Antisocial Scale ($\alpha=.86$, $\alpha=.89$), Distress Scale ($\alpha=.88$, $\alpha=.88$), and Judgment Scale ($\alpha=.84$, $\alpha=.82$). Alpha coefficients in other research reported by the publishers were all above .80.

Validity. In a sample of 3,616 sex offenders, offenders judged to have more severe problems (e.g., multiple offenses) scored higher on the Distress Scale than offenders with one or no sex-related arrests, supporting the discriminant validity of the SAI. Offenders scoring high on one scale tend to score higher on other scales, suggesting that offenders with sexual adjustment problems have other problems not related to sexual concerns. Scores on the SAI identified sex offenders with sex related and non-sex-related problems and risk ranges approximated those predicted from other sources of information, providing support for the predictive validity of the SAI.

Used diskettes are returned to the publisher and the data are downloaded into a database used for the purpose of ongoing research. The publishers provide an overview of reliability and validity studies conducted with the SAI (Professional Online Testing Solutions, Inc.).

Clinical Utility

High. The SAI has been used in assessment and screening of sexual offenders in court, probation, and correctional settings. The SAI has also been used to identify sexually deviate and paraphiliac behavior. Additionally, the SAI has been used to investigate attitudes and behaviors linked with inappropriate and illegal sexual acts (e.g., substance abuse, violent predispositions, antisocial thinking, feelings of distress).

Research Applicability

Moderate. Administration time makes the SAI inefficient in settings where there are time constraints. Additionally, the SAI covers a broad range of attitudes and behaviors. Specific measures relevant to research hypotheses may better provide needed data without the extraneous information obtained from using a more general measure such as the SAI.

Original Citation

Risk & Needs Assessment, Inc 2007. *Sexual Adjustment Inventory.* Retrieved June 28, 2009, from http://www.riskandneeds.com/TestsA_SAI.asp

Source

Risk & Needs Assessment, Inc., P.O. Box 44828, Phoenix, Arizona 85064-4828; Telephone: (602) 234-3506, Fax: (602) 266-8227; skarca@riskandneeds.com.

Cost

$8.00 per test (Diskettes contain 25 or 50 tests), volume discounts available.

Alternative Forms

A Juvenile Form of the SAI is available (SAI-J). The SAI-J contains 195 items that are organized into the same 13 scales as the original SAI. It has been found to possess adequate psychometric properties.

The SAI is available in Spanish.

Reference

Professional Online Testing Solutions, Inc. *Sexual Adjustment Inventory SAI: An inventory of scientific findings*. Retrieved June 2013, from http://www.riskandneeds.com/PDF/TestsA_SAI-Sci.pdf

Sexual Experiences Survey (SES)

Purpose

To assess sexual aggression and victimization from a dimensional viewpoint.

Population

Adults.

Background and Description

The Sexual Experiences Survey (SES) was developed to provide support for a dimensional view of sexual aggression and as a means to assess unreported incidences of rape and sexual aggression. The measure uses behaviorally specific language that has been shown to facilitate respondents' accurate reporting of rape incidents (Koss et al., 2007). The SES was revised by the SES Collaboration, a group of nine scholars with extensive experience using the SES in research. During this review process, four new versions of the SES were developed. Two long versions were created, the SES Long Form Perpetration (SES-LFP) and the SES Long Form Victimization (SES-LFV). Two short versions were also created, the SES Short Form Perpetration (SES-SFP) and the SES Short Form Victimization (SES-SFV). The two short versions of the SES most closely resemble the original SES (Koss, Abbey, Campbell, Cook, Norris, Testa, et al., 2006a; Koss, Abbey, Campbell, Cook, Norris, Testa, et al., 2006b).

The newer versions of the SES retained several characteristics of the original SES that were deemed to be valuable. These included: definitions of rape and attempted rape that were congruent with legal statutes, behavioral specificity, items to assess both perpetration and victimization, scoring to facilitate estimation of prevalence rates and incidence rates, evidence of acceptable psychometric properties, and brevity (Koss et al., 2007). Several items were rewritten to clarify item content and make items more behaviorally specific. Additionally, items were reworded to remove gendered language. Respondents are asked to report how frequently each behavior occurred in the past 12 months, and since the age of 14, using a 4-point scale ranging from 0 to 3. Sample items from the SES-SFV follows:

- Even though it did not happen, someone TRIED to have oral sex with me, or make me have oral sex with them without my consent by:
  - Telling lies, threatening to end the relationship, threatening to spread rumors about me, making promises I knew were untrue, or continually verbally pressuring me after I said I didn't want to.
  - Showing displeasure, criticizing my sexuality or attractiveness, getting angry but not using physical force, after I said I didn't want to.
  - Taking advantage of me when I was too drunk or out of it to stop what was happening.
  - Threatening to physically harm me or someone close to me.
  - Using force, for example holding me down with their body weight, pinning my arms, or having a weapon.

Administration

The SES is estimated to take 10–15 min to complete.

Scoring

Item-level scoring is used to estimate incidence rates. Ordinal level scoring is used to estimate prevalence rates.

Interpretation

Higher scores are indicative of more victimization experiences or more experiences as a sexual aggressor.

Psychometric Properties

Reliability. The SES victimization scales are conceptualized as induced models. In this type of model, observed variables are believed to combine to form a new variable that represents a set of experiences (Koss et al., 2007). The experiences do not necessarily correlate with one another, and thus internal consistency analyses are not appropriate. The SES perpetration scales can be conceptualized as induced models or latent models, depending on the assessment question. If they are conceptualized as latent models, internal consistency analyses would be appropriate. The revised SES scales are considered works in progress, and no reliability information has yet been published on the scales.

Validity. The revised SES scales are considered works in progress, and no validity information has yet been published on the scales. However, the revised SES scales retained many of the positive aspects of the original SES, and thus the validity evidence for the SES may apply to the revised SES scales. Scores on the original SES were used to classify women and men into four levels of victimization (nonvictimized, sexually coerced, sexually abused, and sexually assaulted) and sexual aggression (nonsexually aggressive, sexually coercive, sexually abusive, and sexually assaultive). These levels correlated .73 for women and .61 for men with responses obtained from individual interviews. Other data have shown that women who had experienced

rape gave consistent responses, regardless of the method (interview or self-report) used to obtain the information, whereas men tended to deny behaviors in an interview that they reported engaging in on the self-report SES (Koss, Gidycz, & Wisniewski, 1987).

Clinical Utility

Moderate. The original SES was a quick and efficient way to assess sexual victimization experienced by women. It had been used in a variety of clinical settings as a brief screening tool to identify women in need of further services or to identify risk factors. The new SES scales may fulfill these functions, but information on the psychometric properties of the scales is needed before widespread clinical use.

Research Applicability

Limited to Moderate. The original SES had been extensively used in research settings. It had been used to assess prevalence of rape, and also as a selection tool, predictor variable, and outcome measure in a variety of research settings (Koss et al., 2007). The new SES scales may be useful for these research purposes, but information on the psychometric properties of the scales is needed.

Original Citation

Koss, M. P., & Oros, C. J. (1982). Sexual Experiences Survey: A research instrument investigating sexual aggression and victimization. *Journal of Consulting and Clinical Psychology, 50*(3), 455–457.

Source

Mary P. Koss, Mel and Enid Zuckerman College of Public Health, University of Arizona, 1632 E Lester St, Tuscon, AZ 85719, (520) 626-9502, Fax: (520) 626-9515, mpk@u.arizona.edu.

Cost

Please contact the source (above) for permission to use the SES. There is no cost associated with use, but an agreement must be signed for use with group data collection.

References

Koss, M. P., Gidycz, C. A., & Wisniewski, N. (1987). The scope of rape: Incidence and prevalence of sexual aggression and victimization in a national sample of higher education students. *Journal of Consulting and Clinical Psychology, 55*, 162–170.

Koss, M. P., Abbey, A., Campbell, R., Cook, S., Norris, J., Testa, M., et al. (2006a). *The sexual experiences short form perpetration (SES-SFP)*. Tucson, AZ: University of Arizona.

Koss, M. P., Abbey, A., Campbell, R., Cook, S., Norris, J., Testa, M., et al. (2006b). *The sexual experiences short form victimization (SES-SFV)*. Tucson, AZ: University of Arizona.

Koss, M. P., Abbey, A., Campbell, R., Cook, S., Norris, J., Tessta, M., et al. (2007). Revising the SES: A collaborative process to improve assessment of sexual aggression and victimization. *Psychology of Women Quarterly, 31*, 357–370.

Spousal Assault Risk Assessment (SARA)

Purpose

To assess risk factors associated with re-assault in those committing spousal assault.

Population

Adults.

Background and Description

The Spousal Assault Risk Assessment (SARA) was developed to address concerns that there was a lack of well-validated measures for assessing risk of spousal violence. The 20 factors addressed in the SARA were developed from a review of the literature on risk for violence, risk for recidivistic violence specific to spousal assault, and clinical and legal issues. The authors reported that the SARA was developed as a checklist and is meant to be used as a guide to ensure all pertinent information is considered when assessing risk of re-offense.

The SARA is a manual providing recommendations for assessing risk for spousal abuse (e.g., training of evaluators, nature and extent of information that should be included in the evaluation, 20 risk factors, and recommendations for how to document and communicate judgments of risk). Items on the SARA are the 20 identified risk factors, which are grouped into five content areas: criminal history, psychosocial adjustment, spousal assault history, alleged (current) offense, and other considerations. The SARA consists of two parts. Part 1, which contains Factors 1 to 10, assesses general violence risk. Part 2, consisting of factors 11 to 20, assesses risk of spousal violence. Four options are available for scoring: (1) score the 20 risk factors using a 0–2 rating system (0 = absent, 1 = subthreshold, 2 = present), (2) score the 20 risk factors based on absolute presence (0 = absent, 1 = present), (3) score the 20 risk factors based on an evaluator's judgment of how many risk factors are critical (0 = absent, 1 = present), and (4) give an overall summary risk rating (0 = low, 1 = moderate, 2 = high). To evaluate the risk factors, the authors recommend using multiple sources (e.g., files and collateral contacts) and multiple methods (e.g., clinical and structured interviews, self-report measures). Interviews of offenders to assess factors should cover the following areas: childhood abuse and neglect, occupational and social history, relationship history, physical and mental health history, current mental status, history of assaultive/abusive behavior, criminal history, current life stressors, and current social support network.

Administration

It is recommended that qualified mental health professionals give the SARA, but others with adequate access to psychological reports may also complete the SARA.

Scoring

Four scores may be calculated for the SARA by summing scores for each of four scales. Total scores range from 0 to 40 and are obtained by summing ratings on items 1–20. Scores for number of factors present range from 0 to 20, as does the number of critical items (for these scores, items are coded as 0 = absent or 1 = present). Overall summary risk rating scores are qualitative; overall risk is assessed as low, moderate, or high.

Interpretation

Higher scores are indicative of a greater likelihood of re-assault.

Psychometric Properties

Reliability. Interrater reliability was assessed on 14 spousal assaulters by Kropp and Hart (1997). The authors reported obtaining correlations ranging from .64 to .95 for individual items. Interrater reliabilities (using Pearson *r* correlations) for the four score possibilities of sum of item scores, number of items present, number of critical items, and summary risk level were .92, .86, .66, and .80, respectively. Reliability was also evaluated on 2,681 adult male offenders (Kropp & Hart, 2000). Ratings of risk factors were made by correctional, mental health, and research staff. Internal consistencies, as calculated by Cronbach's alpha coefficients, ranged from .62 to .83 for total scores on the SARA, total scores on factors present and critical items, and total scores on Part 1 and Part 2. Interrater reliabilities ranged from .18 (critical items on Part 1) to .87 (Total score on Part 2). Interrater reliabilities were low for all critical item scores (total score, Part 1 and Part 2).

Validity. Criterion validity was evaluated by comparing offenders with and without histories of spousal assault and by comparing offenders who did and did not recidivate after treatment (Kropp & Hart, 2000). Data indicate that scores on the SARA differentiated between offenders with and without histories of spousal assault. Additionally, data indicated that recidivistic spousal assaulters were more likely to have been considered unsuitable for treatment, and scored higher on critical items and number of factors present than those who did not recidivate.

Concurrent validity was assessed by correlating SARA ratings with the Psychopathy Checklist-Screening Version (PCL:SV, pp. 220–222), Statistical Information on Recidivism (SIR, pp. 247–249), and the Violence Risk Appraisal Guide (VRAG, pp. 258–260). Critical items on the SARA did not correlate with any other measure scores. All measures correlated moderately with total scores on the SARA; specifically, the PCL:SV had moderate scores with Part 1 scores of the SARA and the SIR and VRAG had moderate to high correlations with Part 1 scores of the SARA. The above findings suggest that the SARA has adequate discriminant validity but only moderate construct validity.

The concurrent and predictive validity of the SARA was assessed using 88 male batterers convicted of spousal assault in Sweden (Grann & Wedin, 2002). SARA items found to be significantly related to increased risk of recidivism were past violation of conditional release or community supervisions; personality disorder with anger, impulsivity, or behavioral instability; and extreme minimization or denial of spousal assault history. The authors also reported that use of the SARA was marginally better than relying on chance to predict recidivism.

Clinical Utility

Moderate. The SARA is a comprehensive guide to assessing risk factors of re-assault in those committing spousal assault. Campbell, Sharps, and Glass (2001) reported that the SARA has been used in Canada and Vermont to aid in making probation, supervision, and treatment decisions. Additionally, the authors of the SARA argue that it is appropriate for use in pretrial, presentencing, correctional intake, correctional discharge, and civil justice contexts. Additionally, the authors provide a list of risk management strategies for items on the SARA.

The SARA, however, has some drawbacks. When interviewing in a legal context, information given by the offender is not confidential, and the offender may not give needed information; in such cases, reliance on other sources is crucial. The SARA relies on clinical judgment to assess risk factors, and reported interrater reliabilities have not been good for all items. Finally, without norms, scores are difficult to interpret in a given population.

Research Applicability

Limited. The SARA has not been used extensively for research purposes. Gathering information for the SARA may be a long process, requiring interviews, contact with other sources, and administration and scoring of other instruments.

Original Citation

Kropp, P. R., Hart, S. D., Webster, C. W., & Eaves, D. (1994). *Manual for the Spousal Assault Risk Assessment Guide.* Vancouver, BC: British Columbia Institute on Family Violence.

Kropp, P. R., Hart, S. D., Webster, C. W., & Eaves, D. (1995). *Manual for the Spousal Assault Risk Assessment Guide* (2nd ed.). Vancouver, BC: British Columbia Institute on Family Violence.

Kropp, P. R., Hart, S. D., Webster, C. W., & Eaves, D. (1998). *Spousal Assault Risk Assessment: User's guide.* Toronto: Multi-Health Systems, Inc.

Source

The BC Institute Against Family Violence, Suite 551 - 409 Granville Street, Vancouver, BC V6C 1T2; Telephone: (604) 669-7055' Toll free (Canada): 1-877-755-7055, Fax: (604)

669-7054. The SARA may also be purchased online from Psychcorp: http://www.psychcorp. co.uk/product.aspx?n=1316&s=1322&cat=14 26&skey=3756

Cost

The complete kit, which includes the manual, 25 checklist forms, and 25 Quikscore forms costs $75 (Canadian).

Alternative Forms

The SARA was modified for use by police. Modifications included changing the order in which the SARA is completed, developing an interview guide, eliminating the critical risk factors system, and revising the language to better suit the law enforcement context. The B-SAFER has two sections (spousal assault and psychosocial adjustment) and 10 risk factors (Belfrage, 2008). It has been translated into Swedish and Norwegian (Grann & Wedin, 2002).

References

Belfrage, H. (2008). Police-based structured spousal violence risk assessment: The process of developing a police version of the SARA. In A. C. Baldry & F. W. Winkel (Eds.), *Intimate Partner Violence Prevention and Intervention.* New York: Nova Science Publishers, Inc.

Campbell, J. C., Sharps, P., & Glass, N. (2001). Risk assessment for intimate partner homicide (pp. 136–157). In G. Pinard & L. Pagani (Eds.), *Clinical assessment of dangerousness: Empirical contributions.* Cambridge, UK: Cambridge University Press.

Grann, M., & Wedin, I. (2002). Risk factors for recidivism among spousal assault and spousal homicide offenders. *Psychology Crime & Law Special Issue: Swedish Studies on Psychology, Crime and Law, 8*(1), 5–23.

Kropp, P. R., & Hart, S. D. (2000). The Spousal Assault Risk Assessment (SARA) Guide: Reliability and validity in adult male offenders. *Law and Human Behavior, 24*(1), 101–118.

Kropp, P. R., & Hart, S. D. (1997). Assessing risk of violence in wife assaulters: The Spousal Assault Risk Assessment Guide (pp. 302–325). In C. D. Webster & M. A. Jackson (Eds.), *Impulsivity: Theory, assessment, and treatment.* New York, NY: The Guilford Press.

Stalking Victimization Survey

Purpose

To assess various aspects of stalking

Population

Adults.

Background and Description

Items on the Stalking Victimization Survey were compiled from two sources: the Violence and Threats of Violence Against Women in America Survey (Tjaden & Thoennes, 1998) and the HARASS instrument (Sheridan, 1998). As defined by the authors in the original citation, the Stalking Victimization Survey was designed to answer the following fundamental questions: "How much stalking is there in the United States, who stalks whom, how often do stalkers overtly threaten their victims, how often is stalking reported to the police, and what are the psychological and social consequences of stalking?"

The Stalking Victimization Survey is an 18-item self-report measure of various aspects of stalking. Respondents answer either yes or no to each item. Content of the items address the following topics: being followed or spied on, being sent unsolicited letters or written correspondence, finding the perpetrator standing outside the victim's home, school, or workplace, threats by the abuser to harm children or commit suicide if the woman left the relationship, leaving scary notes on the woman's car, and threatening the family.

Administration

The Stalking Victimization Survey is administered to groups of people and is estimated to take 5–10 min to complete.

Scoring and Interpretation

Items are scored qualitatively and percentages calculated for each item across respondents.

Psychometric Properties

Reliability. In a sample of 100 participants, Cronbach's coefficient alpha for the 18 questions was .83.

Validity. To establish content validity, a panel of experts reviewed items. Stalking was found to be related to physical or sexual assault by the partner who stalked.

Clinical Utility

Limited. The survey is not designed for individual assessment. It is intended for assessment of prevalence and characteristics of stalking in groups of people.

Research Applicability

Moderate. The Stalking Victimization Survey is a time-efficient, easily scored survey that can be used to assess characteristics of stalking, which can provide information in treatment planning and implementation.

Original Citation

Tjaden, P., & Thoennes, N. (1998). *Stalking in America: findings from the National Violence Against Women Survey* (National Institute of Justice and Centers for Disease Control and Prevention Grant No. 93-IJ-CX-0012). Washington, DC: Department of Justice, National Institute of Justice.

Source

National Institute of Justice and Centers for Disease Control and Prevention Grant No. 93-IJ-

CX-0012). Washington, DC: Department of Justice, National Institute of Justice.

Cost

Contact the source (above) for permission to use the Stalking Victimization Survey.

References

Sheridan, D. (1998). *Measuring harassment of battered women: A nursing concern*. Unpublished doctoral dissertation, Oregon Health Science University.

McFarlane, J., Willson, P., Malecha, A., & Lemmey, D. (2000). Intimate partner violence: A gender comparison. *Journal of Interpersonal Violence, 15*(2), 158–169.

Statistical Information on Recidivism (SIR)

Purpose

To predict the likelihood of recidivism of released offenders.

Population

Adult, non-native males.

Background and Description

The Statistical Information on Recidivism (SIR) was developed to aid parole boards in Canada in making parole decisions. The SIR is also referred to as the Recidivism Prediction Score (RPS) or the General Statistical Information on Recidivism (GSIR). The National Parole Board in Canada requested an investigation to determine the factors that parole boards used to make parole decisions. There were concerns that risk prediction involved no clear criteria to guide decision making, resulting in inconsistent decision making.

Using these factors as a guideline, the researchers were asked to develop guidelines for the future. The data indicated individuals at low risk for re-offense were not being granted parole at a rate as high as would be predicted by statistical techniques alone. Such a finding prompted the idea that statistical information on the likelihood of recidivism would be useful in making parole decisions.

Using a sample of 2,475 male inmates who were released from Canadian federal penitentiaries between the years 1970 and 1972, researchers collected re-offense data for a period of 3 years. Using statistical techniques, 15 variables were identified as related to general recidivism. These variables were weighted to create a model for predicting recidivism. The model was cross-validated on a second sample to demonstrate its stability.

The SIR is a statistical technique that combines demographic characteristics and criminal history to predict re-offense rates. Criminal history factors examined include offense type, aggregate sentence length, security classification and escape history, age at first adult conviction, record of previous incarceration and breaches of supervision, previous convictions for assault, violent sex offenses, breaking and entering, and time at risk since last offense. Social background factors that are considered include age, marital status, number of dependents, and employment status at time of last offense.

Scores for each factor are assigned by examining the average base rate of recidivism. For every difference of 5 % from the average base rate, the individual receives a score of ±1 for that factor. Scores on the SIR range from –27 to 30. Score ranges represent categories ranging from Very Good Risk (i.e., low risk of re-offending within 3 years) to Poor Risk (i.e., high risk of re-offending within 3 years).

Administration

The SIR may be completed by interviewing the offender and reviewing the offender's file.

Scoring

Scores on the SIR are calculated by summing scores on individual items.

Interpretation

Higher scores on the SIR are indicative of greater risk of recidivism. Categories associated with score ranges are listed below, along with the probability that the released offender will not re-offend.

Category	Score range	Percentage of those expected to not re-offend
Very good	−6 to −27	80
Good	−1 to −5	66
Fair	0 to 4	50
Fair to Poor	5 to 8	40
Poor	9 to 30	33

Psychometric Properties

Reliability. Agreement rate between the SIR classifications provided by researchers and the decisions made by parole office staff on 202 inmates was 85 %. In a set of scores ranging from −15 to 21, agreement ratings between total scores was 52 %. When scores were grouped into the five probability levels of risk for general recidivism, agreement ratings between scores was 85 %. Low agreement was found on the following items: previous convictions for break and enter, interval at risk, and age at first adult conviction.

Validity. Bonta, Harman, Hann, & Cormier (1996) sought to determine more current base rates to improve the accuracy in prediction using the SIR. Using a sample of 3,267 inmates released from federal penitentiaries between 1983–1984, they collected information on general personal and social demographic factors, and offense data.

The SIR scale was slightly modified for the study, as two items (Number of Dependents and Employment Status) were unavailable. The correlation between SIR scores and recidivism was $r = .42$. Base rates of violent behavior were only slightly higher than in original study. Data revealed that all items predicted recidivism except for Previous Conviction for Violent Sex Offense, which was argued to be retained as it would predict narrowly defined violent recidivism. Analyses supported the original cutoff scores.

Other studies have produced similar patterns of results as the original data and continue to support the ability of the SIR to predict re-offense rates. Additionally, the SIR was compared to four other risk prediction instruments and was found to be equal to or marginally superior to the alternative instruments, with prediction accuracy of the five instruments ranging from 68.8 % to 74.1 % (Duguid & Pawson, 1998; Serin, 1996; Wormith & Goldstone, 1984).

The SIR has not been shown to be reliable for prediction of re-offense in Canadian Natives and women. Particularly for women, the relationship between SIR and post-release recidivism is weaker and less uniform than it is for men.

Clinical Utility

Moderate. The SIR has been criticized because it is not appropriate for women and Canadian Natives, because it provides no data on dynamic risk factors that could be targeted for intervention, and because it was not designed to predict individual behavior (due to its development from aggregate data). However, the SIR has been demonstrated to be a stable predictor of general recidivism and to have the ability to differentiate between low and high-risk inmates. Additionally, studies have found that clinical judgments (i.e., the decisions to grant parole) have generally been in agreement with SIR scores.

Research Applicability

High. The SIR has been used to evaluate programs such as Cognitive Living Skills and vocational training. Additionally, there is potential to expand the SIR by examining dynamic risk factors to improve prediction and to modify the SIR to make it more applicable to women and Canadian Natives.

Original Citation

Nuffield, J. (1982). *Parole decision-making in Canada.* Ottawa, Ontario: Communication Division, Solicitor General Canada.

Source

Joan Nuffield, Solicitor General of Canada, 340 Laurier Avenue West, Ottawa, Ontario K1A 0P8, Canada.

Cost

Please contact the source (above) for permission to use the SIR.

Alternative Forms

The SIR has been revised. The SIR-R1 has been found to be internally reliable and valid at predicting general and violent recidivism in male, adult offenders. The SIR-R1 has also been adapted for use with female offenders and aboriginal offenders in Canada. This adapted measure, the SIR-Proxy, was found to highly correlate with the SIR-R1 and was found to predict post-release outcome in female offenders. However, it was not found to have predictive validity for aboriginal male offenders (Nafekh & Motiuk, 2002).

References

Bonta, J., Harman, W. G., Hann, R. G., & Cormier, R. B. (1996). The prediction of recidivism among federally sentenced offenders: A revalidation of the SIR scale. *Canadian Journal of Criminology, 38*(1), 61–79.

Duguid, S., & Pawson, R. (1998). Education, change, and transformation: The prison experience. *Evaluation Review, 22*(4), 470–495.

Nafekh, M., & Motiuk, L. L. (2002). *The statistical information on recidivism – Revised 1 (SIR-R1) Scale: A psychometric examination.* Ottawa, Ontario: Research Branch Correctional Service of Canada. Retrieved from http://www.csc-scc.gc.ca/text/rsrch/reports/r126/r126_e.pdf

Serin, R. C. (1996). Violent recidivism in criminal psychopaths. *Law and Human Behavior, 20,* 207–217.

Wormith, J. S., & Goldstone, C. S. (1984). The clinical and statistical prediction of recidivism. *Criminal Justice and Behavior, 11*(1), 3–34.

Subtle and Overt Psychological Abuse of Women Scale (SOPAS)

Purpose

To assess instances of psychological abuse committed by men against their female partners.

Population

Adult women.

Background and Description

The Subtle and Overt Psychological Abuse of Women Scale (SOPAS) was designed to measure a variety of forms of psychological abuse previously identified in the literature, but not measured by existing abuse measures. It replaced the Men's Psychological Harm and Abuse in Relationships Measure—Overt scales and Subtle scales (Marshall, 1999). Items were written so that the intent of the male partner in committing the act could be variable (loving, joking, serious, or overtly abusive). An initial item pool comprised of 184 items was administered to a sample of low-income, ethnically diverse women. Items with too high (>50 %) or too low (<15 %) endorsement rates were eliminated. A long and a short version of the SOPAS were developed. The long version contains 65 items measuring overt and subtle forms of psychological abuse, whereas the short form contains 35 items.

Respondents are asked to rate how often their partners engage in the listed behaviors. Several response formats have been used, depending on the assessment question. When using the SOPAS with battered women, a 12-point response format is recommended that ranges from 0 (never) to 11 (several times a day). For other samples, a 6-point scale ranging from 0 (never) to 5 (a great many times) or a 10-point scale ranging from 0 (never) to 9 (almost daily) may be used, depending on the detail in frequency of acts desired. Sample items follow.

- Play games with your head.
- Make you feel guilty about something you have done or have not done.
- Act like he owns you.

Administration

The SOPAS takes approximately 10–15 min to complete.

Scoring

Items are summed.

Interpretation

Higher scores indicate a greater frequency of experiencing psychological abuse.

Psychometric Properties

Factor analysis. Factor analyses were done separately for the overt psychological abuse items and the subtle psychological abuse items for the long version of the SOPAS. Factor analysis of the overt psychological abuse items revealed four interpretable, independent factors: dominate, indifference, monitor, and discredit. A three-factor solution was found for the subtle psychological abuse items: undermine, discount, and isolate.

Principal axis and maximum likelihood analyses with varimax and oblique rotations were used to examine the factor structure of the SOPAS in an independent sample of 172 women. Both analyses identified a one-factor solution. A rational approach was then undertaken wherein experts were asked to sort the items into the seven scales identified by Marshall (1999). Items were successfully placed into six of the seven scales (12 items were deleted because they were unable to be reliably placed into a scale). A maximum likelihood factor analysis was then performed on the reduced scale and indicated a one-factor solution (Jones, Davidson, Bogat, Levendosky, & von Eye, 2005).

Reliability. Test–retest reliability was assessed with 395 women. Two year test–retest reliability ranged from $r = .64$ to $.72$ (wave 1 to wave 2 data) and $r = .51$ to $.61$ (wave 2 to wave 5 data). Four year test–retest reliability ranged from $r = .41$ to $.60$.

In a sample of 172 women, Cronbach's alpha was .98 for the total score of the reduced scale (SOPAS after the elimination of 12 items that could not be reliably categorized into one of the seven theoretical dimensions). Cronbach's alpha for the six subscales of the reduced scale ranged from .80 (monitor) to .97 (dominate) (Jones et al., 2005).

Validity. The SOPAS subscales of the long version were correlated with violent acts and sexual aggression to examine construct validity. The correlations between SOPAS subscales and violent acts ranged from $r = .25$ to $.36$, and the correlations between SOPAS subscales and sexual aggression ranged from $r = .23$ to $.33$. Regression analyses were performed to examine the ability of the SOPAS scales to predict women's state (i.e., self-esteem, stress, health quality, emotional distress, severe depression, suicidal ideation) and relationship well-being. The subtle psychological abuse scale explained the most variance in women's state, and explained more variance in relationship well-being than the overt psychological abuse scale.

A series of hierarchical regressions were conducted that indicated subtle psychological abuse significantly predicted women's state and relationship well-being even after controlling for overt psychological abuse and men's violence and sexual aggression.

The discriminant validity of the SOPAS long version was examined in a sample of 172 women. The SOPAS was intended to measure a form of psychological abuse distinct from that measured by other abuse measures. The SOPAS was significantly related to the dominance and verbal/emotional subscales of the Psychological Maltreatment of Women Inventory (PMWI; pp. 218–220), and the psychological abuse scale of the Severity of Violence Against Women Scale (SVAWS; pp. 235–237), thus failing to provide evidence of discriminant validity. The correlations between the SOPAS and external criteria were expected to have a unique pattern relative to correlations between other abuse measures and external criteria. This was examined by correlating the SOPAS, PMWI and SVAWS with depression, self-esteem, and relationship measures. The results indicated the SOPAS and PMWI had similar correlations with external variables.

Clinical Utility

Moderate. The SOPAS is brief, easy to administer, and may be a useful tool for assessing instances of overt or subtle psychological abuse women experience from their intimate partners. The psychometric properties of the SOPAS have not been extensively researched and available validity data have not consistently supported the SOPAS as measuring a form of abuse distinct from that measured by other abuse measures. Further evidence of validity and reliability would enhance the clinical utility of the measure.

Research Applicability

Moderate. The SOPAS may be useful in exploring the dimensionality of psychological abuse. Further information is needed on the factor structure and psychometric properties of the SOPAS.

Original Citation

Marshall, L. L. (1996). *Subtle and Overt Psychological Abuse Scale.* Unpublished manuscript.

Marshall, L. L. (1999). Effects of men's subtle and overt psychological abuse on low-income women. *Violence and Victims, 14,* 69–88.

Source

Linda L. Marshall, University of North Texas, Department of Psychology, 1155 Union Circle #311280, Denton, TX 76203, (940) 565-2339, linda.marshall@unt.edu.

Cost

Please contact the source (above) for permission to use the SOPAS.

Reference

Jones, S., Davidson II, W. S., Bogat, G. A., Levendosky, A., & von Eye, A. (2005). Validation of the Subtle and Overt Psychological Abuse Scale: An examination of construct validity. *Violence and Victims, 20,* 407–416.

Tolerance Toward Violence Scale

Purpose

To measure tolerance toward violence.

Population

Adults.

Background and Description

The Tolerance Toward Violence Scale was developed to understand the processes and mechanisms that underlie different forms of aggression by the use of constructs that are more specific than aggression. It was an adaptation of a similar measure created in Italian. The measure appears to assess tolerance to varying forms of violence rather than one specific form. The Tolerance Toward Violence Scale is a 29-item scale. Three of the items are control items to avoid response-set effects. Respondents rate how true each statement is of them or their behavior using a 6-point scale ranging from 0 (completely false for me) to 5 (completely true for me). Sample items follow.

- Because of its idealistic motivation, political violence is different from common violence and can be condoned more easily.
- Women who suffer from violence are always at least in part responsible for it.

Administration

The questionnaire takes approximately 10 min to complete.

Scoring

Scores are summed across items for a total score. Scores on individual items can also be evaluated.

Interpretation

Higher scores indicate stronger tolerance toward violence.

Psychometric Properties

Factor analysis. Principal components analysis revealed two factors accounting for 18.9 % and 6.7 % of the total variance, respectively. When examining the latent factorial structure, two rotations were performed on the basis of the two extracted components; neither led to a simple structure.

Reliability. The reliability coefficient calculated using Cronbach's alpha was .81. The reliability

coefficient calculated using split-half reliability was .74.

Validity. Support for the construct validity of the measure was evidenced by the correlations with the Irritability scale ($r =.39$) and Dissipation–Rumination scale ($r =.44$, pp. 121–123). Tolerance toward violence was also associated with a greater history of involvement in violent incidents. These findings were similar to those found for the Italian version of the scale.

Clinical Utility

Limited. This measure has not been widely used within clinical settings and evidence of the measure's psychometric properties is limited.

Research Applicability

Limited. The Tolerance Toward Violence Scale has not been widely studied or used in research investigations. Additional information on the psychometric properties of the measure is needed.

Original Citation

Caprara, G. V., Cinanni, V., & Mazzotti, E. (1989). Measuring attitudes toward violence. *Personality and Individual Differences*, 10(4), 479–481.

Source

Gian V. Caprara, Department of Psychology, Sapienza University of Rome, Piazzale Aldo Moro 5, 00185 Roma, Italia, phone (064) 991-7532, gianvittorio.caprara@uniroma1.it.

Cost

Please contact the source (above) for permission to use the Tolerance Toward Violence Scale.

Alternative Forms

The Tolerance Toward Violence Scale is available in English and Italian.

Victimization Screening Form

Purpose

To assess the risk of future injury at the time of adolescent health maintenance visits.

Population

Adolescents.

Background and Description

The Victimization Screening Form was developed to determine which screening questions used in routine adolescent health care maintenance visits would correlate with subsequent violence-related injury. Data were initially collected based on adolescent health intake forms in medical records. The primary outcome measure, time until first violence-related injury, was determined through identification on chart review of the treatment of any such injuries at the urgent care center at the health clinic in the subsequent 10 years.

The Victimization Screening Form is a 3-item screening instrument used to evaluate the risk of future injury. The measure is a simple screening instrument that consists of items concerning school status, drug use, and fighting history to classify youth into low, moderate, and high risk of violence-related injury during the follow-up period. A sample question is provided:

• In how many fights have you been within the past year?

Administration

It is estimated that the Victimization Screening Form requires less than a minute to complete.

Scoring

Responses are summed.

Interpretation

The classification scheme places individuals who are not in school or in danger of failing school at high risk, as well as those with one of the two risk factors (drug use or any fights in the past year). Individuals with one risk factor are considered to be at moderate risk, and those with no risk factors are at low risk.

Psychometric Properties

Norms. Normative data were collected on 317 adolescent patients visiting an urgent care health center.

Reliability. Reliability data have not been published for the Victimization Screening Form. Internal consistency analysis may not be appropriate for this measure, as it consists of only three items.

Validity. Data were collected on 430 adolescent patients. During the follow-up period, 12 % of these patients had one or more violence-related injuries resulting in an urgent care visit to a health center. Complete data were available for 317 patients, 38 of whom had been treated for an intentional injury (12 %). Of the 113 patients with incomplete data, 11 (9.7 %) had recorded intentional injuries. Male gender, cigarette smoking, alcohol use, other drug use, poor relationships with parents, not being in school or failing school, and history of fighting in the past year predicted violence-related injury within the follow-up period. The incidence of subsequent injury was correlated with the number of fights in the year preceding the office visit. This effect was observed within the first year of follow-up and continued throughout the study period.

Clinical Utility

Moderate. This brief measure has not been widely used in clinical settings or with additional populations. However, it has demonstrated limited predictive validity and may be useful in identifying individuals at high risk of subsequent violence-related injury.

Research Applicability

Limited. This measure has not been widely used in the research literature. Additional information on the psychometric properties of the Victimization Screening Form is needed.

Original Citation

Sege, R., Stringham, P., Short, S., & Griffith, J. (1999). Ten years after: Examination of adolescent screening questions that predict future violence-related injury. *Journal of Adolescent Health, 24*, 395–402.

Source

Dr. Robert Sege, The Institute for Clinical Research and Health Policy Studies, Tufts Medical Center, 800 Washington St, Tufts MC #63, Boston, MA 02111, Robert.-sege@bmc.org.

Cost

Please contact the source (above) for permission to use the Victimization Screening Form.

Video Camera Surveillance

Purpose

To more reliably characterize and classify violent assaults.

Population

Adult inpatients.

Background and Description

The video camera surveillance approach was developed in response to the problem with unreliable characterization and recording of violent events in psychiatric facilities, particularly because such events occur so quickly. The approach was designed to provide a more sensitive method of documenting assaults. A closed circuit television camera with an 8-mm wide-angle lens and a microphone is placed in each of the four corners of a day room. Cables are connected to each of the cameras, to a recorder, and a monitor screen located in the physicians' office. This type of instrumentation allows simultaneous viewing and recording of events in the day room. The videos are then reviewed to identify assaults (violent incidents). Behaviorally, assaults are defined as attacks upon another person including hitting, kicking, slapping, biting, choking, and throwing objects. The degree of hostility of incidents is also rated by taking into account accompanying gestures, verbal threats, and avoidance by the victim. The assailant's intent was not included in the definition, but a method was devised to classify events as demonstrating high or low hostility. The assailant is defined as the person who initiated the physical contact. The victim is the recipient of initial contact, even if he or she responded with physical force. Events are rated dichotomously for the following behaviors of the assailant and the victim: (1) gesturing (pointing, fist shaking) or verbal assault (threat) before contact, (2) gesturing or verbal assault after contact, (3) avoidance (running or evading grasp), (4) pursuit, and (5) close proximity after physical contact.

Administration

Timing of administration varies depending on if assessments are designed to evaluate a single event, daily events, or weekly or monthly observations of violent events.

Scoring

A total hostility score is the sum of the points given for items 1–5. The presence of each of the items 1-4 is scored as 1 point, and 1 point is given for the absence of item 5 for the assailant, or the victim, or both. In addition, the day room staff interventions (separation, verbal counseling, and restraint) are noted for each event.

Crowner, Stepcic, Peric, and Czobor (1994) introduced additional scoring methods for impact, body areas targeted, and staff reactions. Forcefulness and target were dichotomous variables: raters choose between "forceful" or "not forceful" and between "target includes head and face" or "body blows only." The investigators choose one of the following four mutually exclusive classes of staff reactions: "missing" is defined as "no staff in day room at time of incident" or "staff in day room but with backs turned to combatants"; 0 is defined as "staff in day room, can see event, but do not intervene in any way"; 1 is defined as "staff intervene, but don't separate combatants"; 2 is defined as "staff separate combatants." These encompass all possible staff options that are visible on videotape. Additionally, three classes representing seriousness of assault were developed: 0 represents "play," 1 represents intermediate seriousness, and 2 represents "hurt." Initially raters are allowed to assign more than one class to describe how incidents progressed, usually from less to more serious. Later, in an effort to simplify, each event is assigned only one class, 0 for events that did not escalate beyond play, 2 for events that seemed hurtful at any point, 1 for all others.

Interpretation

Events with a total score of 3 or more (the maximum possible score was 5 points) were classified as high-hostility events. Higher scores for staff reactions and seriousness of assault represent a greater need for intervention by staff and intent to hurt, respectively.

Psychometric Properties

Norms. Initial normative data were collected on male and female inpatients that were considered to be too assaultive to be managed elsewhere in the hospital.

Reliability. Reliability between raters in identifying who played the roles of assailant and victim and on classification of events as demonstrating high or low hostility were calculated by means of the intraclass correlation coefficient (ICC). The number of high-hostility assaults detected by the videotape reviewers was compared to the number noted in staff reports obtained over a 2-month period during which the tapes were systematically reviewed. Out of the 24 assaultive episodes, complete agreement was obtained among all three raters in identifying the assailant and the victim in each episode for 20 of the 24 events (ICC = .69). All three raters achieved agreement on 16 of the 24 events with respect to the classification of high versus low hostility (ICC = .62). In official incident reports, only two of the nine (22 %) were noted, while three of the nine (33 %) were reported verbally by staff and four of the nine (44 %) were recorded in the ward journal. Of the 15 low-hostility events, none were reported by any other method, and only one resulted in staff intervention. Videotaped reviewers missed one event, which was reported verbally by a staff member as one patient "playfully wrestling" with another.

Crowner et al. (1994) further examined reliability of the video camera surveillance method. Interrater reliability in detecting assault in 19 unedited 4-h tape segments was calculated using the kappa statistic. The kappa was .88 for two raters. The same raters agreed completely in identifying victim and assailant in 30 assaults. Interrater reliability for the three incident descriptors (forcefulness of assailant blows, target of blows, and staff reactions) ranged from .86 to .96. For target of blows, the raters chose between inclusion of head and face and body blows only. For 27 independently rated assaults, kappa was .92. For forcefulness of blows, the raters chose between forceful and not forceful. For 32 independently rated assaults, kappa was .86. Interrater reliability was also calculated for the four classes of staff reactions. For 33 independently rated events, kappa was .96. The single disagreement was reportedly in discriminating classes 1 and 2. Finally, two experienced raters independently assigned assault classifications to 30 assaults to determine interrater reliability. Kappa was .85. Disagreement occurred in discriminating classes 1 and 2 but not in separating class 0 from either class 1 or class 2. In another study conducted by Crowner, Peric, Stepcic, and Van Oss (1994), interrater reliability was found to be .75 (using the phi statistic).

Validity. Over a 2-month period, the videotape reviewers documented more than twice as many hostile assaults as were documented by other methods of reporting (Brizer, Crowner, Convit, & Volavka, 1988).

Clinical Utility

Moderate. This method has been used primarily in inpatient psychiatric hospitals. The approach is useful for providing behavioral information without bias of respondent self-report or ward staff. However, this method was limited to incidents that occurred in the day room setting. This measure has potential to be used for other populations and settings.

Research Applicability

Moderate. Increasing studies have been conducted demonstrating the utility of using the video camera surveillance method.

Original Citation

Brizer, D. A., Crowner, M. L., Convit, A., & Volavka, J. (1988). Videotape recording of inpatient assaults: A pilot study. *American Journal of Psychiatry*, *145*(6), 751–752.

Source

David A. Brizer, M.D., Psychopharmacology Associates, Warwick, NY, 1-888-593-5370

Cost

Please contact the source (above) for additional information regarding the video camera surveillance method.

References

Crowner, M. L., Peric, G., Stepcic, F., & Van Oss, E. (1994). A comparison of videocameras and official incidents reports in detecting inpatient assaults. *Hospital and Community Psychiatry*, *45*, 1144–1145.

Crowner, M. L., Stepcic, F., Peric, G., & Czobor, P. (1994). Typology of patient-patient assaults detected by videocameras. *American Journal of Psychiatry*, *151*, 1669–1672.

Violence and Suicide Assessment Form (VASA)

Purpose

To assess suicide and violence risk in the psychiatric emergency room.

Population

Adult emergency room patients.

Background and Description

The Violence and Suicide Assessment Form (VASA) was developed to assess violence and suicidal risk in psychiatric emergency rooms. The impetus was to examine the extent to which the newly developed measure would be able to predict certain aspects of subsequent course of hospitalization and for better predicting violent and suicidal behaviors. The VASA is a 10-item instrument that covers 10 areas that include (1) current violent thoughts (during interview), (2) recent violent behaviors (i.e., during the past several weeks), (3) past history of violent/antisocial/disruptive behaviors (lifetime history), (4) current suicidal thoughts, (5) recent suicidal behaviors, (6) past history of suicidal behaviors, (7) support systems, (8) ability to cooperate, (9) substance abuse, and (10) reactions during the interview. Within each of the 10 areas of interest, there are a number of brief descriptions of relevant behaviors varying in degree of severity or degree of psychopathology. Items are weighted accordingly.

The instructions given to clinicians are the following: "Your probability estimate (on a scale from 0 to 100) should refer to the next 3 weeks. In that period, do you expect that this patient will show suicidal ideation or behavior and/or violent ideation or behavior?"

Administration

The instrument is completed by the patient's clinician.

Scoring

Scores are summed across items for a total score and can also be viewed in terms of individual items.

Interpretation

Lower scores indicate lower violence or suicidal potential/risk.

Psychometric Properties

Norms. Normative data were collected on emergency room patients (50 discharged patients and 45 patients admitted to inpatient wards).

Reliability. For the first three items, which are concerned with violence, the internal reliability as measured by coefficient alpha was .68. The internal consistency reliability of the next three items concerned with suicide was .73. When the entire group of 10 items was considered as a scale, the internal reliability was .79, demonstrating a high degree of interrelation among the violence items, the suicide items, and the social support and motivational items. The authors purport that the total score can be conceptualized as a psychosocial distress index.

Validity. In terms of predictive validity, significant product–moment correlations obtained described short-term predictions. The presence of suicidal ideation at the time of admission to the emergency room was highly correlated with suicide precautions taken on the ward ($r=.63$) and with the number of days on suicide precautions ($r=-.32$). The number of prior suicide attempts was highly correlated ($r=.61$) with the harassment of others on the wards and was also highly correlated with the risk of violence in the hospital ($r=.60$). The risk of violence in the hospital was also highly correlated with a history of substance abuse ($r=.63$). Some degree of prediction of acting out aggressive behavior is possible over relatively short time periods.

Sensitivity and specificity of the VASA was evaluated to determine if the measure could discriminate between those emergency room patients who were admitted to the inpatient services and those who were not. The optimum cutoff score for maximum sensitivity and specificity was found to be 11. A score of this value reportedly produced a sensitivity and specificity of approximately 82 %. The VASA was able to discriminate between those who were admitted and discharged as emergency room patients.

Clinical Utility

Limited. The VASA has not been widely used in other clinical settings. However, preliminary evidence seems to suggest the potential use of the VASA as a useful tool for clinicians in emergency rooms to guide interviews and to help identify patients who need increased supervision.

Research Applicability

Limited. The VASA has not been extensively used in research studies.

Original Citation

Feinstein, R., & Plutchik, R. (1990). Violence and suicide risk assessment in the psychiatric emergency room. *Comprehensive Psychiatry, 31*(4), 337–343.

Source

Robert Feinstein, MD., University of Colorado Denver, Department of Psychiatry, (303) 724-7734, Robert.feinstein@ucdenver.edu

Cost

Please contact the source (above) for permission to use the VASA.

Violence Risk Appraisal Guide (VRAG)

Purpose

To assess risk of violent recidivism.

Population

Adult offenders.

Background and Description

The Violence Risk Appraisal Guide (VRAG) is an actuarial instrument designed to aid in the prediction of violent recidivism in convicted offenders. Recidivism was defined as any new criminal charge for a violent offense. The following offenses were considered "violent": homicide, attempted homicide, kidnapping, forcible confinement,

wounding, assault causing bodily harm, rape, sexual assaults involving physical contact, and armed robbery. An item pool was created be examining violence and criminal behavior literature for predictor variables with empirical support, examining variables predictive of rehospitalization for a mental disorder, and examining variables believed to be predictive of recidivism by clinicians but lacking empirical support (e.g., expressions of remorse). The correlation of the items with violent recidivism was examined and items without a significant correlation were excluded. Some of the items were highly correlated with each other; in such cases the item with the highest correlation with violent recidivism was retained. Then a series of regression analyses were conducted to further narrow down the item pool. This resulted in 12 predictor variables that were included in the VRAG. Sample predictor variables are as follows:

- Revised Psychopathy Checklist Score (PCL-R, pp. 220–222)
- Age at the time of the index offense
- Alcohol abuse score

Administration

The VRAG is completed by thoroughly reviewing offenders' files. The time required varies depending on the amount of information contained in the offender's file.

Scoring

Items are weighted based on how much the recidivism rate for individuals with the item differs from the base rate. If there was a difference of 5 % or greater from the mean overall recidivism rate, then a weight of one was added or subtracted. For example, in the initial study the base rate for overall violent recidivism was 31 %, but offenders who had married had a violent recidivism rate of 21 %. Since this was two 5 % increments below the base rate, the item "married" was weighted as −2. Missing items are scored as 0. Scores are summed for all items.

Interpretation

Higher scores reflect a greater risk of violently recidivating.

Psychometric Properties

Norms. Normative data are available and can be found in the original citation.

Reliability. All of the items in the VRAG were found to be highly reliable, with kappas of .70 or higher for categorical variables, and Pearson correlations of .80 or higher for continuous variables. Two raters independently rated a sample of 20 offenders. The VRAG scores for the two raters correlated .90.

Validity. The predictor variables that comprise the VRAG were correlated with violent recidivism. Some of the variables were inversely related to violent recidivism, with correlations ranging from -.26 (age at the time of the index offense) to -.11 (female victim in the index offense). The remaining variables were positively related to violent recidivism, with correlations ranging from .13 (alcohol abuse score) to .34 (PCL-R score). A Relative Operating Characteristic was computed to determine the predictive ability of the VRAG. The area under the curve was .76, indicating there was a 76 % chance that a randomly selected individual that recidivated scored higher on the VRAG than a randomly selected individual that did not recidivate. The effect size for the VRAG was quite large (Cohen's $d = 1.06$). This indicates scores on the VRAG are positively related to the probability of at least one re-offense occurring. The VRAG was also found to positively correlate with severity of re-offenses that occurred and negatively correlate with the length of time until the re-offense occurred.

The VRAG has been assessed using diverse samples with varying base rates, and has been found to adequately predict violent recidivism in these samples with ROC areas ranging from .73 to .77. The VRAG has been found to predict violent misconduct in offenders in a maximum security prison (Kroner & Mills, 1997). The VRAG has also been found to predict violent recidivism in a sample of male and female offenders with an intellectual disability as well as the PCL-SV (pp. 220–222), and was able to predict violent recidivism in a sample of male and female offenders without an intellectual disability better than the HCR-20 (pp. 194–196) and the PCL-SV (pp. 220–222) (Gray et al., 2007).

Clinical Utility

High. The VRAG has been shown to accurately predict violent recidivism in convicted male offenders. It has been shown to predict violent recidivism in female offenders, but at a lower rate (ROC area = .65, Coid et al., 2009). It may be a useful tool in making parole and probation decisions, but the authors caution that it should not be used exclusively to make such decisions. It may also be used to identify the risk level of offenders so that the most intensive resources (i.e., supervision, treatment, etc.) are given to the highest risk offenders.

Research Applicability

High. The VRAG is a useful tool for indentifying persons at risk of committing violent acts. The thorough risk assessment can be used to aid in the identification of other risk factors and psychological correlates of violence and aggression.

Original Citation

Quinsey, V. L., Harris, G. T., Rice, M. E., & Cormier, C. A. (1998). *Violent offenders appraising and managing risk*. Washington, DC: American Psychological Association.

Source

Dr. Vernon L. Quinsey, Department of Psychology, Queen's University, Kingston, Ontario, Canada K7L 3N6, (613) 533-2881, Fax: (613) 533-2499, vern.quinsey@queensu.ca

Cost

Please contact the source (above) for permission to use the VRAG.

Alternative Forms

The VRAG has been slightly modified for use with sex offenders. The Sex Offender Risk Appraisal Guide (SORAG) has been found to predict violent recidivism in sex offenders slightly better than the VRAG and has also been shown to predict sexual recidivism.

References

Coid, J., Yang, M., Ullrich, S., Zhang, T., Sizmur, S., Roberts, C., et al. (2009). Gender differences in structured risk assessment: Comparing the accuracy of five instruments. *Journal of Consulting and Clinical Psychology, 77*, 337–348.

Gray, N. S., Fitzgerald, S., Taylor, J., MacCulloch, M. J., & Snowden, R. J. (2007). Predicting future reconviction in offenders with intellectual disabilities: The predictive efficacy of VRAG, PCL-SV, and the HCR-20. *Psychological Assessment, 19*, 474–479.

Kroner, D. G., & Mills, J. F. (1997). *The VRAG: Predicting institutional misconduct in violent offenders.* Paper presented at the Annual Convention of the Ontario Psychological Association, Toronto, Canada.

Violence Scale

Purpose

To measure aggression and violent behaviors in hospital settings.

Population

Adult psychiatric inpatients.

Background and Description

The Violence Scale (VS) was developed in response to the lack of an adequate research scale to measure violence in institutional settings. The measure was designed to index aggressive and violent behavior specifically in hospital settings. The VS was developed in a two-stage process in which current theoretical and measurement approaches to violence were reviewed. The VS was designed out of a response to the problems with self-report, scale rating formats, and incidence measures. Items for the scale were generated using 11 psychiatric nurses' responses to an interview about observed violent incidents in inpatient psychiatric settings which suggested three types of aggression and violence (self, others, and property). Subsequently, three subscales were developed to measure each type of violence.

The VS is an 18-item, behavioral rating scale which measures aggressive and violent behavior toward self, others, and property. The instrument requires nurses to rate each patient for the frequency of aggressive behaviors since admission and at the time of discharge. Each item is rated on a Likert-type scale for frequency of aggressive behaviors. The Likert-type format technique used five response alternatives, ranging from 0 (never) to 4 (frequently). The total range of possible scores is 0–60.

Administration

The completion of the VS is estimated to take 10–20 min.

Scoring

Items are summed.

Interpretation

Higher scores represent greater frequency of observed aggression.

Psychometric Properties

Norms. The VS has been tested in three independent studies of psychiatric inpatients.

Factor analysis. The items met criteria for loading onto the three predicted factors (others, self, and property).

Reliability. Internal consistency of the three sub-scales (violence to self, others, and property) is adequate with Cronbach's alphas ranging from .68 to .91. Interrater reliability was tested using the vignette method and was modest (.50 to .70). Test–retest reliability was $r = .79$.

Validity. Factor analysis and predictive model testing were used to measure construct validity. In studies one and three, both confirmatory and exploratory factor analyses were conducted, resulting in the presence of the significant theoretical factors, explaining over 70 % of the variance.

Clinical Utility

Limited. The VS has been increasingly used with psychiatric inpatients to track aggressive behavior. Additional normative, reliability and validity information would increase the utility of this measure.

Research Applicability

Limited to Moderate. Studies using the VS have been limited but the measure has the potential for research purposes due to its brevity, ease in administration, and scoring.

Original Citation(s)

Morrison, E. F. (1993). The measurement of aggression and violence in hospitalized psychiatric patients. *International Journal of Nursing Studies, 30,* 51–64.

Source

Morrison, E. F. (1993). The measurement of aggression and violence in hospitalized psychiatric patients. *International Journal of Nursing Studies, 30,* 51–64.

Cost

Unavailable.

Appendix: Reprinted Measures

Abuse Assessment Screen

Nursing Network on Violence Against Women, International (n.d.). *The Abuse Assessment Screen.* Retrieved June 1, 2010, from http://www.nnvawi.org

1. **WITHIN THE LAST YEAR,** have you been hit, slapped, kicked, or   YES   NO
   otherwise physically hurt by someone?

   If YES, by whom? _____

   Total number of times _____

2. **SINCE YOU'VE BEEN PREGNANT,** have you been hit, slapped,
   kicked, or otherwise physically hurt by someone?   YES   NO

   If YES, by whom? _____

   Total number of times _____

   **MARK THE AREA OF INJURY ON THE BODY MAP SCORE EACH INCIDENT
   ACCORDING TO THE FOLLOWING SCALE:**

                                             SCORE

   1 = Threats of abuse including use of a weapon   _____

   2 = Slapping, pushing; no injuries and/or lasting pain   _____

   3 = Punching, kicking, bruises, cuts and/or continuing pain   _____

   4 = Beating up, severe contusions, burns, broken bones   _____

   5 = Head injury, internal injury, permanent injury   _____

   6 = Use of weapon; wound from weapon   _____

   If any of the descriptions for the higher number apply, use the higher number.

3. **WITHIN THE LAST YEAR,** has anyone forced you to have   YES   NO
   sexual activities?

   If YES, by whom? _____

   Total number of times _____

   Developed by the Nursing Research Consortium on Violence and Abuse.
   Readers are encouraged to reproduce and use this assessment tool.

G.F. Ronan et al., *Practitioner's Guide to Empirically Supported Measures of Anger, Aggression, and Violence,* ABCT Clinical Assessment Series, DOI 10.1007/978-3-319-00245-3, © Springer International Publishing Switzerland 2014

1. **DURANTE EL ÚLTIMO AÑO**, fué golpeada, bofeteada, pateada, o   SI   NO
   lastimada fisicamente de alguna otra manera por alguien?

   Si la respuesta es "SI" por
   quien(es) _____

   Cuantas

2. **DESDE QUE SALIO EMBARAZADA,** ha sido golpeada,   SI   NO
   bofeteada, pateada, o lastimada fisicamente de alguna otra manera
   por alguien?

   Si la respuesta es "SI" por quien(es)   _____

   Cuantas veces?_____

EN EL DIAGRAMA, ANATÓMICO MARQUE LAS PARTES DE SU CUERPO QUE
HAN SIDO LASTIMADAS. VALORE CADA INCIDENTE USANDO LAS
SIGUIENTE ESCALA:

GRADO

1=Amenazas de maltrato que incluyen el use de un arma   _____

2=Bofeteadas, empujones sin lesiones fisicas o dolor permanente   _____

3=Moquestes, patadas, moretones, heridas, y/o dolor continuo   _____

4=Molida a palos, contusiones several, quemaduras, fracturas de huesos   _____

5=Heridas en la cabeza, lesiones internal, lesiones permanents   _____

6=Uso de armas; herida por arma   _____

Si cualquiera de las situaciones valora un numero alto en la escala,
uselo.

3. **DURANTE EL ÚLTIMO AÑO**, fué forzada a tener relaciones   SI   NO
   sexuales?

   Si la respuesta es "SI" por quien(es) _____

   Cuantas veces? _____

Abusive Behavior Inventory

Reprinted with permission from the author (Shepard, M.F. and Campbell, J.A., 1992).

Here is a list of behaviors that many women report have been used by their partners or former partners. Circle a number from the list below for each item to show your closest estimate of how often the behavior happened in your relationship with your partner of former partner during the past six months.

1. Never
2. Rarely
3. Occasionally
4. Frequently
5. Very Frequently

1	2	3	4	5	Called you names and/or criticized you.
1	2	3	4	5	Tried to keep you from doing something you wanted to do (e.g., going out with friends, going to meetings, leaving a room, etc.)
1	2	3	4	5	Screamed at you.
1	2	3	4	5	Pressured you to have sex when you didn't want to.
1	2	3	4	5	Ended a discussion with you and made the decision himself.
1	2	3	4	5	Threatened to hit or throw something at you.
1	2	3	4	5	Put down your family and friends.
1	2	3	4	5	Accused you of paying too much attention to someone or something else.
1	2	3	4	5	Gave you angry stares or looks.

1	2	3	4	5	Gave you angry stares or looks.
1	2	3	4	5	Slapped, hit or punched you.
1	2	3	4	5	Bossed you around.
1	2	3	4	5	Pushed, grabbed or shoved you.
1	2	3	4	5	Said things to scare you. (e.g., told you something "bad" would happen; threatened to commit suicide)
1	2	3	4	5	Checked up on you (e.g., listened to your phone calls, checked the mileage on your car, called you repeatedly at work)
1	2	3	4	5	Used the children to threaten you (e.g., told you that you would lose custody, said he would leave town with the children)
1	2	3	4	5	Drove recklessly when you were in the car.
1	2	3	4	5	Pressured you to have sex in a way that you didn't like or want to.
1	2	3	4	5	Refused to do housework or child care.
1	2	3	4	5	Injured you by causing bruises, cuts, broken bones, etc.
1	2	3	4	5	Put you down in front of others.
1	2	3	4	5	Stopped or tried to stop you from going to work or school.
1	2	3	4	5	Threw, hit, kicked or smashed something.

1   2   3   4   5   Physically forced you to have sex.

1   2   3   4   5   Became very upset because dinner, housework or laundry was not ready when he wanted it or done the way he thought it should be.

1   2   3   4   5   Made you do something humiliating or degrading. (e.g., begging for forgiveness, having to ask his permission to use the car or do something)

1   2   3   4   5   Threatened you with a knife, gun or other weapon.

1   2   3   4   5   Kicked or bit you.

1   2   3   4   5   Threw you around.

1   2   3   4   5   Choked or strangled you.

1   2   3   4   5   Used a knife, gun or other weapon.

Accountability Scale

Reprinted with permission from the author (Babcock, J., et al., 2007).

Please answer as carefully and accurately as you can by circling a number for each of
the items below.

How much do you agree with each of the following statements about your abusive behavior toward your partner?				
1. I have acknowledged to my partner that I committed acts of violence against her/him.	Agree Strongly 1	Agree Mildly 2	Disagree Mildly 3	Disagree Strongly 4
2. I realized that my pattern of abusive control harmed her/him.	Agree Strongly 1	Agree Mildly 2	Disagree Mildly 3	Disagree Strongly 4
3. My behavior was provoked.	Agree Strongly 1	Agree Mildly 2	Disagree Mildly 3	Disagree Strongly 4
4. My behavior was a criminal act.	Agree Strongly 1	Agree Mildly 2	Disagree Mildly 3	Disagree Strongly 4
5. My behavior was caused by stress, alcohol or other outside factors.	Agree Strongly 1	Agree Mildly 2	Disagree Mildly 3	Disagree Strongly 4
6. I was out of control when I was abusive toward my partner.	Agree Strongly 1	Agree Mildly 2	Disagree Mildly 3	Disagree Strongly 4
7. I admit that I intended to control or punish my partner.	Agree Strongly 1	Agree Mildly 2	Disagree Mildly 3	Disagree Strongly 4
8. I recognize that my partner may remain afraid of me forever.	Agree Strongly 1	Agree Mildly 2	Disagree Mildly 3	Disagree Strongly 4
9. There is nothing in the relationship or in my partner that caused me to be abusive.	Agree Strongly 1	Agree Mildly 2	Disagree Mildly 3	Disagree Strongly 4
10. I have admitted to my partner's friends and family that I was violent toward her/him.	Agree Strongly 1	Agree Mildly 2	Disagree Mildly 3	Disagree Strongly 4
11. I accept full responsibility for my actions.	Agree Strongly 1	Agree Mildly 2	Disagree Mildly 3	Disagree Strongly 4

Scoring Key:
Factor 1, Acknowledging Harm: Sum of items 1, 2, 4, 7, 8, 10.
Factor 2, Internalizing Responsibility: Sum of items 3, 5, 6, 9, 11.

Antisocial Behavior Scale – Teacher Rating Scale

Reprinted with permission from the author (Brown, K., Atkins, M., Osborne, M., and Milnamow, M., 1996).

Teacher _____   Child's Name

Grade _____   Date

Please indicate the degree to which the statements below is true by circling one of the numbers to the right of the statement.

		never	sometimes	very often
1.	Has good sense of humor	0	1	2
2.	Gets mad when corrected	0	1	2
3.	Deliberately plays mean tricks on other students	0	1	2
4.	Misbehaves when the teacher's back is turned	0	1	2
5.	Takes things from other students with their knowledge	0	1	2
6.	Need to be the leader all the time	0	1	2
7.	Picks on kids smaller than he/she	0	1	2
8.	Is a leader of playground games	0	1	2
9.	Causes trouble but doesn't get caught	0	1	2
10.	Blames others when he/she gets into trouble	0	1	2
11.	Gets mad when he/she doesn't get his/her own way	0	1	2
12.	Says mean things about other children behind their backs	0	1	2
13.	Invites classmates to join games or activities	0	1	2
14.	Fights with other children for no good reason	0	1	2
15.	Changes the rules of the game to help him/her win	0	1	2
16.	Stays calm when little things go wrong	0	1	2

	never	sometimes	very often
17. Gets mad for no good reason	0	1	2
18. Does sneaky things	0	1	2
19. Has hurt others to win a game or contest	0	1	2
20. Poor loser	0	1	2
21. Gets others to gang up on children	0	1	2
22. Volunteers to help classmates in class or on the playground	0	1	2
23. Shares things with others	0	1	2
24. Tells people things that aren't true	0	1	2
25. Writes things on the walls	0	1	2
26. Won't admit that anything is ever his/her fault	0	1	2
27. Threaten others	0	1	2
28. Makes friends easily	0	1	2

Antisocial Personality Questionnaire

Reprinted with permission, ©1996 R. Blackburn and D.J. Fawcett

1. Did you like school?
2. Do you sometimes feel full of energy?
3. Are you the sort of person who rarely strikes back, even if someone hits you first?
4. Do you like parties and socials?
5. Are you easily beaten in an argument?
6. Is your daily life full of things that keep you interested?
7. Have you at times very much wanted to leave home?
8. Do you feel that no one understands you?
9. Do you sometimes feel like swearing?
10. Are you a good mixer?
11. Would you have been more successful if people hadn't had it in for you?
12. Do you sometimes feel like smashing things?
13. Do you always tell the truth?
14. Would you rather pass by someone you hadn't seen for a long time if they didn't speak to you first?
15. Do you think that the police treat people badly?
16. Nowadays, do you tend to given up hope of amounting to something?
17. Do you very much lack self confidence?
18. Do you mind being made fun of?
19. Do you sometimes have a strong urge to do something harmful or shocking?
20. Do you like to go to parties or other affairs where there is lots of loud fun?
21. Do you feel happy most of the time?
22. Are the people who run things usually against you?
23. Do people sometimes bother you just by being around?
24. Has anyone got it in for you?
25. Have you ever done anything dangerous just for the thrill of it?
26. Do you frequently find it necessary to stand up for what you believe is right?
27. At school, were you sometimes sent to the head for misbehaving?
28. Do you ever get the feeling that you are being plotted against?
29. Do you often find it hard to understand why you've been so bad tempered?
30. Have your thoughts sometimes raced ahead faster than you could speak them?
31. If you could get into a cinema without paying, and be sure you weren't seen, would you probably do it?
32. Do you ever get the feeling that you are being followed?
33. Is your home life as pleasant as that of most people you know?
34. Do you often wonder what hidden reason a person may have for doing something nice for you?
35. Is your behaviour controlled largely by the habits of those around you?
36. Do you sometimes feel extremely useless?
37. Is your weight about the same as it has always been?
38. Do you think that police and magistrates will tell you one thing and do another?
39. Are you irritated a great deal more than people realise?
40. Do you feel that the only way to settle anything is to make sure you beat the other fellow?
41. Does it make you uncomfortable to put on a stunt at a party even when others are doing the same sort of thing?
42. Do you find it hard to make conversation when you meet strangers?
43. When you get bored, do you like to stir up some excitement?
44. Are there people you know whom you don't like?
45. Do you often wish you weren't so shy?

46. Do you enjoy many different kinds of play and recreation?
47. Do you like to flirt?
48. Have you ever used alcohol excessively?
49. Do you feel that there is little love and friendship in your family as compared to other homes?
50. Have your parents often objected to the kind of people you mix with?
51. Do you gossip a little at times?
52. Do you like to talk about sex?
53. Do you lose you temper easily and then get over it soon?
54. Do you brood a great deal?
55. Have you been disappointed in love?
56. Are people inclined to misunderstand your way of doing things?
57. Do your parents and family find more fault with you than they should?
58. Do you have difficulty in starting to do things?
59. Do you feel that it's safer to trust nobody?
60. When you are in a group of people, do you have trouble thinking of the right things to talk about?
61. If someone hits you first, do you let him have it?
62. Have you often felt that strangers were looking at you critically?
63. Do you think that most people make friends because friends are likely to be useful to them?
64. Do you feel that you are being talked about?
65. Do you feel that you are always patient with others?
66. Do you tend to avoid using strong language, even when you are angry?
67. Are you likely not to speak to people until they speak to you?
68. Have you ever been in trouble with the law?
69. Is life a strain for you a lot of the time?
70. In school, did you find it very hard to talk in front of the class?
71. Even when you are with people, do you feel lonely much of the time?
72. Do you seem to make friends about as quickly as other people?
73. Do you feel that most people inwardly dislike going out of their way to help others?
74. Are you easily embarrassed?
75. Do you easily get impatient with people?
76. Have you often crossed the street so as not to meet someone you see?
77. When you lose your temper, are you capable of slapping someone?
78. Have you any enemies who wish to harm you?
79. Do you have more trouble concentrating than others seem to have?
80. When you get angry, do you say nasty things?
81. At a party, are you more likely to sit by yourself or with just one other person than to join in with the crowd?
82. When someone says silly or ignorant things about something you know about, do you try to put them right?
83. Are you often said to be hotheaded?
84. Do you often wish you could get over worrying about things you have said that might have injured other people's feelings?
85. Do people often disappoint you?
86. Do you feel that you can't tell anyone all about yourself?
87. Have you frequently had to give up your plans because they seemed so full of difficulties?

88. Have you often felt badly over being misunderstood when you try to stop someone making a mistake?
89. Do you enjoy going to dances or discos?
90. Would you say that you do not easily get angry?
91. Does it make you feel like a failure when you hear of the success of someone you know well?
92. Have you often met people who were supposed to be experts who were no better than you?
93. Are you inclined to take disappointments so seriously that you can't put them out of your mind?
94. Do you often get so annoyed when someone tries to get ahead of you in a queue that you speak to them about it?
95. Do you sometimes feel you are no good at all?
96. Have you sometimes felt it necessary to be rough with people who were rude or annoying?
97. Would you like to be a motor racing driver?
98. Would you resort to violence to defend your rights?
99. Are you inclined to go out of your way to win a point against someone who has opposed you?
100. Have you been bothered by people outside, in buses or in shops, watching you?
101. Do you enjoy social gatherings just to be with people?
102. Have you several times had a change of heart about the job you do?
103. When you were a youngster did you ever indulge in petty stealing?
104. Have you often found people jealous of your good ideas just because they hadn't thought of them first?
105. Do you try to avoid being in a crowd whenever possible?
106. Do you mind meeting strangers?
107. Can you remember playing sick to get out of something?
108. Have you known people who pushed you so far that you came to blows?
109. When you are on trains and buses do you often talk to strangers?
110. Do you feel like giving up when things go wrong?
111. Do you find yourself being a bit rude to people you dislike?
112. Have you frequently worked under people who seem to take all the credit for good work but pass off mistakes on to those under them?
113. Do you sometimes find it hard to stick up for your rights because you are so reserved?
114. Do some of your family have quick tempers?
115. Do you strongly defend your own opinions as a rule?
116. Do you shrink from facing a crisis or difficulty?
117. Are you very careful about the way you dress?
118. Do you believe that a large number of people are guilty of bad sexual behaviour?
119. Have you often had to take orders from someone who didn't know as much as you?
120. Do you feel that there is someone who is responsible for most of your troubles?
121. Have you ever been in trouble over your sexual behaviour?
122. Do you frequently wish you could be as happy as others seem to be?
123. Do you get angry sometimes?
124. Do you often find yourself disagreeing with people?
125. Do you feel that you haven't lived the right kind of life?

ANSWER SHEET FOR THE PERSONAL REACTION QUESTIONNAIRE (APQ)

Name _____

Date _____

Age _____

1	26	51	76	101
2	27	52	77	102
3	28	53	78	103
4	29	54	79	104
5	30	55	80	105
6	31	56	81	106
7	32	57	82	107
8	33	58	83	108
9	34	59	84	109
10	35	60	85	110
11	36	61	86	111
12	37	62	87	112
13	38	63	88	113
14	39	64	89	114
15	40	65	90	115
16	41	66	91	116
17	42	67	92	117
18	43	68	93	118
19	44	69	94	119
20	45	70	95	120
21	46	71	96	121
22	47	72	97	122
23	48	73	98	123
24	49	74	99	124
25	50	75	100	125

Anger Response Inventory – Adolescent Version

Reprinted with permission from the author (Tangney, J., et al., 1991).

ARI-ADOL

On each of these pages, you will find a description of a situation. Then
will see several statements about different ways that people might think
feel.

As you read each situation, *really imagine* that you are in that situation now.
Imagine how you might think or feel. Then read each statement. Put an X
in the circle that describes how likely it is that the statement would be
for you. The largest circle means that you are very likely to think or
that way, and the smallest circle means that you are not at all likely
think or feel that way.

SAMPLE:

You wake up very early one morning on a school day.

	Never	One Time	A Few Times	Often	Very Often
a) I would eat breakfast right	○	○	○	○	○
b) I would try to finish my homework before I left for school.	○	○	○	○	○
c) I would feel like staying in	○	○	○	○	○
d) I would wonder why I woke up so early.	○	○	○	○	○

There are no right or wrong answers to these   We're simply interested
in your own thoughts and ideas about these

1. You find out a "friend" was talking about you behind your back

<u>Section 1</u>

	not at all angry	a little angry	fairly angry	very angry	very, very angry
a) How angry would you be if this happened to you?	○	○	○	○	○

<u>Section 2</u>

The next 3 questions are about how you would <u>feel</u>, not necessarily what you would <u>do</u>.

	not at all	a little	somewhat (half & half)	pretty much	very much
b) How much would you <u>feel</u> like getting back at the friend? Or getting even?	○	○	○	○	○
c) How much would you <u>feel</u> like fixing the situation? Or making it better?	○	○	○	○	○
d) How much would you <u>feel</u> like letting off steam?	○	○	○	○	○

<u>Section 3</u>

The next 7 questions are about what you would <u>really</u> do.

	not at all likely	unlikely	maybe (half & half)	likely	very likely
e) I'd slam down the phone the next time the friend called.	○	○	○	○	○
f) I'd go do something I enjoy to get my mind off it.	○	○	○	○	○
g) I'd tell all our friends this person can't be trusted.	○	○	○	○	○
h) I wouldn't really care what they think. We weren't good friends anyway.	○	○	○	○	○
i) I'd be angry with myself for trusting the friend.	○	○	○	○	○
j) I'd ask the friend why we couldn't talk to <u>each other</u> about things that are bothering us.	○	○	○	○	○
k) I'd take it out on another friend by being short-tempered.	○	○	○	○	○

<u>Section 4</u>

The next 3 questions are about the long-term consequences of how you would handle the situation. Looking back over what you would really do, how do you think things would turn out in the long run.

	terrible	pretty bad	OK	pretty good	wonderful
l) How do you think things would turn out for YOU in the long run?	○	○	○	○	○
m) How do you think thinkg would turn out for YOUR FRIEND in the long run	○	○	○	○	○
n) How do you think things would turn out in the long run for your RELATIONSHIP with your friend.	○	○	○	○	○

2. Your friends make fun of you in front of someone you like.

Section 1

	not at all angry	a little angry	fairly angry	very angry	very, very angry
a) How angry would you be if this happened to you?	○	○	○	○	○

Section 2

The next 3 questions are about how you would feel, not necessarily what you would do.

	not at all	a little	somewhat (half & half)	pretty much	very much
b) How much would you feel like getting back at your friends? Or getting even?	○	○	○	○	○
c) How much would you feel like fixing the situation? Or making it better?	○	○	○	○	○
d) How much would you feel like letting off steam?	○	○	○	○	○

Section 3

The next 7 questions are about what you would really do.

	not at all likely	unlikely	maybe (half & half)	likely	very likely
e) I'd hit one of them.	○	○	○	○	○
f) I'd be nice on the outside, but deep down I'd hate those friends.	○	○	○	○	○
g) I'd think that I shouldn't let it bother me.	○	○	○	○	○
h) I'd walk away from them all.	○	○	○	○	○
i) I'd kick something - really hard.	○	○	○	○	○
j) I'd tell my friends that it bothers me when they tease me like that.	○	○	○	○	○
k) I'd tell everyone something bad about those friends.	○	○	○	○	○

Section 4

The next 3 questions are about the long-term consequences of how you would handle the situation. Looking back over what you would really do, how do you think things would turn out in the long run.

	terrible	pretty bad	OK	pretty good	wonderful
l) How do you think things would turn out for YOU in the long run?	○	○	○	○	○
m) How do you think thinkg would turn out for YOUR FRIENDS in the long run?	○	○	○	○	○
n) How do you think things would turn out in the long run for your RELATIONSHIP with those friends?	○	○	○	○	○

---

3. You try to explain something to your best friend, and they keep interrupting you.

Section 1

a) How angry would you be if this happened to you?

not at all angry	a little angry	fairly angry	very angry	very, very angry
◯	◯	◯	◯	◯

Section 2

The next 3 questions are about how you would <u>feel</u>, not necessarily what you would <u>do</u>.

	not at all	a little	somewhat (half & half)	pretty much	very much
b) How much would you <u>feel</u> like getting back at your friend? Or getting even?	◯	◯	◯	◯	◯
c) How much would you <u>feel</u> like fixing the situation? Or making it better?	◯	◯	◯	◯	◯
d) How much would you <u>feel</u> like letting off steam?	◯	◯	◯	◯	◯

Section 3

The next 7 questions are about what you would <u>really</u> do.

	not at all likely	unlikely	maybe (half & half)	likely	very likely
e) I'd leave the room so I wouldn't lose my temper.	◯	◯	◯	◯	◯
f) I'd go in the other room and break something.	◯	◯	◯	◯	◯
g) I'd threaten my friend with my fist.	◯	◯	◯	◯	◯
h) It doesn't matter. I'll get my chance to talk eventually.	◯	◯	◯	◯	◯
i) I'd give the friend the silent treatment.	◯	◯	◯	◯	◯
j) I'd think mabe my friend didn't realize he or she was interrupting me.	◯	◯	◯	◯	◯
k) I'd be angry with myself for even trying to discuss it.	◯	◯	◯	◯	◯

Section 4

The next 3 questions are about the long-term consequences of how you would handle the situation. Looking back over what you would really do, how do you think things would turn out in the long run.

	terrible	pretty bad	OK	pretty good	wonderful
l) How do you think things would turn out for YOU in the long run?	◯	◯	◯	◯	◯
m) How do you think thinkg would turn out for YOUR FRIEND in the long run?	◯	◯	◯	◯	◯
n) How do you think things would turn out in the long run for your RELATIONSHIP with your friend?	◯	◯	◯	◯	◯

4. Your friend makes planes to meet you after school, but doesn't show up.

<u>Section 1</u>

	not at all angry	a little angry	fairly angry	very angry	very, very angry
a) How angry would you be if this happened to you?	○	○	○	○	○

<u>Section 2</u>

The next 3 questions are about how you would <u>feel</u>, not necessarily what you would <u>do</u>.

	not at all	a little	somewhat (half & half)	pretty much	very much
b) How much would you <u>feel</u> like getting back at that friend? Or getting even?	○	○	○	○	○
c) How much would you <u>feel</u> like fixing the situation? Or making it better?	○	○	○	○	○
d) How much would you <u>feel</u> like letting off steam?	○	○	○	○	○

<u>Section 3</u>

The next 7 questions are about what you would <u>really</u> do.

	not at all likely	unlikely	maybe (half & half)	likely	very likely
e) I'd think that something serious must have come up for the friend not to show up.	○	○	○	○	○
f) I'd stop speaking to that friend.	○	○	○	○	○
g) I'd be angry with myself for waiting around.	○	○	○	○	○
h) I'd just forget about it.	○	○	○	○	○
i) I'd snarl at another friend.	○	○	○	○	○
j) I'd call my friends to yell at them for being so thoughtless.	○	○	○	○	○
k) I'd call my friends and ask what had happened.	○	○	○	○	○

<u>Section 4</u>

The next 3 questions are about the long-term consequences of how you would handle the situation. Looking back over what you would really do, how do you think things would turn out in the long run.

	terrible	pretty bad	OK	pretty good	wonderful
l) How do you think things would turn out for YOU in the long run?	○	○	○	○	○
m) How do you think thinkg would turn out for YOUR FRIEND in the long run	○	○	○	○	○
n) How do you think things would turn out in the long run for your RELATIONSHIP with your friend.	○	○	○	○	○

> **5. You are waiting in line for a movie, and someone cuts in front of you.**

<u>Section 1</u>

	not at all <u>angry</u>	a little <u>angry</u>	fairly <u>angry</u>	very <u>angry</u>	very, very <u>angry</u>
a) How angry would you be if this happened to you?	○	○	○	○	○

<u>Section 2</u>

The next 3 questions are about how you would <u>feel</u>, not necessarily what you would <u>do</u>.

	not at all	a little	somewhat (half & half)	pretty much	very much
b) How much would you <u>feel</u> like getting back at that person? Or getting even?	○	○	○	○	○
c) How much would you <u>feel</u> like fixing the situation? Or making it better?	○	○	○	○	○
d) How much would you <u>feel</u> like letting off steam?	○	○	○	○	○

<u>Section 3</u>

The next 7 questions are about what you would <u>really</u> do.

	not at all likely	unlikely	maybe (half & half)	likely	very likely
e) I'd ask the manager to speak to the person.	○	○	○	○	○
f) I'd tell the other people in the line how rude the person was.	○	○	○	○	○
g) I'd just ignore it.	○	○	○	○	○
h) I'd snap at the ticket clerk.	○	○	○	○	○
i) I'd tell myself that it's no big deal. There are plenty of seats.	○	○	○	○	○
j) I wouldn't say anything, but I'd be so angry I couldn't enjoy the movie.	○	○	○	○	○
k) I'd shove the person back out of the line.	○	○	○	○	○

<u>Section 4</u>

The next 2 questions are about the long-term consequences of how you would handle the situation. Looking back over what you would really do, how do you think things would turn out in the long run.

	terrible	pretty bad	OK	pretty good	wonderful
l) How do you think things would turn out for YOU in the long run?	○	○	○	○	○
m) How do you think thinkg would turn out for THAT PERSON in the long run?	○	○	○	○	○

6. While arguing with your brother, he pushes you.

Section 1

	not at all angry	a little angry	fairly angry	very angry	very, very angry
a) How angry would you be if this happened to you?	○	○	○	○	○

Section 2

The next 3 questions are about how you would <u>feel</u>, not necessarily what you would <u>do</u>.

	not at all	a little	somewhat (half & half)	pretty much	very much
b) How much would you <u>feel</u> like getting back at your brother? Or getting even?	○	○	○	○	○
c) How much would you <u>feel</u> like fixing the situation? Or making it better?	○	○	○	○	○
d) How much would you <u>feel</u> like letting off steam?	○	○	○	○	○

Section 3

The next 7 questions are about what you would <u>really</u> do.

	not at all likely	unlikely	maybe (half & half)	likely	very likely
e) I'd hit him as hard as I could.	○	○	○	○	○
f) I'd be angry with myself for getting into it. I should know better than to argue with him.	○	○	○	○	○
g) I'd walk away.	○	○	○	○	○
h) I'd think I shouldn't have gotten him so angry.	○	○	○	○	○
i) I'd hit a younger brother or sister later.	○	○	○	○	○
j) I'd think my brother was really having a bad day.	○	○	○	○	○
k) I'd destroy something important to him.	○	○	○	○	○

Section 4

The next 3 questions are about the long-term consequences of how you would handle the situation. Looking back over what you would really do, how do you think things would turn out in the long run.

	terrible	pretty bad	OK	pretty good	wonderful
l) How do you think things would turn out for YOU in the long run?	○	○	○	○	○
m) How do you think thinkg would turn out for YOUR BROTHER in the long run	○	○	○	○	○
n) How do you think things would turn out in the long run for your RELATIONSHIP with your brother.	○	○	○	○	○

7. You are using the last of your change to buy a soda from a machine. It keeps your moeny without giving you a soda

Section 1

	not at all angry	a little angry	fairly angry	very angry	very, very angry
a) How angry would you be if this happened to you?	◯	◯	◯	◯	◯

Section 2

The next 3 questions are about how you would <u>feel</u>, not necessarily what you would <u>do</u>.

	not at all	a little	somewhat (half & half)	pretty much	very much
b) How much would you <u>feel</u> like getting back at someone or something? Or getting even?	◯	◯	◯	◯	◯
c) How much would you <u>feel</u> like fixing the situation? Or making it better?	◯	◯	◯	◯	◯
d) How much would you <u>feel</u> like letting off steam?	◯	◯	◯	◯	◯

Section 3

The next 7 questions are about what you would <u>really</u> do.

	not at all likely	unlikely	maybe (half & half)	likely	very likely
e) I'd take a deep breath and try to cool down.	◯	◯	◯	◯	◯
f) I'd slam my fist against the wall.	◯	◯	◯	◯	◯
g) I'd wonder if I put the right change in.	◯	◯	◯	◯	◯
h) I'd be angry at myself for losing the last of my change.	◯	◯	◯	◯	◯
i) I'd request a refund.	◯	◯	◯	◯	◯
j) I'd yell at the next person I saw.	◯	◯	◯	◯	◯
k) I'd think, "Well, I wasn't that thirsty anyway."	◯	◯	◯	◯	◯

Section 4

The next question is about the long-term consequences of how you would handle the situation. Looking back over what you would really do, how do you think things would turn out in the long run.

	terrible	pretty bad	OK	pretty good	wonderful
l) Over all, how do you think things would turn out in the long run?	◯	◯	◯	◯	◯

8. Your teacher refuses to listen to your point of view.

<u>Section 1</u>

	not at all angry	a little angry	fairly angry	very angry	very, very angry
a) How angry would you be if this happened to you?	◯	◯	◯	◯	◯

<u>Section 2</u>

The next 3 questions are about how you would <u>feel</u>, not necessarily what you would <u>do</u>.

	not at all	a little	somewhat (half & half)	pretty much	very much
b) How much would you <u>feel</u> like getting back at your teacher? Or getting even?	◯	◯	◯	◯	◯
c) How much would you <u>feel</u> like fixing the situation? Or making it better?	◯	◯	◯	◯	◯
d) How much would you <u>feel</u> like letting off steam?	◯	◯	◯	◯	◯

<u>Section 3</u>

The next 7 questions are about what you would <u>really</u> do.

	not at all likely	unlikely	maybe (half & half)	likely	very likely
e) I'd be so angry I couldn't concentrate on anything all day.	◯	◯	◯	◯	◯
f) I'd think it doesn't reall matter. Teachers do this all the time.	◯	◯	◯	◯	◯
g) I'd walk away so I wouldn't lose my temper.	◯	◯	◯	◯	◯
h) If any classmates got in my way, I'd shove them aside.	◯	◯	◯	◯	◯
i) I'd grab my teacher by the arm and make him or her listen.	◯	◯	◯	◯	◯
j) I'd think the teacher was having a bad day.	◯	◯	◯	◯	◯
k) I'd destroy some papers on the teacher's desk in front of him or her.	◯	◯	◯	◯	◯

<u>Section 4</u>

The next 3 questions are about the long-term consequences of how you would handle the situation. Looking back over what you would really do, how do you think things would turn out in the long run.

	terrible	pretty bad	OK	pretty good	wonderful
l) How do you think things would turn out for YOU in the long run?	◯	◯	◯	◯	◯
m) How do you think thinkg would turn out for YOUR TEACHER in the long run?	◯	◯	◯	◯	◯
n) How do you think things would turn out in the long run for your RELATIONSHIP with your teacher?	◯	◯	◯	◯	◯

9. You tell a good friend a secret, and the friend tells everyone.

<u>Section 1</u>

	not at all <u>angry</u>	a little <u>angry</u>	fairly <u>angry</u>	very <u>angry</u>	very, very <u>angry</u>
a) How angry would you be if this happened to you?	○	○	○	○	○

<u>Section 2</u>

The next 3 questions are about how you would <u>feel</u>, not necessarily what you would <u>do</u>.

	not at all	a little	somewhat (half & half)	pretty much	very much
b) How much would you <u>feel</u> like getting back at the friend? Or getting even?	○	○	○	○	○
c) How much would you <u>feel</u> like fixing the situation? Or making it better?	○	○	○	○	○
d) How much would you <u>feel</u> like letting off steam?	○	○	○	○	○

<u>Section 3</u>

The next 7 questions are about what you would <u>really</u> do.

	not at all likely	unlikely	maybe (half & half)	likely	very likely
e) I'd yell at my parents to leave me alone when I got home.	○	○	○	○	○
f) I'd yell at the friend, "I hate you!"	○	○	○	○	○
g) I'd tell everyone a secret that the friend had told me.	○	○	○	○	○
h) I'd be really angry with myself for trusting that friend.	○	○	○	○	○
i) I'd go do something to get my mind off it.	○	○	○	○	○
j) I'd be so mad I'd break something.	○	○	○	○	○
k) I'd give the friend a dirty look the next time we saw each other.	○	○	○	○	○

<u>Section 4</u>

The next 3 questions are about the long-term consequences of how you would handle the situation. Looking back over what you would really do, how do you think things would turn out in the long run.

	terrible	pretty bad	OK	pretty good	wonderful
l) How do you think things would turn out for YOU in the long run?	○	○	○	○	○
m) How do you think thinkg would turn out for YOUR FRIEND in the long run?	○	○	○	○	○
n) How do you think things would turn out in the long run for your RELATIONSHIP with your friend?	○	○	○	○	○

10. You're in a hurry to get to school and you spill something on yourself

Section 1

| | not at all angry | a little angry | fairly angry | very angry | very, very angry |

a) How angry would you be if this happened to you?

Section 2

The next 3 questions are about how you would feel, not necessarily what you would do.

| | not at all | a little | somewhat (half & half) | pretty much | very much |

b) How much would you feel like getting back at someone or something? Or getting even?

c) How much would you feel like fixing the situation? Or making it better?

d) How much would you feel like letting off steam?

Section 3

The next 7 questions are about what you would really do.

| | not at all likely | unlikely | maybe (half & half) | likely | very likely |

e) I'd change my clothes.

f) I'd smack my brother or sister.

g) I'd be furious about it all morning.

h) I'd think I should have taken my time.

i) I'd take several deep breaths and try to relax.

j) I'd just pretend it didn't happen.

k) I'd be so angry with myself for be so careless.

Section 4

The next question is about the long-term consequences of how you would handle the situation. Looking back over what you would really do, how do you think things would turn out in the long run.

| | terrible | pretty bad | OK | pretty good | wonderful |

l) Overall, how do you think things would turn out in the long run?

11. You tell a friend about a problem, and your friend doesn't take it seriously

<u>Section 1</u>

	not at all angry	a little angry	fairly angry	very angry	very, very angry
a) How angry would you be if this happened to you?	◯	◯	◯	◯	◯

<u>Section 2</u>

The next 3 questions are about how you would <u>feel</u>, not necessarily what you would <u>do</u>.

	not at all	a little	somewhat (half & half)	pretty much	very much
b) How much would you <u>feel</u> like getting back at the friend? Or getting even?	◯	◯	◯	◯	◯
c) How much would you <u>feel</u> like fixing the situation? Or making it better?	◯	◯	◯	◯	◯
d) How much would you <u>feel</u> like letting off steam?	◯	◯	◯	◯	◯

<u>Section 3</u>

The next 7 questions are about what you would <u>really</u> do.

	not at all likely	unlikely	maybe (half & half)	likely	very likely
e) I'd be nice to the friend but my anger would build inside.	◯	◯	◯	◯	◯
f) I'd pound on the wall.	◯	◯	◯	◯	◯
g) I'd never speak to them again.	◯	◯	◯	◯	◯
h) I'd shove the frined aside.	◯	◯	◯	◯	◯
i) I'd make a joke to lighten up the conversation.	◯	◯	◯	◯	◯
j) I'd think maybe I'm taking it too seriously.	◯	◯	◯	◯	◯
k) I'd tell my problem to someone who would take it seriously.	◯	◯	◯	◯	◯

<u>Section 4</u>

The next 3 questions are about the long-term consequences of how you would handle the situation. Looking back over what you would really do, how do you think things would turn out in the long run.

	terrible	pretty bad	OK	pretty good	wonderful
l) How do you think things would turn out for YOU in the long run?	◯	◯	◯	◯	◯
m) How do you think thinkg would turn out for YOUR FRIEND in the long run?	◯	◯	◯	◯	◯
n) How do you think things would turn out in the long run for your RELATIONSHIP with your friend?	◯	◯	◯	◯	◯

12. Someone you have just met treats you like you are not good enough.

Section 1

	not at all angry	a little angry	fairly angry	very angry	very, very angry
a) How angry would you be if this happened to you?	◯	◯	◯	◯	◯

Section 2

The next 3 questions are about how you would <u>feel</u>, not necessarily what you would <u>do</u>.

	not at all	a little	somewhat (half & half)	pretty much	very much
b) How much would you <u>feel</u> like getting back at that person? Or getting even?	◯	◯	◯	◯	◯
c) How much would you <u>feel</u> like fixing the situation? Or making it better?	◯	◯	◯	◯	◯
d) How much would you <u>feel</u> like letting off steam?	◯	◯	◯	◯	◯

Section 3

The next 7 questions are about what you would <u>really</u> do.

	not at all likely	unlikely	maybe (half & half)	likely	very likely
e) I'd make a nasty gesture in the person's face.	◯	◯	◯	◯	◯
f) I'd tell everyone what a snob that person is.	◯	◯	◯	◯	◯
g) I'd calmly explain that I didn't appreciate how he or she was treating me.	◯	◯	◯	◯	◯
h) I'd keep thinking about how rude the person was until I was ready to explode.	◯	◯	◯	◯	◯
i) I'd walk away.	◯	◯	◯	◯	◯
j) I'd hit the next person I saw.	◯	◯	◯	◯	◯
k) I'd wonder if I was being too sensitive.	◯	◯	◯	◯	◯

Section 4

The next 3 questions are about the long-term consequences of how you would handle the situation. Looking back over what you would really do, how do you think things would turn out in the long run.

	terrible	pretty bad	OK	pretty good	wonderful
l) How do you think things would turn out for YOU in the long run?	◯	◯	◯	◯	◯
m) How do you think thinkg would turn out for THAT PERSONin the long run?	◯	◯	◯	◯	◯
n) How do you think things would turn out in the long run for your RELATIONSHIP with that person?	◯	◯	◯	◯	◯

13. During an argument, a friend calls you "stupid."

Section 1

	not at all angry	a little angry	fairly angry	very angry	very, very angry

a) How angry would you be if this happened
to you?

Section 2

The next 3 questions are about how you would <u>feel</u>, not necessarily what you would <u>do</u>.

	not at all	a little	somewhat (half & half)	pretty much	very much

b) How much would you <u>feel</u> like getting back
at the friend? Or getting even?

c) How much would you <u>feel</u> like fixing the
situation? Or making it better?

d) How much would you <u>feel</u> like letting off
steam?

Section 3

The next 7 questions are about what you would <u>really</u> do.

	not at all likely	unlikely	maybe (half & half)	likely	very likely

e) I'd think about it over and over until I was
sick.

f) I'd be so angry I would just walk away.

g) I'd explain that I don't like being called,
"stupid".

h) I'd think it wasn't worth worrying about.

i) I'd shove the friend against the wall.

j) I'd think that my friend was having a bad
day.

k) I'd shove the next person who got in my way.

Section 4

**The next 3 questions are about the long-term consequences of how you would handle
the situation. Looking back over what you would really do, how do you think things
would turn out in the long run.**

	terrible	pretty bad	OK	pretty good	wonderful

l) How do you think things would turn out for
YOU in the long run?

m) How do you think thinkg would turn out for
YOUR FRIEND in the long run?

n) How do you think things would turn out in
the long run for your RELATIONSHIP with
your friend?

14. Your parents blame you for something that was not your fault.

Section 1

	not at all angry	a little angry	fairly angry	very angry	very, very angry
a) How angry would you be if this happened to you?	○	○	○	○	○

Section 2

The next 3 questions are about how you would <u>feel</u>, not necessarily what you would <u>do</u>.

	not at all	a little	somewhat (half & half)	pretty much	very much
b) How much would you <u>feel</u> like getting back at your parents? Or getting even?	○	○	○	○	○
c) How much would you <u>feel</u> like fixing the situation? Or making it better?	○	○	○	○	○
d) How much would you <u>feel</u> like letting off steam?	○	○	○	○	○

Section 3

The next 7 questions are about what you would <u>really</u> do.

	not at all likely	unlikely	maybe (half & half)	likely	very likely
e) I'd throw things around in my room.	○	○	○	○	○
f) I'd go to my room to cool off.	○	○	○	○	○
g) I'd yell at my parents at the top of my lungs.	○	○	○	○	○
h) I'd think my parents were in a bad mood.	○	○	○	○	○
i) I'd try to explain to my parents what really happened.	○	○	○	○	○
j) I'd break something that belonged to them.	○	○	○	○	○
k) I'd give them a really dirty look.	○	○	○	○	○

Section 4

The next 3 questions are about the long-term consequences of how you would handle the situation. Looking back over what you would really do, how do you think things would turn out in the long run.

	terrible	pretty bad	OK	pretty good	wonderful
l) How do you think things would turn out for YOU in the long run?	○	○	○	○	○
m) How do you think thinkg would turn out for YOUR PARENTS in the long run?	○	○	○	○	○
n) How do you think things would turn out in the long run for your RELATIONSHIP with your parents?	○	○	○	○	○

15. You tell the truth about something, but your parents don't believe you.

Section 1

	not at all angry	a little angry	fairly angry	very angry	very, very angry

a) How angry would you be if this happened to you?

Section 2

The next 3 questions are about how you would <u>feel</u>, not necessarily what you would <u>do</u>.

	not at all	a little	somewhat (half & half)	pretty much	very much

b) How much would you <u>feel</u> like getting back at your parents? Or getting even?

c) How much would you <u>feel</u> like fixing the situation? Or making it better?

d) How much would you <u>feel</u> like letting off steam?

Section 3

The next 7 questions are about what you would <u>really</u> do.

	not at all likely	unlikely	maybe (half & half)	likely	very likely

e) I'd go do something fun to get my mind off what happened.

f) I'd kick the wall in my room.

g) I'd try to get some proof that I was telling the truth.

h) I'd think I didn't explain myself very well.

i) I'd try to explain the truth to them again.

j) I'd slam my bedroom door so they could hear it.

k) I'd just try to forget it.

Section 4

The next 3 questions are about the long-term consequences of how you would handle the situation. Looking back over what you would really do, how do you think things would turn out in the long run.

	terrible	pretty bad	OK	pretty good	wonderful

l) How do you think things would turn out for YOU in the long run?

m) How do you think thinkg would turn out for YOUR PARENTS in the long run?

n) How do you think things would turn out in the long run for your RELATIONSHIP with your parents?

> **16. You're struggling to carry four large sodas to your table in a cafeteria. Someone bumps into you, spilling the sodas.**

<u>Section 1</u>

	not at all angry	a little angry	fairly angry	very angry	very, very angry
a) How angry would you be if this happened to you?	O	O	O	O	O

<u>Section 2</u>

The next 3 questions are about how you would <u>feel</u>, not necessarily what you would <u>do</u>.

	not at all	a little	somewhat (half & half)	pretty much	very much
b) How much would you <u>feel</u> like getting back at that person? Or getting even?	O	O	O	O	O
c) How much would you <u>feel</u> like fixing the situation? Or making it better?	O	O	O	O	O
d) How much would you <u>feel</u> like letting off steam?	O	O	O	O	O

<u>Section 3</u>

The next 7 questions are about what you would <u>really</u> do.

	not at all likely	unlikely	maybe (half & half)	likely	very likely
e) I'd get more sodas.	O	O	O	O	O
f) I'd be angry with myself for trying to carry so many sodas.	O	O	O	O	O
g) I'd kick the chair.	O	O	O	O	O
h) I'd think I should have watched where I was going.	O	O	O	O	O
i) I'd think it must have been an accident. I'm sure the person didn't mean it.	O	O	O	O	O
j) I'd bump the person back and make sure he or she spilled something.	O	O	O	O	O
k) I'd forget about it and go about my business.	O	O	O	O	O

<u>Section 4</u>

The next 2 questions are about the long-term consequences of how you would handle the situation. Looking back over what you would really do, how do you think things would turn out in the long run.

	terrible	pretty bad	OK	pretty good	wonderful
l) How do you think things would turn out for YOU in the long run?	O	O	O	O	O
m) How do you think thinkg would turn out for THE OTHER PERSON in the long run?	O	O	O	O	O

---

17. Your brother or sister takes something that's yours without asking.

Section 1

	not at all angry	a little angry	fairly angry	very angry	very, very angry
a) How angry would you be if this happened to you?	○	○	○	○	○

Section 2

The next 3 questions are about how you would feel, not necessarily what you would do.

	not at all	a little	somewhat (half & half)	pretty much	very much
b) How much would you feel like getting back at your brother or sister? Or getting even?	○	○	○	○	○
c) How much would you feel like fixing the situation? Or making it better?	○	○	○	○	○
d) How much would you feel like letting off steam?	○	○	○	○	○

Section 3

The next 7 questions are about what you would really do.

	not at all likely	unlikely	maybe (half & half)	likely	very likely
e) I'd yell at my mother for letting them get away with it.	○	○	○	○	○
f) I'd yell at my brother or sister for "stealing" my stuff.	○	○	○	○	○
g) I'd be angry with myself for not keeping an eye on my things.	○	○	○	○	○
h) I'd take something of theirs without asking.	○	○	○	○	○
i) I wouldn't do anything. I'd just ignore it.	○	○	○	○	○
j) I'd punch my brother or sister really hard.	○	○	○	○	○
k) I'd go in my room and break something.	○	○	○	○	○

Section 4

The next 3 questions are about the long-term consequences of how you would handle the situation. Looking back over what you would really do, how do you think things would turn out in the long run.

	terrible	pretty bad	OK	pretty good	wonderful
l) How do you think things would turn out for YOU in the long run?	○	○	○	○	○
m) How do you think thinkg would turn out for YOUR BROTHER OR SISTER in the long run?	○	○	○	○	○
n) How do you think things would turn out in the long run for your RELATIONSHIP with your brother or sister?	○	○	○	○	○

18. You are walking down the hall, and a group of people laugh as you walk by.

<u>Section 1</u>

	not at all angry	a little angry	fairly angry	very angry	very, very angry
a) How angry would you be if this happened to you?	○	○	○	○	○

<u>Section 2</u>

The next 3 questions are about how you would <u>feel</u>, not necessarily what you would <u>do</u>.

	not at all	a little	somewhat (half & half)	pretty much	very much
b) How much would you <u>feel</u> like getting back at those students? Or getting even?	○	○	○	○	○
c) How much would you <u>feel</u> like fixing the situation? Or making it better?	○	○	○	○	○
d) How much would you <u>feel</u> like letting off steam?	○	○	○	○	○

<u>Section 3</u>

The next 7 questions are about what you would <u>really</u> do.

	not at all likely	unlikely	maybe (half & half)	likely	very likely
e) I'd tell a teacher they were harrassing me.	○	○	○	○	○
f) I don't know them, and I don't care what they think anyway.	○	○	○	○	○
g) I'd snap at the next person I spoke to.	○	○	○	○	○
h) I wouldn't say anything, but I'd be furious, thinking over and over about what I should have said.	○	○	○	○	○
i) I'd yell at them to shut up.	○	○	○	○	○
j) I'd ignore them.	○	○	○	○	○
k) I'd be angry with myself for letting it bother me.	○	○	○	○	○

<u>Section 4</u>

The next 2 questions are about the long-term consequences of how you would handle the situation. Looking back over what you would really do, how do you think things would turn out in the long run.

	terrible	pretty bad	OK	pretty good	wonderful
l) How do you think things would turn out for YOU in the long run?	○	○	○	○	○
m) How do you think thinkg would turn out for THOSE STUDENTSin the long run?	○	○	○	○	○

19. A friend accuses you of something and doesn't let you tell your side of the story.

<u>Section 1</u>

	not at all angry	a little angry	fairly angry	very angry	very, very angry
a) How angry would you be if this happened to you?	◯	◯	◯	◯	◯

<u>Section 2</u>

The next 3 questions are about how you would <u>feel</u>, not necessarily what you would <u>do</u>.

	not at all	a little	somewhat (half & half)	pretty much	very much
b) How much would you <u>feel</u> like getting back at the friend? Or getting even?	◯	◯	◯	◯	◯
c) How much would you <u>feel</u> like fixing the situation? Or making it better?	◯	◯	◯	◯	◯
d) How much would you <u>feel</u> like letting off steam?	◯	◯	◯	◯	◯

<u>Section 3</u>

The next 7 questions are about what you would <u>really</u> do.

	not at all likely	unlikely	maybe (half & half)	likely	very likely
e) I'd go out and get into a fist fight with a stranger.	◯	◯	◯	◯	◯
f) I'd give that friend the silent treatment.	◯	◯	◯	◯	◯
g) I'd write my friend a letter explaining my side of the story.	◯	◯	◯	◯	◯
h) I'd go out later to get my mind off it.	◯	◯	◯	◯	◯
i) I'd yell at the friend to shut up and listen.	◯	◯	◯	◯	◯
j) I'd think that something else must be bothering the friend.	◯	◯	◯	◯	◯
k) I'd hold my anger inside, and it would make me sick.	◯	◯	◯	◯	◯

<u>Section 4</u>

The next 3 questions are about the long-term consequences of how you would handle the situation. Looking back over what you would really do, how do you think things would turn out in the long run.

	terrible	pretty bad	<u>OK</u>	pretty good	wonderful
l) How do you think things would turn out for YOU in the long run?	◯	◯	◯	◯	◯
m) How do you think thinkg would turn out for THAT FRIEND in the long run?	◯	◯	◯	◯	◯
n) How do you think things would turn out in the long run for your RELATIONSHIP with that friend?	◯	◯	◯	◯	◯

20. Your parents criticize you in front of your friends for something you've done.

Section 1

	not at all angry	a little angry	fairly angry	very angry	very, very angry
a) How angry would you be if this happened to you?	○	○	○	○	○

Section 2

The next 3 questions are about how you would feel, not necessarily what you would do.

	not at all	a little	somewhat (half & half)	pretty much	very much
b) How much would you feel like getting back at your parents? Or getting even?	○	○	○	○	○
c) How much would you feel like fixing the situation? Or making it better?	○	○	○	○	○
d) How much would you feel like letting off steam?	○	○	○	○	○

Section 3

The next 7 questions are about what you would really do.

	not at all likely	unlikely	maybe (half & half)	likely	very likely
e) I'd ignore my parents' comments and just go back to whatever I was doing.	○	○	○	○	○
f) I'd shove one of my friends.	○	○	○	○	○
g) I'd complain to one of our relatives.	○	○	○	○	○
h) I'd wonder if I was taking it too hard.	○	○	○	○	○
i) I'd tell my parents off.	○	○	○	○	○
j) I'd try to do better next time.	○	○	○	○	○
k) I'd figure what they did was just part of being a parent.	○	○	○	○	○

Section 4

The next 3 questions are about the long-term consequences of how you would handle the situation. Looking back over what you would really do, how do you think things would turn out in the long run.

	terrible	pretty bad	OK	pretty good	wonderful
l) How do you think things would turn out for YOU in the long run?	○	○	○	○	○
m) How do you think thinkg would turn out for YOUR PARENTS in the long run?	○	○	○	○	○
n) How do you think things would turn out in the long run for your RELATIONSHIP with your parents?	○	○	○	○	○

Anger Response Inventory – Adult Version

Reprinted with permission from the author (Tangney, J., et al., 1991).

Below are situations that people are likely to encounter in day-to-day life, followed by several common reactions to those situations.

As you read each scenario, try to imagine yourself in that situation. Then indicate how likely you would be to react in each of the ways described. We ask you to rate <u>all</u> responses because people may feel or react more than one way to the same situation, or they may react different ways at different times.

For example:

> **You wake up early one Saturday morning. It is cold and rainy outside.**

	not likely	very likely
a) You would telephone a friend to catch up on news.	①- - 2 - - - 3 - - - 4 - - - 5
b) You would take the extra time to read the paper.	1 - - - 2 - - - 3 - - - 4 - -⑤
c) You would feel disappointed that it's raining.	1 - - - 2 - -③- - 4 - - - 5
d) You would wonder why you woke up so early.	1 - - - 2 - - - 3 - -④- - 5

In the above example, I've rated <u>ALL</u> of the answers by <u>circling a number</u>. I circled a "1" for answer (a) because I wouldn't want to wake up a friend very early on a Saturday morning - - so it's not at all likely that I would do that. I circled a "5" for answer (b) because I almost always read the paper if I have time in the morning (very likely). I circled a "3" for answer (c) because for me it's about half and half. Sometimes I would be disappointed about the rain and sometimes I wouldn't - - it would depend on what I had planned. Also, I circled a "4" for answer (d) because I would probably wonder why I had awakened so early.

Please do not skip any items - - rate all responses.

> **1. You are waiting to be served at a restaurant. Fifteen minutes have gone by, and you still haven't even received a menu.**

	not at all angry				extremely angry

a) How angry would you be in this situation?   1 --- 2 --- 3 --- 4 --- 5

The next 3 questions are about how you would <u>feel</u>, not necessarily what you would <u>do</u>:

	not at all				very much

b) How much would you <u>feel</u> like getting back at the waitress or restaurant?   1 --- 2 --- 3 --- 4 --- 5

c) How much would you <u>feel</u> like fixing the situation?   1 --- 2 --- 3 --- 4 --- 5

d) How much would you <u>feel</u> like letting off steam?   1 --- 2 --- 3 --- 4 --- 5

The next 7 questions are about what you would <u>actually</u> <u>do</u>:

	not likely				very likely

e) I wouldn't leave a tip.   1 --- 2 --- 3 --- 4 --- 5

f) I'd go get a menu myself.   1 --- 2 --- 3 --- 4 --- 5

g) I'd just sit there and wait.   1 --- 2 --- 3 --- 4 --- 5

h) The longer I sat there, the more I would think about how angry I was.   1 --- 2 --- 3 --- 4 --- 5

i) I'd pound a knife on the table as the waitress walked by.   1 --- 2 --- 3 --- 4 --- 5

j) I'd think the waitress must be new.   1 --- 2 --- 3 --- 4 --- 5

k) I'd snap at the person sitting with me.   1 --- 2 --- 3 --- 4 --- 5

The next question is about the <u>long-term</u> consequences of how you would handle the situation. Looking back over what you would actually do, how do you think things would turn out in the long-run?

	harmful				beneficial

l) Would the long-term effect be harmful or beneficial?   1 --- 2 --- 3 --- 4 --- 5

---

2. You get pulled over for speeding when you were driving at the speed limit.

---

	not at all angry	extremely angry
a) How angry would you be in this situation?	1 - - - 2 - - - 3 - - - 4 - - - 5	

The next 3 questions are about how you would <u>feel</u>, not necessarily what you would <u>do</u>:

	not at all	very much
b) How much would you <u>feel</u> like getting back at the policeman?	1 - - - 2 - - - 3 - - - 4 - - - 5	
c) How much would you <u>feel</u> like fixing the situation?	1 - - - 2 - - - 3 - - - 4 - - - 5	
d) How much would you <u>feel</u> like letting off steam?	1 - - - 2 - - - 3 - - - 4 - - - 5	

The next 7 questions are about what you would <u>actually do</u>:

	not likely	very likely
e) I'd wonder if I was going faster than I thought.	1 - - - 2 - - - 3 - - - 4 - - - 5	
f) I'd go to court.	1 - - - 2 - - - 3 - - - 4 - - - 5	
g) Afterwards, I'd turn on the radio to take my mind off it.	1 - - - 2 - - - 3 - - - 4 - - - 5	
h) I'd take down the policeman's badge number and report him.	1 - - - 2 - - - 3 - - - 4 - - - 5	
i) I'd tell the policeman off.	1 - - - 2 - - - 3 - - - 4 - - - 5	
j) I'd pay the ticket, but I would steam over it for days.	1 - - - 2 - - - 3 - - - 4 - - - 5	

The next 2 questions are about the <u>long-term</u> consequences of how you would handle the situation. Looking back over what you would actually do, how do you think things would turn out in the long-run?

	harmful	beneficial
k) Would the long-term effect be harmful or beneficial for <u>you</u>, personally?	1 - - - 2 - - - 3 - - - 4 - - - 5	
l) Would the long-term effect be harmful or beneficial for the policeman, personally?	1 - - - 2 - - - 3 - - - 4 - - - 5	

> **3. You are trying to rest or read, but there are children nearby who are making a lot of noise while playing.**

	not at all angry	extremely angry
a) How angry would you be in this situation?	1 - - - 2 - - - 3 - - - 4 - - - 5	

The next 3 questions are about how you would feel, not necessarily what you would do:

	not at all	very much
b) How much would you feel like getting back at the children?	1 - - - 2 - - - 3 - - - 4 - - - 5	
c) How much would you feel like fixing the situation?	1 - - - 2 - - - 3 - - - 4 - - - 5	
d) How much would you feel like letting off steam?	1 - - - 2 - - - 3 - - - 4 - - - 5	

The next 7 questions are about what you would actually do:

	not likely	very likely
e) I'd watch TV until I calmed down.	1 - - - 2 - - - 3 - - - 4 - - - 5	
f) I'd be angry with myself for not being able to ignore it.	1 - - - 2 - - - 3 - - - 4 - - - 5	
g) I'd think, "They're only children. They don't know better."	1 - - - 2 - - - 3 - - - 4 - - - 5	
h) I'd yell at them to shut up.	1 - - - 2 - - - 3 - - - 4 - - - 5	
i) I'd take their toys away.	1 - - - 2 - - - 3 - - - 4 - - - 5	
j) I'd snap at someone else in the house.	1 - - - 2 - - - 3 - - - 4 - - - 5	
k) I'd move to a quieter room.	1 - - - 2 - - - 3 - - - 4 - - - 5	

The next 3 questions are about the long-term consequences of how you would handle the situation. Looking back over what you would actually do, how do you think things would turn out in the long-run?

	harmful	beneficial
l) Would the long-term effect be harmful or beneficial for you, personally?	1 - - - 2 - - - 3 - - - 4 - - - 5	
m) Would the long-term effect be harmful or beneficial for the children, personally?	1 - - - 2 - - - 3 - - - 4 - - - 5	
n) Would the long-term effect be harmful or beneficial for your relationship with the children?	1 - - - 2 - - - 3 - - - 4 - - - 5	

4.   Your boss implies that you're lying when you are really telling the truth.

	not at all angry	extremely angry
a) How angry would you be in this situation?	1 - - - 2 - - - 3 - - - 4 - - - 5	

The next 3 questions are about how you would <u>feel</u>, not necessarily what you would <u>do</u>:

	not at all	very much
b) How much would you <u>feel</u> like getting back at the boss?	1 - - - 2 - - - 3 - - - 4 - - - 5	
c) How much would you <u>feel</u> like fixing the situation?	1 - - - 2 - - - 3 - - - 4 - - - 5	
d) How much would you <u>feel</u> like letting off steam?	1 - - - 2 - - - 3 - - - 4 - - - 5	

The next 7 questions are about what you would <u>actually</u> <u>do</u>:

	not likely	very likely
e) I'd slam something on the boss's desk.	1 - - - 2 - - - 3 - - - 4 - - - 5	
f) For the next several days, I wouldn't do any more work than I had to.	1 - - - 2 - - - 3 - - - 4 - - - 5	
g) I'd think the boss probably just misunderstood.	1 - - - 2 - - - 3 - - - 4 - - - 5	
h) I'd get into a fist-fight with another co-worker.	1 - - - 2 - - - 3 - - - 4 - - - 5	
i) I'd think maybe I should have been clearer.	1 - - - 2 - - - 3 - - - 4 - - - 5	
j) I'd calmly explain to my boss that I was telling the truth.	1 - - - 2 - - - 3 - - - 4 - - - 5	
k) I'd walk away before I lost my temper.	1 - - - 2 - - - 3 - - - 4 - - - 5	

The next 3 questions are about the <u>long-term</u> consequences of how you would handle the situation. Looking back over what you would actually do, how do you think things would turn out in the long-run?

	harmful	beneficial
l) Would the long-term effect be harmful or beneficial for <u>you</u>, personally?	1 - - - 2 - - - 3 - - - 4 - - - 5	
m) Would the long-term effect be harmful or beneficial for your boss, personally?	1 - - - 2 - - - 3 - - - 4 - - - 5	
n) Would the long-term effect be harmful or beneficial for your <u>relationship</u> with your boss?	1 - - - 2 - - - 3 - - - 4 - - - 5	

---

5. During an argument, a friend calls you "stupid".

	not at all angry	extremely angry
a) How angry would you be in this situation?	1 - - - 2 - - - 3 - - - 4 - - - 5	

The next 3 questions are about how you would <u>feel</u>, not necessarily what you would <u>do</u>:

	not at all	very much
b) How much would you <u>feel</u> like getting back at the friend?	1 - - - 2 - - - 3 - - - 4 - - - 5	
c) How much would you <u>feel</u> like fixing the situation?	1 - - - 2 - - - 3 - - - 4 - - - 5	
d) How much would you <u>feel</u> like letting off steam?	1 - - - 2 - - - 3 - - - 4 - - - 5	

The next 7 questions are about what you would <u>actually</u> <u>do</u>:

	not likely	very likely
e) I'd be so angry I would just walk away.	1 - - - 2 - - - 3 - - - 4 - - - 5	
f) I'd explain that I don't like being called "stupid".	1 - - - 2 - - - 3 - - - 4 - - - 5	
g) I wouldn't speak to the friend for at least a week.	1 - - - 2 - - - 3 - - - 4 - - - 5	
h) I'd think it wasn't worth worrying about.	1 - - - 2 - - - 3 - - - 4 - - - 5	
i) I'd shove the friend against the wall.	1 - - - 2 - - - 3 - - - 4 - - - 5	
j) I'd think that the friend was having a bad day.	1 - - - 2 - - - 3 - - - 4 - - - 5	
k) I'd shove the next person that got in my way.	1 - - - 2 - - - 3 - - - 4 - - - 5	

The next 3 questions are about the <u>long-term</u> consequences of how you would handle the situation. Looking back over what you would actually do, how do you think things would turn out in the long-run?

	harmful	beneficial
l) Would the long-term effect be harmful or beneficial for <u>you</u>, personally?	1 - - - 2 - - - 3 - - - 4 - - - 5	
m) Would the long-term effect be harmful or beneficial for the friend, personally?	1 - - - 2 - - - 3 - - - 4 - - - 5	
n) Would the long-term effect be harmful or beneficial for your <u>relationship</u> with the friend?	1 - - - 2 - - - 3 - - - 4 - - - 5	

---

6. Your brother borrows you car and leaves you with an empty gas tank.

	not at all angry	extremely angry
a) How angry would you be in this situation?	1 - - - 2 - - - 3 - - - 4 - - - 5	

The next 3 questions are about how you would <u>feel</u>, not necessarily what you would <u>do</u>:

	not at all	very much
b) How much would you <u>feel</u> like getting back at your brother?	1 - - - 2 - - - 3 - - - 4 - - - 5	
c) How much would you <u>feel</u> like fixing the situation?	1 - - - 2 - - - 3 - - - 4 - - - 5	
d) How much would you <u>feel</u> like letting off steam?	1 - - - 2 - - - 3 - - - 4 - - - 5	

The next 7 questions are about what you would <u>actually do</u>:

	not likely	very likely
e) I'd just forget about it.	1 - - - 2 - - - 3 - - - 4 - - - 5	
f) I'd borrow his car and return it with no gas.	1 - - - 2 - - - 3 - - - 4 - - - 5	
g) I wouldn't say anything, but I'd get more angry every time I thought about it.	1 - - - 2 - - - 3 - - - 4 - - - 5	
h) I'd hit him.	1 - - - 2 - - - 3 - - - 4 - - - 5	
i) I'd calmly ask him to put more gas in the car.	1 - - - 2 - - - 3 - - - 4 - - - 5	
j) I'd think it's no problem, I can just get gas next time I go out.	1 - - - 2 - - - 3 - - - 4 - - - 5	
k) When I saw the gas gauge, I'd slam my fist on the dashboard.	1 - - - 2 - - - 3 - - - 4 - - - 5	

The next 3 questions are about the <u>long-term</u> consequences of how you would handle the situation. Looking back over what you would actually do, how do you think things would turn out in the long-run?

	harmful	beneficial
l) Would the long-term effect be harmful or beneficial for <u>you</u>, personally?	1 - - - 2 - - - 3 - - - 4 - - - 5	
m) Would the long-term effect be harmful or beneficial for your brother, personally?	1 - - - 2 - - - 3 - - - 4 - - - 5	
n) Would the long-term effect be harmful or beneficial for your <u>relationship</u> with your brother?	1 - - - 2 - - - 3 - - - 4 - - - 5	

---

7. You're struggling to carry four cups of coffee to your table at a cafeteria. Someone bumps into you, spilling the coffee.

	not at all angry	extremely angry
a) How angry would you be in this situation?	1 - - - 2 - - - 3 - - - 4 - - - 5	

The next 3 questions are about how you would <u>feel</u>, not necessarily what you would <u>do</u>:

	not at all	very much
b) How much would you <u>feel</u> like getting back at him or her?	1 - - - 2 - - - 3 - - - 4 - - - 5	
c) How much would you <u>feel</u> like fixing the situation?	1 - - - 2 - - - 3 - - - 4 - - - 5	
d) How much would you <u>feel</u> like letting off steam?	1 - - - 2 - - - 3 - - - 4 - - - 5	

The next 8 questions are about what you would <u>actually</u> <u>do</u>:

	not likely	very likely
e) I'd some more coffee.	1 - - - 2 - - - 3 - - - 4 - - - 5	
f) I'd be angry with myself for trying to carry so many cups of coffee	1 - - - 2 - - - 3 - - - 4 - - - 5	
g) I'd kick a chair.	1 - - - 2 - - - 3 - - - 4 - - - 5	
h) I'd think I should have watched where I was going.	1 - - - 2 - - - 3 - - - 4 - - - 5	
i) I'd spill something on that person's coat on the way out.	1 - - - 2 - - - 3 - - - 4 - - - 5	
j) I'd think it must have been an accident, I'm sure the person didn't mean it.	1 - - - 2 - - - 3 - - - 4 - - - 5	
k) I'd bump the person back and make sure he or she spilled something.	1 - - - 2 - - - 3 - - - 4 - - - 5	
l) I'd forget about it and go about my business.	1 - - - 2 - - - 3 - - - 4 - - - 5	

The next 2 questions are about the <u>long-term</u> consequences of how you would handle the situation. Looking back over what you would actually do, how do you think things would turn out in the long-run?

	harmful	beneficial
m) Would the long-term effect be harmful or beneficial for <u>you</u>, personally?	1 - - - 2 - - - 3 - - - 4 - - - 5	
n) Would the long-term effect be harmful or beneficial for the other person, personally?	1 - - - 2 - - - 3 - - - 4 - - - 5	

8. You see a friend being bullied by another person.

		not at all angry	extremely angry
a)	How angry would you be in this situation?	1 - - - 2 - - - 3 - - - 4 - - - 5	

The next 3 questions are about how you would <u>feel</u>, not necessarily what you would <u>do</u>:

		not at all	very much
b)	How much would you <u>feel</u> like getting back at that other person?	1 - - - 2 - - - 3 - - - 4 - - - 5	
c)	How much would you <u>feel</u> like fixing the situation?	1 - - - 2 - - - 3 - - - 4 - - - 5	
d)	How much would you <u>feel</u> like letting off steam?	1 - - - 2 - - - 3 - - - 4 - - - 5	

The next 6 questions are about what you would <u>actually</u> do:

		not likely	very likely
e)	I'd snap at a bystander to do something.	1 - - - 2 - - - 3 - - - 4 - - - 5	
f)	I'd walk away and keep my cool.	1 - - - 2 - - - 3 - - - 4 - - - 5	
g)	I'd kick myself for doing nothing.	1 - - - 2 - - - 3 - - - 4 - - - 5	
h)	I'd make a threatening gesture.	1 - - - 2 - - - 3 - - - 4 - - - 5	
i)	I'd think maybe I was overreacting.	1 - - - 2 - - - 3 - - - 4 - - - 5	
j)	I'd take the friend's arm and get him to walk away.	1 - - - 2 - - - 3 - - - 4 - - - 5	

The next 3 questions are about the <u>long-term</u> consequences of how you would handle the situation. Looking back over what you would actually do, how do you think things would turn out in the long-run?

		harmful	beneficial
k)	Would the long-term effect be harmful or beneficial for <u>you</u>, personally?	1 - - - 2 - - - 3 - - - 4 - - - 5	
l)	Would the long-term effect be harmful or beneficial for the other person, personally?	1 - - - 2 - - - 3 - - - 4 - - - 5	
m)	Would the long-term effect be harmful or beneficial for your <u>relationship</u> with the other person?	1 - - - 2 - - - 3 - - - 4 - - - 5	

9. Your friend makes plans to meet you for lunch, but doesn't show up.

	not at all angry	extremely angry
a) How angry would you be in this situation?	1 - - - 2 - - - 3 - - - 4 - - - 5	

The next 3 questions are about how you would <u>feel</u>, not necessarily what you would <u>do</u>:

	not at all	very much
b) How much would you <u>feel</u> like getting back at the friend?	1 - - - 2 - - - 3 - - - 4 - - - 5	
c) How much would you <u>feel</u> like fixing the situation?	1 - - - 2 - - - 3 - - - 4 - - - 5	
d) How much would you <u>feel</u> like letting off steam?	1 - - - 2 - - - 3 - - - 4 - - - 5	

The next 7 questions are about what you would <u>actually do</u>:

	not likely	very likely
e) I'd wonder if I'd made a mistake about the time or the place.	1 - - - 2 - - - 3 - - - 4 - - - 5	
f) I'd think that something serious must have come up to make the friend miss lunch.	1 - - - 2 - - - 3 - - - 4 - - - 5	
g) I'd stop speaking to that friend.	1 - - - 2 - - - 3 - - - 4 - - - 5	
h) I'd be angry with myself for waiting around.	1 - - - 2 - - - 3 - - - 4 - - - 5	
i) I'd just forget about it.	1 - - - 2 - - - 3 - - - 4 - - - 5	
j) I'd snarl at the waiter.	1 - - - 2 - - - 3 - - - 4 - - - 5	
k) I'd call the friend to yell at him or her for being so thoughtless.	1 - - - 2 - - - 3 - - - 4 - - - 5	

The next 3 questions are about the <u>long-term</u> consequences of how you would handle the situation. Looking back over what you would actually do, how do you think things would turn out in the long-run?

	harmful	beneficial
l) Would the long-term effect be harmful or beneficial for <u>you</u>, personally?	1 - - - 2 - - - 3 - - - 4 - - - 5	
m) Would the long-term effect be harmful or beneficial for the friend, personally?	1 - - - 2 - - - 3 - - - 4 - - - 5	
n) Would the long-term effect be harmful or beneficial for your <u>relationship</u> with the friend?	1 - - - 2 - - - 3 - - - 4 - - - 5	

---

10. You are driving to the airport to pick up a friend and get stuck in traffic.

---

	not at all angry	extremely angry
a) How angry would you be in this situation?	1 - - - 2 - - - 3 - - - 4 - - - 5	

The next 3 questions are about how you would <u>feel</u>, not necessarily what you would <u>do</u>:

	not at all	very much
b) How much would you <u>feel</u> like getting back at someone or something?	1 - - - 2 - - - 3 - - - 4 - - - 5	
c) How much would you <u>feel</u> like fixing the situation?	1 - - - 2 - - - 3 - - - 4 - - - 5	
d) How much would you <u>feel</u> like letting off steam?	1 - - - 2 - - - 3 - - - 4 - - - 5	

The next 5 questions are about what you would <u>actually</u> <u>do</u>:

	not likely	very likely
e) I'd turn on my favorite radio station to relax.	1 - - - 2 - - - 3 - - - 4 - - - 5	
f) I'd honk my horn repeatedly.	1 - - - 2 - - - 3 - - - 4 - - - 5	
g) I'd think the plane will probably be late anyway.	1 - - - 2 - - - 3 - - - 4 - - - 5	
h) I'd shove people out of my way once I got to the airport.	1 - - - 2 - - - 3 - - - 4 - - - 5	
i) I'd be angry with myself for not having left earlier.	1 - - - 2 - - - 3 - - - 4 - - - 5	

The next question is about the <u>long-term</u> consequences of how you would handle the situation. Looking back over what you would actually do, how do you think things would turn out in the long-run?

	harmful	beneficial
j) Would the long-term effect be harmful or beneficial?	1 - - - 2 - - - 3 - - - 4 - - - 5	

> **11. You are driving along at the speed limit, and the person behind you is right on your bumper.**

	not at all angry	extremely angry
a) How angry would you be in this situation?	1 - - - 2 - - - 3 - - - 4 - - - 5	

The next 3 questions are about how you would <u>feel</u>, not necessarily what you would <u>do</u>:

	not at all	very much
b) How much would you <u>feel</u> like getting back at him or her?	1 - - - 2 - - - 3 - - - 4 - - - 5	
c) How much would you <u>feel</u> like fixing the situation?	1 - - - 2 - - - 3 - - - 4 - - - 5	
d) How much would you <u>feel</u> like letting off steam?	1 - - - 2 - - - 3 - - - 4 - - - 5	

The next 7 questions are about what you would <u>actually do</u>:

	not likely	very likely
e) I'd be angry at myself for letting it bother me.	1 - - - 2 - - - 3 - - - 4 - - - 5	
f) I'd wonder if I was going slower than I thought.	1 - - - 2 - - - 3 - - - 4 - - - 5	
g) I'd make some nasty gesture at that driver.	1 - - - 2 - - - 3 - - - 4 - - - 5	
h) I'd change lanes and let the car go by.	1 - - - 2 - - - 3 - - - 4 - - - 5	
i) I'd just keep going the speed limit and I'd ignore it.	1 - - - 2 - - - 3 - - - 4 - - - 5	
j) I'd pound the dashboard.	1 - - - 2 - - - 3 - - - 4 - - - 5	
k) I'd take down the driver's license plate number and report it to the police.	1 - - - 2 - - - 3 - - - 4 - - - 5	

The next 2 questions are about the <u>long-term</u> consequences of how you would handle the situation. Looking back over what you would actually do, how do you think things would turn out in the long-run?

	harmful	beneficial
l) Would the long-term effect be harmful or beneficial for <u>you</u>, personally?	1 - - - 2 - - - 3 - - - 4 - - - 5	
m) Would the long-term effect be harmful or beneficial for the driver, personally?	1 - - - 2 - - - 3 - - - 4 - - - 5	

12. While arguing with your brother, he pushes you.

	not at all angry	extremely angry
a) How angry would you be in this situation?	1 - - - 2 - - - 3 - - - 4 - - - 5	

The next 3 questions are about how you would <u>feel</u>, not necessarily what you would <u>do</u>:

	not at all	very much
b) How much would you <u>feel</u> like getting back at your brother?	1 - - - 2 - - - 3 - - - 4 - - - 5	
c) How much would you <u>feel</u> like fixing the situation?	1 - - - 2 - - - 3 - - - 4 - - - 5	
d) How much would you <u>feel</u> like letting off steam?	1 - - - 2 - - - 3 - - - 4 - - - 5	

The next 7 questions are about what you would <u>actually</u> <u>do</u>:

	not likely	very likely
e) I'd hit him as hard as I could.	1 - - - 2 - - - 3 - - - 4 - - - 5	
f) I'd be angry with myself for getting into it. I should know better than to argue with him.	1 - - - 2 - - - 3 - - - 4 - - - 5	
g) I'd tell my brother he'd hurt me, and ask if we could talk about what was bothering him.	1 - - - 2 - - - 3 - - - 4 - - - 5	
h) I'd walk away.	1 - - - 2 - - - 3 - - - 4 - - - 5	
i) I'd hit my younger brother or sister later.	1 - - - 2 - - - 3 - - - 4 - - - 5	
j) I'd think my brother was having a bad day.	1 - - - 2 - - - 3 - - - 4 - - - 5	
k) I'd destroy something important to him.	1 - - - 2 - - - 3 - - - 4 - - - 5	

The next 3 questions are about the <u>long-term</u> consequences of how you would handle the situation. Looking back over what you would actually do, how do you think things would turn out in the long-run?

	harmful	beneficial
l) Would the long-term effect be harmful or beneficial for <u>you</u>, personally?	1 - - - 2 - - - 3 - - - 4 - - - 5	
m) Would the long-term effect be harmful or beneficial for your brother, personally?	1 - - - 2 - - - 3 - - - 4 - - - 5	
n) Would the long-term effect be harmful or beneficial for your <u>relationship</u> with your brother?	1 - - - 2 - - - 3 - - - 4 - - - 5	

13. A co-worker makes a mistake and blames it on you.

		not at all angry			extremely angry

a) How angry would you be in this situation?   1 --- 2 --- 3 --- 4 --- 5

The next 3 questions are about how you would <u>feel</u>, not necessarily what you would <u>do</u>:

		not at all			very much

b) How much would you <u>feel</u> like getting back at the co-worker?   1 --- 2 --- 3 --- 4 --- 5

c) How much would you <u>feel</u> like fixing the situation?   1 --- 2 --- 3 --- 4 --- 5

d) How much would you <u>feel</u> like letting off steam?   1 --- 2 --- 3 --- 4 --- 5

The next 7 questions are about what you would <u>actually do</u>:

		not likely			very likely

e) I'd shove the next person that spoke to me.   1 --- 2 --- 3 --- 4 --- 5

f) I'd corner the co-worker and yell at him or her for being such a liar.   1 --- 2 --- 3 --- 4 --- 5

g) I'd start a rumor that would ruin that co-worker's reputation.   1 --- 2 --- 3 --- 4 --- 5

h) I'd talk it over with the co-worker to try to clear things up.   1 --- 2 --- 3 --- 4 --- 5

i) I'd go home early.   1 --- 2 --- 3 --- 4 --- 5

j) I'd think about the co-worker over and over and really come to hate the person.   1 --- 2 --- 3 --- 4 --- 5

k) I'd wonder if maybe I <u>did</u> have something to do with it.   1 --- 2 --- 3 --- 4 --- 5

The next 3 questions are about the <u>long-term</u> consequences of how you would handle the situation. Looking back over what you would actually do, how do you think things would turn out in the long-run?

		harmful			beneficial

l) Would the long-term effect be harmful or beneficial for <u>you</u>, personally?   1 --- 2 --- 3 --- 4 --- 5

m) Would the long-term effect be harmful or beneficial for the co-worker, personally?   1 --- 2 --- 3 --- 4 --- 5

n) Would the long-term effect be harmful or beneficial for your <u>relationship</u> with the co-worker?   1 --- 2 --- 3 --- 4 --- 5

14. You are arguing with your spouse or partner and a friend tries to interfere.

	not at all angry	extremely angry
a) How angry would you be in this situation?	1 --- 2 --- 3 --- 4 --- 5	

The next 3 questions are about how you would <u>feel</u>, not necessarily what you would <u>do</u>:

	not at all	very much
b) How much would you <u>feel</u> like getting back at the friend?	1 --- 2 --- 3 --- 4 --- 5	
c) How much would you <u>feel</u> like fixing the situation?	1 --- 2 --- 3 --- 4 --- 5	
d) How much would you <u>feel</u> like letting off steam?	1 --- 2 --- 3 --- 4 --- 5	

The next 7 questions are about what you would <u>actually do</u>:

	not likely	very likely
e) I'd yell at the friend to mind their own business.	1 --- 2 --- 3 --- 4 --- 5	
f) The more I'd think about the friend's interruption, the angrier I'd get.	1 --- 2 --- 3 --- 4 --- 5	
g) I'd stop speaking to the friend.	1 --- 2 --- 3 --- 4 --- 5	
h) I'd leave the room to calm myself down.	1 --- 2 --- 3 --- 4 --- 5	
i) I'd go into the kitchen and break something.	1 --- 2 --- 3 --- 4 --- 5	
j) I'd tell the friend I appreciate the concern, but I'd like to keep this between me and my partner.	1 --- 2 --- 3 --- 4 --- 5	
k) I'd decide it's OK if the friend wants to put in a word or two.	1 --- 2 --- 3 --- 4 --- 5	

The next 3 questions are about the <u>long-term</u> consequences of how you would handle the situation. Looking back over what you would actually do, how do you think things would turn out in the long-run?

	harmful	beneficial
l) Would the long-term effect be harmful or beneficial for <u>you</u>, personally?	1 --- 2 --- 3 --- 4 --- 5	
m) Would the long-term effect be harmful or beneficial for the friend, personally?	1 --- 2 --- 3 --- 4 --- 5	
n) Would the long-term effect be harmful or beneficial for your <u>relationship</u> with the friend?	1 --- 2 --- 3 --- 4 --- 5	

15. You are walking along on a rainy day, and a car speeds past, splashing you with muddy water.

	not at all angry				extremely angry
a) How angry would you be in this situation?	1 - - - 2 - - - 3 - - - 4 - - - 5

The next 3 questions are about how you would _feel_, not necessarily what you would _do_:

	not at all				very much
b) How much would you _feel_ like getting back at the driver?	1 - - - 2 - - - 3 - - - 4 - - - 5
c) How much would you _feel_ like fixing the situation?	1 - - - 2 - - - 3 - - - 4 - - - 5
d) How much would you _feel_ like letting off steam?	1 - - - 2 - - - 3 - - - 4 - - - 5

The next 7 questions are about what you would _actually_ _do_:

	not likely				very likely
e) I'd take down the license plate number and report the driver for reckless driving.	1 - - - 2 - - - 3 - - - 4 - - - 5
f) I'd figure it was just an accident. The driver didn't see me.	1 - - - 2 - - - 3 - - - 4 - - - 5
g) I'd go home, wash up, and change clothes.	1 - - - 2 - - - 3 - - - 4 - - - 5
h) I'd just shrug it off. Worse things happen.	1 - - - 2 - - - 3 - - - 4 - - - 5
i) I'd make a joke about it being "just one of those days".	1 - - - 2 - - - 3 - - - 4 - - - 5
j) I'd throw down my umbrella.	1 - - - 2 - - - 3 - - - 4 - - - 5
k) I'd be furious with myself for walking so close to the road.	1 - - - 2 - - - 3 - - - 4 - - - 5

The next 2 questions are about the _long-term_ consequences of how you would handle the situation. Looking back over what you would actually do, how do you think things would turn out in the long-run?

	harmful				beneficial
l) Would the long-term effect be harmful or beneficial for _you_, personally?	1 - - - 2 - - - 3 - - - 4 - - - 5
m) Would the long-term effect be harmful or beneficial for the driver, personally?	1 - - - 2 - - - 3 - - - 4 - - - 5

---

16. You find out a "friend" was talking about you behind your back.

	not at all angry	extremely angry
a) How angry would you be in this situation?	1 - - - 2 - - - 3 - - - 4 - - - 5	

The next 3 questions are about how you would _feel_, not necessarily what you would _do_:

	not at all	very much
b) How much would you _feel_ like getting back at him or her?	1 - - - 2 - - - 3 - - - 4 - - - 5	
c) How much would you _feel_ like fixing the situation?	1 - - - 2 - - - 3 - - - 4 - - - 5	
d) How much would you _feel_ like letting off steam?	1 - - - 2 - - - 3 - - - 4 - - - 5	

The next 7 questions are about what you would _actually_ _do_:

	not likely	very likely
e) I'd slam the door in the friend's face next time he or she came by.	1 - - - 2 - - - 3 - - - 4 - - - 5	
f) I'd do something I enjoy to get my mind off of it.	1 - - - 2 - - - 3 - - - 4 - - - 5	
g) I'd tell all our friends this person can't be trusted.	1 - - - 2 - - - 3 - - - 4 - - - 5	
h) I'd think maybe the friend just slipped, and the whole thing was blown out of proportion.	1 - - - 2 - - - 3 - - - 4 - - - 5	
i) I wouldn't really care what he or she thinks. It wasn't a good friend anyway.	1 - - - 2 - - - 3 - - - 4 - - - 5	
j) I'd ask the friend why we couldn't talk to _each other_ about things that are bothering us.	1 - - - 2 - - - 3 - - - 4 - - - 5	
k) I'd take it out on another friend by being short-tempered.	1 - - - 2 - - - 3 - - - 4 - - - 5	

The next 3 questions are about the _long-term_ consequences of how you would handle the situation. Looking back over what you would actually do, how do you think things would turn out in the long-run?

	harmful	beneficial
l) Would the long-term effect be harmful or beneficial for _you_, personally?	1 - - - 2 - - - 3 - - - 4 - - - 5	
m) Would the long-term effect be harmful or beneficial for the friend, personally?	1 - - - 2 - - - 3 - - - 4 - - - 5	
n) Would the long-term effect be harmful or beneficial for your _relationship_ with the friend?	1 - - - 2 - - - 3 - - - 4 - - - 5	

---

17. You find out from your boss that a fellow co-worker has complained about your work.

---

	not at all angry	extremely angry
a) How angry would you be in this situation?	1 --- 2 --- 3 --- 4 --- 5	

The next 3 questions are about how you would <u>feel</u>, not necessarily what you would <u>do</u>:

	not at all	very much
b) How much would you <u>feel</u> like getting back at the co-worker?	1 --- 2 --- 3 --- 4 --- 5	
c) How much would you <u>feel</u> like fixing the situation?	1 --- 2 --- 3 --- 4 --- 5	
d) How much would you <u>feel</u> like letting off steam?	1 --- 2 --- 3 --- 4 --- 5	

The next 7 questions are about what you would <u>actually</u> <u>do</u>:

	not likely	very likely
e) I'd try to look calm, but inside I'd be furious for a long time.	1 --- 2 --- 3 --- 4 --- 5	
f) I'd think that the co-worker didn't mean to cause trouble.	1 --- 2 --- 3 --- 4 --- 5	
g) I'd make a point to tell other co-workers about what he or she had done.	1 --- 2 --- 3 --- 4 --- 5	
h) I'd shove the co-worker up against a wall.	1 --- 2 --- 3 --- 4 --- 5	
i) Once alone, I'd throw something across the room.	1 --- 2 --- 3 --- 4 --- 5	
j) I'd calmly discuss the situation with the co-worker and ask him/her to speak with me first when there are complaints.	1 --- 2 --- 3 --- 4 --- 5	
k) I'd just ignore the situation and go about work as usual.	1 --- 2 --- 3 --- 4 --- 5	

The next 3 questions are about the <u>long-term</u> consequences of how you would handle the situation. Looking back over what you would actually do, how do you think things would turn out in the long-run?

	harmful	beneficial
l) Would the long-term effect be harmful or beneficial for <u>you</u>, personally?	1 --- 2 --- 3 --- 4 --- 5	
m) Would the long-term effect be harmful or beneficial for the co-worker, personally?	1 --- 2 --- 3 --- 4 --- 5	
n) Would the long-term effect be harmful or beneficial for your <u>relationship</u> with the co-worker?	1 --- 2 --- 3 --- 4 --- 5	

18. You are waiting in line for a movie, and someone cuts in front of you.

	not at all angry	extremely angry
a) How angry would you be in this situation?	1 - - - 2 - - - 3 - - - 4 - - - 5	

The next 3 questions are about how you would <u>feel</u>, not necessarily what you would <u>do</u>:

	not at all	very much
b) How much would you <u>feel</u> like getting back at him or her?	1 - - - 2 - - - 3 - - - 4 - - - 5	
c) How much would you <u>feel</u> like fixing the situation?	1 - - - 2 - - - 3 - - - 4 - - - 5	
d) How much would you <u>feel</u> like letting off steam?	1 - - - 2 - - - 3 - - - 4 - - - 5	

The next 7 questions are about what you would <u>actually do</u>:

	not likely	very likely
e) I'd ask the manager to speak to the person.	1 - - - 2 - - - 3 - - - 4 - - - 5	
f) I'd tell the other people in the line how rude the person was.	1 - - - 2 - - - 3 - - - 4 - - - 5	
g) I'd just ignore it.	1 - - - 2 - - - 3 - - - 4 - - - 5	
h) I'd snap at the ticket clerk.	1 - - - 2 - - - 3 - - - 4 - - - 5	
i) I'd remind myself that it's no big deal. There will be plenty of seats.	1 - - - 2 - - - 3 - - - 4 - - - 5	
j) I wouldn't say anything, but I'd be so angry I couldn't enjoy the movie.	1 - - - 2 - - - 3 - - - 4 - - - 5	
k) I'd shove the person back out of line.	1 - - - 2 - - - 3 - - - 4 - - - 5	

The next 2 questions are about the <u>long-term</u> consequences of how you would handle the situation. Looking back over what you would actually do, how do you think things would turn out in the long-run?

	harmful	beneficial
l) Would the long-term effect be harmful or beneficial for <u>you</u>, personally?	1 - - - 2 - - - 3 - - - 4 - - - 5	
m) Would the long-term effect be harmful or beneficial for that person, personally?	1 - - - 2 - - - 3 - - - 4 - - - 5	

---

19. Someone you have just met treats you like you are not good enough.

	not at all angry	extremely angry
a) How angry would you be in this situation?	1 - - - 2 - - - 3 - - - 4 - - - 5	

The next 3 questions are about how you would <u>feel</u>, not necessarily what you would <u>do</u>:

	not at all	very much
b) How much would you <u>feel</u> like getting back at that person?	1 - - - 2 - - - 3 - - - 4 - - - 5	
c) How much would you <u>feel</u> like fixing the situation?	1 - - - 2 - - - 3 - - - 4 - - - 5	
d) How much would you <u>feel</u> like letting off steam?	1 - - - 2 - - - 3 - - - 4 - - - 5	

The next 7 questions are about what you would <u>actually do</u>:

	not likely	very likely
e) I'd make a nasty gesture in the person's face.	1 - - - 2 - - - 3 - - - 4 - - - 5	
f) I'd tell everyone what a snob that person is.	1 - - - 2 - - - 3 - - - 4 - - - 5	
g) I'd calmly explain that I didn't appreciate how he or she was treating me.	1 - - - 2 - - - 3 - - - 4 - - - 5	
h) I'd excuse myself from the conversation.	1 - - - 2 - - - 3 - - - 4 - - - 5	
i) I'd think the person doesn't realize how he or she is coming across.	1 - - - 2 - - - 3 - - - 4 - - - 5	
j) I'd hit the next person I saw.	1 - - - 2 - - - 3 - - - 4 - - - 5	
k) I'd wonder if I was being too sensitive.	1 - - - 2 - - - 3 - - - 4 - - - 5	

The next 3 questions are about the <u>long-term</u> consequences of how you would handle the situation. Looking back over what you would actually do, how do you think things would turn out in the long-run?

	harmful	beneficial
l) Would the long-term effect be harmful or beneficial for <u>you</u>, personally?	1 - - - 2 - - - 3 - - - 4 - - - 5	
m) Would the long-term effect be harmful or beneficial for that person, personally?	1 - - - 2 - - - 3 - - - 4 - - - 5	
n) Would the long-term effect be harmful or beneficial for your <u>relationship</u> with that person, personally?	1 - - - 2 - - - 3 - - - 4 - - - 5	

20. A person who has kept you waiting before is late again for an appointment.

	not at all angry	extremely angry

a) How angry would you be in this situation?   1 - - - 2 - - - 3 - - - 4 - - - 5

The next 3 questions are about how you would <u>feel</u>, not necessarily what you would <u>do</u>:

	not at all	very much

b) How much would you <u>feel</u> like getting back at him or her?   1 - - - 2 - - - 3 - - - 4 - - - 5

c) How much would you <u>feel</u> like fixing the situation?   1 - - - 2 - - - 3 - - - 4 - - - 5

d) How much would you <u>feel</u> like letting off steam?   1 - - - 2 - - - 3 - - - 4 - - - 5

The next 7 questions are about what you would <u>actually</u> <u>do</u>:

	not likely	very likely

e) I'd ask the person to call next time he or she is going to be late.   1 - - - 2 - - - 3 - - - 4 - - - 5

f) I wouldn't show up for our next appointment.   1 - - - 2 - - - 3 - - - 4 - - - 5

g) I'd be furious with myself for waiting.   1 - - - 2 - - - 3 - - - 4 - - - 5

h) I'd kick something near by.   1 - - - 2 - - - 3 - - - 4 - - - 5

i) I'd read something to calm down.   1 - - - 2 - - - 3 - - - 4 - - - 5

j) I'd wonder if I'd made a mistake about the time of our   1 - - - 2 - - - 3 - - - 4 - - - 5
     appointment.

k) I'd yell at the person for being so inconsiderate.   1 - - - 2 - - - 3 - - - 4 - - - 5

The next 3 questions are about the <u>long-term</u> consequences of how you would handle the situation. Looking back over what you would actually do, how do you think things would turn out in the long-run?

	harmful	beneficial

l) Would the long-term effect be harmful or beneficial for <u>you</u>,   1 - - - 2 - - - 3 - - - 4 - - - 5
     personally?

m) Would the long-term effect be harmful or beneficial for   1 - - - 2 - - - 3 - - - 4 - - - 5
     that person, personally?

n) Would the long-term effect be harmful or beneficial for   1 - - - 2 - - - 3 - - - 4 - - - 5
     your <u>relationship</u> with that person, personally?

21. You see an older person pushed aside by someone in a hurry.

	not at all angry	extremely angry
a) How angry would you be in this situation?	1 - - - 2 - - - 3 - - - 4 - - - 5	

The next 3 questions are about how you would <u>feel</u>, not necessarily what you would <u>do</u>:

	not at all	very much
b) How much would you <u>feel</u> like getting back at that person?	1 - - - 2 - - - 3 - - - 4 - - - 5	
c) How much would you <u>feel</u> like fixing the situation?	1 - - - 2 - - - 3 - - - 4 - - - 5	
d) How much would you <u>feel</u> like letting off steam?	1 - - - 2 - - - 3 - - - 4 - - - 5	

The next 7 questions are about what you would <u>actually do</u>:

	not likely	very likely
e) I'd talk loudly about how I hate people who push and shove.	1 - - - 2 - - - 3 - - - 4 - - - 5	
f) I'd yell at the person and call him or her names.	1 - - - 2 - - - 3 - - - 4 - - - 5	
g) I'd think it was just a little bump.	1 - - - 2 - - - 3 - - - 4 - - - 5	
h) I'd make sure the older person was all right.	1 - - - 2 - - - 3 - - - 4 - - - 5	
i) I'd trip the next person that ran by in a hurry.	1 - - - 2 - - - 3 - - - 4 - - - 5	
j) I'd be steamed all day about the incident.	1 - - - 2 - - - 3 - - - 4 - - - 5	
k) I'd just ignore it.	1 - - - 2 - - - 3 - - - 4 - - - 5	

The next 2 questions are about the <u>long-term</u> consequences of how you would handle the situation. Looking back over what you would actually do, how do you think things would turn out in the long-run?

	harmful	beneficial
l) Would the long-term effect be harmful or beneficial for <u>you</u>, personally?	1 - - - 2 - - - 3 - - - 4 - - - 5	
m) Would the long-term effect be harmful or beneficial for that person, personally?	1 - - - 2 - - - 3 - - - 4 - - - 5	

22. A neighbor's dog barks all night while you are trying to sleep.

		not at all angry	extremely angry
a)	How angry would you be in this situation?	1 - - - 2 - - - 3 - - - 4 - - - 5	

The next 3 questions are about how you would <u>feel</u>, not necessarily what you would <u>do</u>:

		not at all	very much
b)	How much would you <u>feel</u> like getting back at someone or something?	1 - - - 2 - - - 3 - - - 4 - - - 5	
c)	How much would you <u>feel</u> like fixing the situation?	1 - - - 2 - - - 3 - - - 4 - - - 5	
d)	How much would you <u>feel</u> like letting off steam?	1 - - - 2 - - - 3 - - - 4 - - - 5	

The next 7 questions are about what you would <u>actually do</u>:

		not likely	very likely
e)	I'd go to work the next day and be grumpy with my fellow workers.	1 - - - 2 - - - 3 - - - 4 - - - 5	
f)	I'd just lay there until I fell asleep.	1 - - - 2 - - - 3 - - - 4 - - - 5	
g)	I'd think I'm just a light sleeper.	1 - - - 2 - - - 3 - - - 4 - - - 5	
h)	I'd complain to the other neighbors about the problem with the dog.	1 - - - 2 - - - 3 - - - 4 - - - 5	
i)	The more the dog barked, the more it would get on my nerves and the angrier I would get.	1 - - - 2 - - - 3 - - - 4 - - - 5	
j)	I'd ask the neighbor to try to keep the dog quiet during the night.	1 - - - 2 - - - 3 - - - 4 - - - 5	
k)	I'd call the neighbor and yell at him to shut his dog up.	1 - - - 2 - - - 3 - - - 4 - - - 5	

The next 3 questions are about the <u>long-term</u> consequences of how you would handle the situation. Looking back over what you would actually do, how do you think things would turn out in the long-run?

		harmful	beneficial
l)	Would the long-term effect be harmful or beneficial for <u>you</u>, personally?	1 - - - 2 - - - 3 - - - 4 - - - 5	
m)	Would the long-term effect be harmful or beneficial for the neighbor, personally?	1 - - - 2 - - - 3 - - - 4 - - - 5	
n)	Would the long-term effect be harmful or beneficial for your <u>relationship</u> with the neighbor, personally?	1 - - - 2 - - - 3 - - - 4 - - - 5	

---

23. You tell a friend about a problem, and your friend doesn't take it seriously.

	not at all angry	extremely angry
a) How angry would you be in this situation?	1 - - - 2 - - - 3 - - - 4 - - - 5	

The next 3 questions are about how you would <u>feel</u>, not necessarily what you would <u>do</u>:

	not at all	very much
b) How much would you <u>feel</u> like getting back at him or her?	1 - - - 2 - - - 3 - - - 4 - - - 5	
c) How much would you <u>feel</u> like fixing the situation?	1 - - - 2 - - - 3 - - - 4 - - - 5	
d) How much would you <u>feel</u> like letting off steam?	1 - - - 2 - - - 3 - - - 4 - - - 5	

The next 7 questions are about what you would <u>actually do</u>:

	not likely	very likely
e) I'd be nice to the friend but my anger would build inside.	1 - - - 2 - - - 3 - - - 4 - - - 5	
f) I'd pound on the wall.	1 - - - 2 - - - 3 - - - 4 - - - 5	
g) I'd never speak to the friend again.	1 - - - 2 - - - 3 - - - 4 - - - 5	
h) I'd grab the friend and force him or her out the door.	1 - - - 2 - - - 3 - - - 4 - - - 5	
i) I'd think maybe the friend is making light of this problem to cheer me up.	1 - - - 2 - - - 3 - - - 4 - - - 5	
j) I'd make a joke to lighten up the conversation.	1 - - - 2 - - - 3 - - - 4 - - - 5	
k) I'd tell my problem to someone else who would take it seriously.	1 - - - 2 - - - 3 - - - 4 - - - 5	

The next 3 questions are about the <u>long-term</u> consequences of how you would handle the situation. Looking back over what you would actually do, how do you think things would turn out in the long-run?

	harmful	beneficial
l) Would the long-term effect be harmful or beneficial for <u>you</u>, personally?	1 - - - 2 - - - 3 - - - 4 - - - 5	
m) Would the long-term effect be harmful or beneficial for the friend, personally?	1 - - - 2 - - - 3 - - - 4 - - - 5	
n) Would the long-term effect be harmful or beneficial for your <u>relationship</u> with the friend, personally?	1 - - - 2 - - - 3 - - - 4 - - - 5	

Anger Response Inventory – Child Version

Reprinted with permission from the author (Tangney, J., et al., 1991).

ARI-C

Here are some situations that might happen to you once in a while.
And here are some different ways that people might think or feel.

Really imagine that you are in the situation now. Imagine how you
might think or feel. Then read each statement. Put an X in the circle
which describes how likely it is that the statement would be true for you.
The largest circle means that you are very likely to think or feel that
way, and the smallest circle means that you are not at all likely to think
or feel that way.

SAMPLE

You wake up very early one morning on a school day.

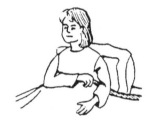

	not at all likely	unlikely	maybe (half&half)	likely	very likely
a) I would eat breakfast right away.	⊗	○	○	○	○
b) I would try to finish my homework before I left for school.	○	○	⊗	○	○
c) I would feel like staying in bed.	○	○	○	⊗	○

Remember that everyone has good days and bad days. Everyone sometimes
does things that they would not usually do. There are no right or wrong
answers to these questions.

IMAGINE --

'. It's Saturday and you want to go out and play, but your mother says you
   have to clean your room.

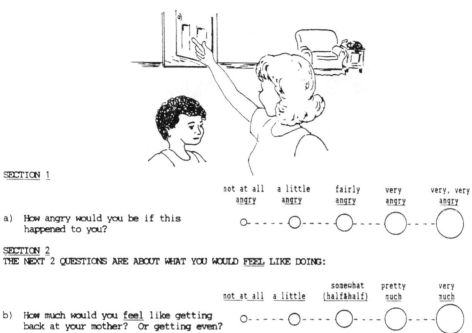

SECTION 1

	not at all angry	a little angry	fairly angry	very angry	very, very angry

a) How angry would you be if this
    happened to you?

SECTION 2
THE NEXT 2 QUESTIONS ARE ABOUT WHAT YOU WOULD FEEL LIKE DOING:

	not at all	a little	somewhat (half&half)	pretty much	very much

b) How much would you feel like getting
    back at your mother? Or getting even?

c) How much would you feel like making
    the situation better?

SECTION 3
THE NEXT 6 QUESTIONS ARE ABOUT WHAT YOU WOULD REALLY DO:

	not at all likely	unlikely	maybe (half&half)	likely	very likely

e) I'd play a game in my room until I
    felt better.

f) It's no big deal. My room won't take
    that long to clean.

g) I'd be angry with myself for not
    having picked up the room the day
    before.

h) I'd punch my little brother or
    sister.

i) I wouldn't speak to my mother for the
    rest of the day.

j) I'd slam my bedroom door so my mother
    could hear it.

SECTION 4
NOW THINK AGAIN ABOUT WHAT YOU WOULD REALLY DO IF THIS HAPPENED.

	terrible	pretty bad	OK	pretty good	wonderful

k) How do you think things would turn
    out for YOU in the long run?

l) How do you think things would turn
    out for YOUR MOTHER in the long run?

IMAGINE --

2.   You know you are right about something, but your teacher insists that
     you are wrong.

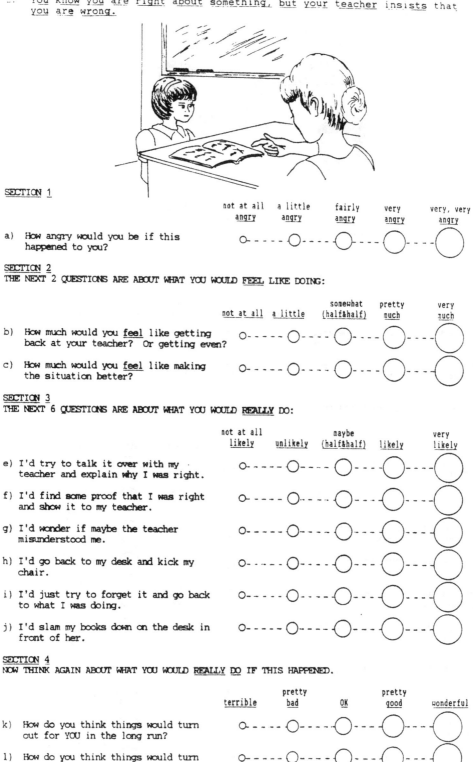

SECTION 1

	not at all angry	a little angry	fairly angry	very angry	very, very angry

a)   How angry would you be if this
     happened to you?

SECTION 2
THE NEXT 2 QUESTIONS ARE ABOUT WHAT YOU WOULD FEEL LIKE DOING:

	not at all	a little	somewhat (half&half)	pretty much	very much

b)   How much would you feel like getting
     back at your teacher? Or getting even?

c)   How much would you feel like making
     the situation better?

SECTION 3
THE NEXT 6 QUESTIONS ARE ABOUT WHAT YOU WOULD REALLY DO:

	not at all likely	unlikely	maybe (half&half)	likely	very likely

e)   I'd try to talk it over with my
     teacher and explain why I was right.

f)   I'd find some proof that I was right
     and show it to my teacher.

g)   I'd wonder if maybe the teacher
     misunderstood me.

h)   I'd go back to my desk and kick my
     chair.

i)   I'd just try to forget it and go back
     to what I was doing.

j)   I'd slam my books down on the desk in
     front of her.

SECTION 4
NOW THINK AGAIN ABOUT WHAT YOU WOULD REALLY DO IF THIS HAPPENED.

	terrible	pretty bad	OK	pretty good	wonderful

k)   How do you think things would turn
     out for YOU in the long run?

l)   How do you think things would turn
     out for YOUR TEACHER in the long run?

IMAGINE --

3.   You are trying to tell a friend something important, and the friend
     won't listen to you.

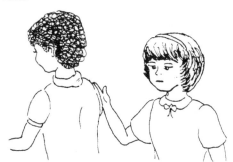

SECTION 1

	not at all angry	a little angry	fairly angry	very angry	very, very angry

a) How angry would you be if this
    happened to you?

SECTION 2
THE NEXT 2 QUESTIONS ARE ABOUT WHAT YOU WOULD FEEL LIKE DOING:

	not at all	a little	somewhat (half&half)	pretty much	very much

b) How much would you feel like getting
    back at that friend? Or getting even?

c) How much would you feel like making
    the situation better?

SECTION 3
THE NEXT 6 QUESTIONS ARE ABOUT WHAT YOU WOULD REALLY DO:

	not at all likely	unlikely	maybe (half&half)	likely	very likely

e) I'd walk away so I wouldn't lose my
    temper.

f) I'd figure I can always talk to
    someone else about it.

g) I'd ask my friend to please listen to
    me because it's REALLY important.

h) I'd yell at another friend.

i) I'd yell at the friend to shut up and
    listen.

j) I'd be mad at myself for
    trying to talk to that friend.

SECTION 4
NOW THINK AGAIN ABOUT WHAT YOU WOULD REALLY DO IF THIS HAPPENED.

	terrible	pretty bad	OK	pretty good	wonderful

k) How do you think things would turn
    out for YOU in the long run?

l) How do you think things would turn
    out for THAT FRIEND in the long run?

IMAGINE --

4. <u>Your</u> <u>parents</u> <u>blame</u> <u>you</u> <u>for</u> <u>something</u> <u>that</u> <u>was</u> <u>not</u> <u>your</u> <u>fault.</u>

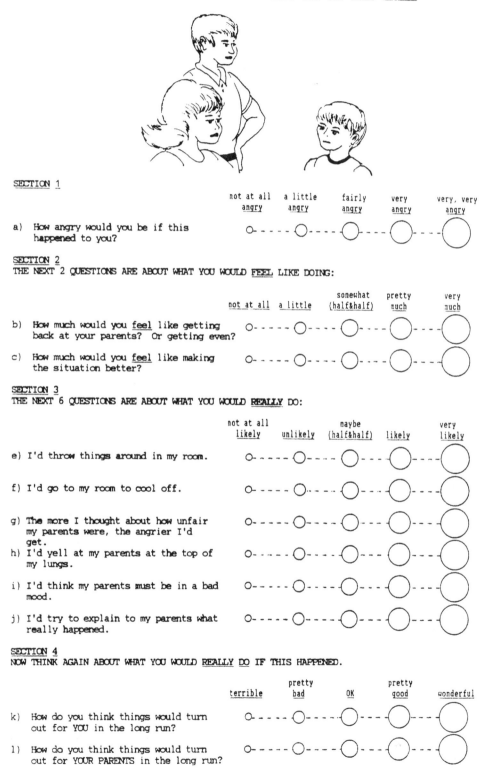

SECTION 1

	not at all angry	a little angry	fairly angry	very angry	very, very angry
a) How angry would you be if this happened to you?	O	O	O	O	O

SECTION 2
THE NEXT 2 QUESTIONS ARE ABOUT WHAT YOU WOULD <u>FEEL</u> LIKE DOING:

	not at all	a little	somewhat (half&half)	pretty much	very much
b) How much would you <u>feel</u> like getting back at your parents? Or getting even?	O	O	O	O	O
c) How much would you <u>feel</u> like making the situation better?	O	O	O	O	O

SECTION 3
THE NEXT 6 QUESTIONS ARE ABOUT WHAT YOU WOULD <u>REALLY</u> DO:

	not at all likely	unlikely	maybe (half&half)	likely	very likely
e) I'd throw things around in my room.	O	O	O	O	O
f) I'd go to my room to cool off.	O	O	O	O	O
g) The more I thought about how unfair my parents were, the angrier I'd get.	O	O	O	O	O
h) I'd yell at my parents at the top of my lungs.	O	O	O	O	O
i) I'd think my parents must be in a bad mood.	O	O	O	O	O
j) I'd try to explain to my parents what really happened.	O	O	O	O	O

SECTION 4
NOW THINK AGAIN ABOUT WHAT YOU WOULD <u>REALLY</u> <u>DO</u> IF THIS HAPPENED.

	terrible	pretty bad	OK	pretty good	wonderful
k) How do you think things would turn out for YOU in the long run?	O	O	O	O	O
l) How do you think things would turn out for YOUR PARENTS in the long run?	O	O	O	O	O

IMAGINE --

5. Someone in your class acts up, so the whole class has to stay in for
    recess.

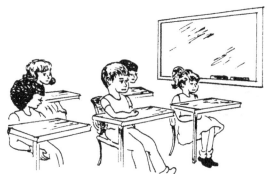

SECTION 1

	not at all angry	a little angry	fairly angry	very angry	very, very angry

a) How angry would you be if this
    happened to you?

SECTION 2
THE NEXT 2 QUESTIONS ARE ABOUT WHAT YOU WOULD FEEL LIKE DOING:

	not at all	a little	somewhat (half&half)	pretty much	very much

b) How much would you feel like getting
    back at that kid? Or getting even?

c) How much would you feel like making
    the situation better?

SECTION 3
THE NEXT 6 QUESTIONS ARE ABOUT WHAT YOU WOULD REALLY DO:

	not at all likely	unlikely	maybe (half&half)	likely	very likely

e) I'd get everyone in the class to
    ignore that kid.

f) It's not a problem. I didn't feel
    like going out for recess anyway.

g) I'd push someone else aside on my way
    to my seat.

h) I'd keep giving the kid dirty looks.

i) I'd try to think of something else to
    take my mind off it.

j) I wouldn't do anything, but while we
    were sitting there I'd be getting
    angrier and angrier.

SECTION 4
NOW THINK AGAIN ABOUT WHAT YOU WOULD REALLY DO IF THIS HAPPENED.

	terrible	pretty bad	OK	pretty good	wonderful

k) How do you think things would turn
    out for YOU in the long run?

l) How do you think things would turn
    out for THAT KID in the long run?

IMAGINE --

6. Your best friend says he or she will come over to your house after
   school, but never shows up.

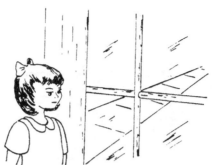

SECTION 1

	not at all angry	a little angry	fairly angry	very angry	very, very angry

a) How angry would you be if this happened to you?

SECTION 2
THE NEXT 2 QUESTIONS ARE ABOUT WHAT YOU WOULD FEEL LIKE DOING:

	not at all	a little	somewhat (half&half)	pretty much	very much

b) How much would you feel like getting back at your friend? Or getting even?

c) How much would you feel like making the situation better?

SECTION 3
THE NEXT 6 QUESTIONS ARE ABOUT WHAT YOU WOULD REALLY DO:

	not at all likely	unlikely	maybe (half&half)	likely	very likely

e) I'd give the friend a really dirty look the next time I saw him or her.

f) I'd ignore the friend at school the next day.

g) I'd just try to forget about it.

h) I'd yell at my mother.

i) I'd act like nothing was wrong, but I'd be mad about it for days.

j) I wouldn't care. My friend can always come over another day.

SECTION 4
NOW THINK AGAIN ABOUT WHAT YOU WOULD REALLY DO IF THIS HAPPENED.

	terrible	pretty bad	OK	pretty good	wonderful

k) How do you think things would turn out for YOU in the long run?

l) How do you think things would turn out for YOUR FRIEND in the long run?

IMAGINE --

7. You tell a good friend a secret, and the friend tells everyone.

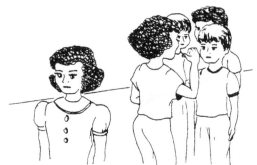

SECTION 1

	not at all angry	a little angry	fairly angry	very angry	very, very angry
a) How angry would you be if this happened to you?	○	○	○	○	○

SECTION 2
THE NEXT 2 QUESTIONS ARE ABOUT WHAT YOU WOULD **FEEL** LIKE DOING:

	not at all	a little	somewhat (half&half)	pretty much	very much
b) How much would you **feel** like getting back at your friend? Or getting even?	○	○	○	○	○
c) How much would you **feel** like making the situation better?	○	○	○	○	○

SECTION 3
THE NEXT 6 QUESTIONS ARE ABOUT WHAT YOU WOULD **REALLY** DO:

	not at all likely	unlikely	maybe (half&half)	likely	very likely
e) I'd yell at my parents to leave me alone when I got home.	○	○	○	○	○
f) I'd yell at the friend "I hate you!"	○	○	○	○	○
g) I'd tell everyone a secret that the friend had told me.	○	○	○	○	○
h) I'd be really angry with myself for trusting that friend.	○	○	○	○	○
i) I'd think I shouldn't have told the friend the secret.	○	○	○	○	○
j) I'd go play to get my mind off it.	○	○	○	○	○

SECTION 4
NOW THINK AGAIN ABOUT WHAT YOU WOULD **REALLY** DO IF THIS HAPPENED.

	terrible	pretty bad	OK	pretty good	wonderful
k) How do you think things would turn out for YOU in the long run?	○	○	○	○	○
l) How do you think things would turn out for YOUR FRIEND in the long run?	○	○	○	○	○

IMAGINE --

3. You are playing a game, and someone on the other side tries to cheat.

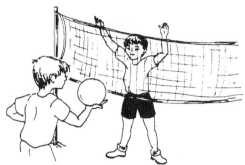

SECTION 1

	not at all angry	a little angry	fairly angry	very angry	very, very angry
a) How angry would you be if this happened to you?	O	O	O	O	O

SECTION 2
THE NEXT 2 QUESTIONS ARE ABOUT WHAT YOU WOULD **FEEL** LIKE DOING:

	not at all	a little	somewhat (half&half)	pretty much	very much
b) How much would you **feel** like getting back at that kid? Or getting even?	O	O	O	O	O
c) How much would you **feel** like making the situation better?	O	O	O	O	O

SECTION 3
THE NEXT 6 QUESTIONS ARE ABOUT WHAT YOU WOULD **REALLY** DO:

	not at all likely	unlikely	maybe (half&half)	likely	very likely
e) I'd shove one of the other players.	O	O	O	O	O
f) I'd just keep playing and ignore it.	O	O	O	O	O
g) I'd be angry with myself for letting the kid play.	O	O	O	O	O
h) I'd think maybe the kid didn't know the rules.	O	O	O	O	O
i) I'd throw something at the kid.	O	O	O	O	O
j) I'd tell all the other kids that the kid cheats.	O	O	O	O	O

SECTION 4
NOW THINK AGAIN ABOUT WHAT YOU WOULD **REALLY DO** IF THIS HAPPENED.

	terrible	pretty bad	OK	pretty good	wonderful
k) How do you think things would turn out for YOU in the long run?	O	O	O	O	O
l) How do you think things would turn out for THAT KID in the long run?	O	O	O	O	O

IMAGINE --

9. You are trying to do your schoolwork, and a classmate bumps your desk
   so that you mess up.

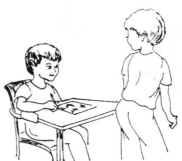

SECTION 1

	not at all angry	a little angry	fairly angry	very angry	very, very angry

a) How angry would you be if this
   happened to you?

SECTION 2
THE NEXT 2 QUESTIONS ARE ABOUT WHAT YOU WOULD **FEEL** LIKE DOING:

	not at all	a little	somewhat (half&half)	pretty much	very much

b) How much would you **feel** like getting
   back at that kid? Or getting even?

c) How much would you **feel** like making
   the situation better?

SECTION 3
THE NEXT 6 QUESTIONS ARE ABOUT WHAT YOU WOULD **REALLY** DO:

	not at all likely	unlikely	maybe (half&half)	likely	very likely

e) I'd bump the kid's desk on purpose.

f) I'd move my desk back out of the way.

g) I'd tell the teacher the kid bumped
   my desk on purpose.

h) I'd walk to the other side of the
   room to calm down.

i) I'd figure maybe it was an accident.
   The kid didn't do it on purpose.

j) I'd slam the desk with my fist.

SECTION 4
NOW THINK AGAIN ABOUT WHAT YOU WOULD **REALLY DO** IF THIS HAPPENED.

	terrible	pretty bad	OK	pretty good	wonderful

k) How do you think things would turn
   out for YOU in the long run?

l) How do you think things would turn
   out for THAT KID in the long run?

IMAGINE --

℃. Your brother or sister takes something that's yours without asking.

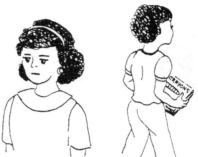

SECTION 1

	not at all angry	a little angry	fairly angry	very angry	very, very angry

a) How angry would you be if this
   happened to you?

SECTION 2
THE NEXT 2 QUESTIONS ARE ABOUT WHAT YOU WOULD FEEL LIKE DOING:

	not at all	a little	somewhat (half&half)	pretty much	very much

b) How much would you feel like getting
   back at your brother or sister?
   Or getting even?
c) How much would you feel like making
   the situation better?

SECTION 3
THE NEXT 6 QUESTIONS ARE ABOUT WHAT YOU WOULD REALLY DO:

	not at all likely	unlikely	maybe (half&half)	likely	very likely

e) I'd yell at my mom for letting them
   get away with it.

f) I'd yell at my brother or sister for
   "stealing" my stuff.

g) I'd be angry with myself for not
   keeping an eye on my things.

h) I'd think maybe my brother or sister
   thought I wouldn't mind.

i) I'd take something of theirs without
   asking.

j) I wouldn't do anything. I'd just
   ignore it.

SECTION 4
NOW THINK AGAIN ABOUT WHAT YOU WOULD REALLY DO IF THIS HAPPENED.

	terrible	pretty bad	OK	pretty good	wonderful

k) How do you think things would turn
   out for YOU in the long run?

l) How do you think things would turn
   out for YOUR BROTHER OR SISTER in
   the long run?

IMAGE --

'. Your mom or dad promises you something, but later they change their mind.

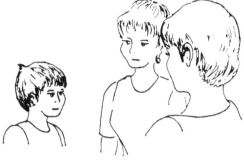

SECTION 1

	not at all angry	a little angry	fairly angry	very angry	very, very angry

a) How angry would you be if this happened to you?

SECTION 2
THE NEXT 2 QUESTIONS ARE ABOUT WHAT YOU WOULD FEEL LIKE DOING:

	not at all	a little	somewhat (half&half)	pretty much	very much

b) How much would you feel like getting back at your mom or dad? Or getting even?

c) How much would you feel like making the situation better?

SECTION 3
THE NEXT 6 QUESTIONS ARE ABOUT WHAT YOU WOULD REALLY DO:

	not at all likely	unlikely	maybe (half&half)	likely	very likely

e) I'd push my brother or sister.

f) I'd tell my parents that I'm unhappy about it.

g) I'd shout at them for lying to me.

h) I'd be angry with myself for trusting my parents.

i) I'd go do something else I enjoyed to get my mind off it.

j) I'd wonder if I did something wrong.

SECTION 4
NOW THINK AGAIN ABOUT WHAT YOU WOULD REALLY DO IF THIS HAPPENED.

	terrible	pretty bad	OK	pretty good	wonderful

k) How do you think things would turn out for YOU in the long run?

l) How do you think things would turn out for YOUR MOM OR DAD in the long run?

IMAGINE --

2. Your mother says you can't play with certain friends.

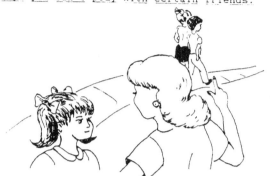

SECTION 1

	not at all angry	a little angry	fairly angry	very angry	very, very angry

a) How angry would you be if this
   happened to you?

SECTION 2
THE NEXT 2 QUESTIONS ARE ABOUT WHAT YOU WOULD FEEL LIKE DOING:

	not at all	a little	somewhat (half&half)	pretty much	very much

b) How much would you feel like getting
   back at your mother? Or getting even?

c) How much would you feel like making
   the situation better?

SECTION 3
THE NEXT 6 QUESTIONS ARE ABOUT WHAT YOU WOULD REALLY DO:

	not at all likely	unlikely	maybe (half&half)	likely	very likely

e) I'd go to my room and break
   something.

f) I wouldn't say anything, but every
   time I saw my mother I'd get very
   mad.

g) I'd talk it over with my mother and
   try to get her to change her mind.

h) I'd yell at my mother and tell her
   she's mean.

i) I wouldn't care that much. I have
   other friends I can play with.

j) I'd leave the house for a while to
   calm down.

SECTION 4
NOW THINK AGAIN ABOUT WHAT YOU WOULD REALLY DO IF THIS HAPPENED.

	terrible	pretty bad	OK	pretty good	wonderful

k) How do you think things would turn
   out for YOU in the long run?

l) How do you think things would turn
   out for YOUR MOTHER in the long run?

IMAGINE --

'3. You tell the truth about something, but your parents don't believe you.

SECTION 1

	not at all angry	a little angry	fairly angry	very angry	very, very angry
a) How angry would you be if this happened to you?	O	O	O	O	O

SECTION 2
THE NEXT 2 QUESTIONS ARE ABOUT WHAT YOU WOULD FEEL LIKE DOING:

	not at all	a little	somewhat (half&half)	pretty much	very much
b) How much would you feel like getting back at your parents? Or getting even?	O	O	O	O	O
c) How much would you feel like making the situation better?	O	O	O	O	O

SECTION 3
THE NEXT 6 QUESTIONS ARE ABOUT WHAT YOU WOULD REALLY DO:

	not at all likely	unlikely	maybe (half&half)	likely	very likely
e) I'd go do something fun to get my mind off what happened.	O	O	O	O	O
f) I'd kick the wall in my room.	O	O	O	O	O
g) I'd try to get some proof that I was telling the truth.	O	O	O	O	O
h) I'd grab my mother's arm to make her listen.	O	O	O	O	O
i) I'd think I didn't explain myself very well.	O	O	O	O	O
j) I'd try to explain the truth to them again.	O	O	O	O	O

SECTION 4
NOW THINK AGAIN ABOUT WHAT YOU WOULD REALLY DO IF THIS HAPPENED.

	terrible	pretty bad	OK	pretty good	wonderful
k) How do you think things would turn out for YOU in the long run?	O	O	O	O	O
l) How do you think things would turn out for YOUR PARENTS in the long run?	O	O	O	O	O

IMAGINE --

'4. A friend is picking people to be on a team, and he or she picks you
   last.

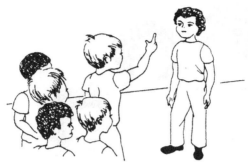

SECTION 1

	not at all angry	a little angry	fairly angry	very angry	very, very angry

a) How angry would you be if this
   happened to you?

SECTION 2
THE NEXT 2 QUESTIONS ARE ABOUT WHAT YOU WOULD **FEEL** LIKE DOING:

	not at all	a little	somewhat (half&half)	pretty much	very much

b) How much would you _feel_ like getting
   back at that friend? Or getting even?

c) How much would you _feel_ like making
   the situation better?

SECTION 3
THE NEXT 6 QUESTIONS ARE ABOUT WHAT YOU WOULD **REALLY** DO:

	not at all likely	unlikely	maybe (half&half)	likely	very likely

e) I would push someone on the other
   team.

f) I'd concentrate on the game to forget
   about being picked last.

g) I'd play badly on purpose.

h) I wouldn't care about being picked
   last.

i) I'd throw the ball in the friend's
   face.

j) I'd play the game the best I could.

SECTION 4
NOW THINK AGAIN ABOUT WHAT YOU WOULD **REALLY** DO IF THIS HAPPENED.

	terrible	pretty bad	OK	pretty good	wonderful

k) How do you think things would turn
   out for YOU in the long run?

l) How do you think things would turn
   out for THAT FRIEND in the long run?

IMAGINE --

5. A <u>friend</u> <u>breaks</u> <u>your</u> <u>favorite</u> <u>game</u> <u>after</u> <u>you</u> <u>asked</u> <u>them</u> <u>not</u> <u>to</u> <u>play</u>
   <u>with</u> <u>it.</u>

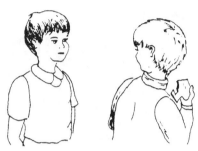

<u>SECTION</u> 1

	not at all angry	a little angry	fairly angry	very angry	very, very angry
a) How angry would you be if this happened to you?	O	O	O	O	O

<u>SECTION</u> 2
THE NEXT 2 QUESTIONS ARE ABOUT WHAT YOU WOULD <u>FEEL</u> LIKE DOING:

	not at all	a little	somewhat (half&half)	pretty much	very much
b) How much would you <u>feel</u> like getting back at that friend? Or getting even?	O	O	O	O	O
c) How much would you <u>feel</u> like making the situation better?	O	O	O	O	O

<u>SECTION</u> 3
THE NEXT 6 QUESTIONS ARE ABOUT WHAT YOU WOULD <u>REALLY</u> DO:

	not at all likely	unlikely	maybe (half&half)	likely	very likely
e) I'd hit the friend real hard.	O	O	O	O	O
f) I wouldn't care that much. It's only a game.	O	O	O	O	O
g) I'd be angry with myself for not putting the toy away in the first place.	O	O	O	O	O
h) I'd throw the game against a wall.	O	O	O	O	O
i) I'd leave the room before I got really angry.	O	O	O	O	O
j) I'd tell the friend's mother what he or she did.	O	O	O	O	O

<u>SECTION</u> 4
NOW THINK AGAIN ABOUT WHAT YOU WOULD <u>REALLY</u> DO IF THIS HAPPENED.

	terrible	pretty bad	OK	pretty good	wonderful
k) How do you think things would turn out for YOU in the long run?	O	O	O	O	O
l) How do you think things would turn out for THAT FRIEND in the long run?	O	O	O	O	O

IMAGINE --

16. In the cafeteria, the kid behind you knocks your lunch out of your hands.

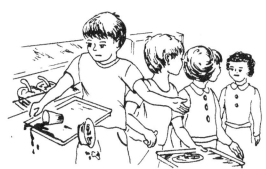

SECTION 1

	not at all angry	a little angry	fairly angry	very angry	very, very angry
a) How angry would you be if this happened to you?	O	O	O	O	O

SECTION 2
THE NEXT 2 QUESTIONS ARE ABOUT WHAT YOU WOULD FEEL LIKE DOING:

	not at all	a little	somewhat (half&half)	pretty much	very much
b) How much would you feel like getting back at that kid? Or getting even?	O	O	O	O	O
c) How much would you feel like making the situation better?	O	O	O	O	O

SECTION 3
THE NEXT 6 QUESTIONS ARE ABOUT WHAT YOU WOULD REALLY DO:

	not at all likely	unlikely	maybe (half&half)	likely	very likely
e) I'd talk to my friends to get my mind off it.	O	O	O	O	O
f) I'd push another kid in the line.	O	O	O	O	O
g) I'd go back and get another lunch.	O	O	O	O	O
h) I'd wonder if it was my own fault for standing too close.	O	O	O	O	O
i) I'd tell everyone how stupid the kid is.	O	O	O	O	O
j) I'd knock the kid's lunch out of his or her hands.	O	O	O	O	O

SECTION 4
NOW THINK AGAIN ABOUT WHAT YOU WOULD REALLY DO IF THIS HAPPENED.

	terrible	pretty bad	OK	pretty good	wonderful
k) How do you think things would turn out for YOU in the long run?	O	O	O	O	O
l) How do you think things would turn out for THAT KID in the long run?	O	O	O	O	O

IMAGINE --

17. While <u>arguing</u> with <u>your</u> brother, he <u>pushes</u> you.

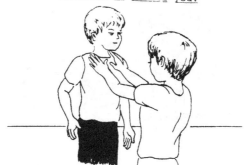

<u>SECTION 1</u>

	not at all angry	a little angry	fairly angry	very angry	very, very angry

a) How angry would you be if this
   happened to you?

<u>SECTION 2</u>
THE NEXT 2 QUESTIONS ARE ABOUT WHAT YOU WOULD <u>FEEL</u> LIKE DOING:

	not at all	a little	somewhat (half&half)	pretty much	very much

b) How much would you <u>feel</u> like getting
   back at your brother? Or getting even?

c) How much would you <u>feel</u> like making
   the situation better?

<u>SECTION 3</u>
THE NEXT 6 QUESTIONS ARE ABOUT WHAT YOU WOULD <u>REALLY</u> DO:

	not at all likely	unlikely	maybe (half&half)	likely	very likely

e) I'd get madder and madder the more I
   thought about how my brother pushed
   me.

f) I'd shake my fist at him.

g) I'd think I shouldn't have gotten him
   so angry.

h) I'd walk away.

i) I'd go to another room and throw
   things around.

j) I'd destroy something important to
   him.

<u>SECTION 4</u>
NOW THINK AGAIN ABOUT WHAT YOU WOULD <u>REALLY DO</u> IF THIS HAPPENED.

	terrible	pretty bad	OK	pretty good	wonderful

k) How do you think things would turn
   out for YOU in the long run?

l) How do you think things would turn
   out for YOUR BROTHER in the long run?

IMAGINE --

'?. You are walking down the hall, and a group of kids laugh as you walk by.

SECTION 1

	not at all angry	a little angry	fairly angry	very angry	very, very angry

a) How angry would you be if this
    happened to you?

SECTION 2
THE NEXT 2 QUESTIONS ARE ABOUT WHAT YOU WOULD FEEL LIKE DOING:

	not at all	a little	somewhat (half&half)	pretty much	very much

b) How much would you feel like getting
    back at those kids? Or getting even?

c) How much would you feel like making
    the situation better?

SECTION 3
THE NEXT 6 QUESTIONS ARE ABOUT WHAT YOU WOULD REALLY DO:

	not at all likely	unlikely	maybe (half&half)	likely	very likely

e) I'd give those kids a mean look.

f) I'd yell at the next person who spoke
    to me.

g) I'd wonder if I'd done something to
    look silly.

h) I'd ignore them and keep walking.

i) I'd get them in trouble with a
    teacher.

j) I'd be angry with myself for letting
    them bother me.

SECTION 4
NOW THINK AGAIN ABOUT WHAT YOU WOULD REALLY DO IF THIS HAPPENED.

	terrible	pretty bad	OK	pretty good	wonderful

k) How do you think things would turn
    out for YOU in the long run?

l) How do you think things would turn
    out for THOSE KIDS in the long run?

IMAGINE --

20. You are waiting in the lunch line, and someone cuts in front of you.

SECTION 1

	not at all angry	a little angry	fairly angry	very angry	very, very angry
a) How angry would you be if this happened to you?	O	O	O	O	O

SECTION 2
THE NEXT 2 QUESTIONS ARE ABOUT WHAT YOU WOULD FEEL LIKE DOING:

	not at all	a little	somewhat (half&half)	pretty much	very much
b) How much would you feel like getting back at that kid? Or getting even?	O	O	O	O	O
c) How much would you feel like making the situation better?	O	O	O	O	O

SECTION 3
THE NEXT 6 QUESTIONS ARE ABOUT WHAT YOU WOULD REALLY DO:

	not at all likely	unlikely	maybe (half&half)	likely	very likely
e) I'd yell at the lunch lady to hurry up.	O	O	O	O	O
f) I'd just ignore it.	O	O	O	O	O
g) I'd think that maybe someone was saving a place for the kid.	O	O	O	O	O
h) I'd shove the kid back out of the line.	O	O	O	O	O
i) I'd calmly ask the kid to move to the end of the line.	O	O	O	O	O
j) I wouldn't say anything, but I'd be angry all afternoon.	O	O	O	O	O

SECTION 4
NOW THINK AGAIN ABOUT WHAT YOU WOULD REALLY DO IF THIS HAPPENED.

	terrible	pretty bad	OK	pretty good	wonderful
k) How do you think things would turn out for YOU in the long run?	O	O	O	O	O
l) How do you think things would turn out for THAT KID in the long run?	O	O	O	O	O

Driving Anger Expression Inventory

Reprinted with permission from the author (Deffenbacher, J., et al., 2002)

<u>Directions</u>: Everyone feels angry or furious from time to time <u>when driving</u>, but people differ in the ways that they react when they are angry <u>while driving.</u> A number of statements are listed below which people have used to describe their reactions when they feel <u>angry</u> or <u>furious</u>. Read each statement and then fill in the bubble to the right of the statement indicating how <u>often</u> you <u>generally</u> react or behave in the manner described <u>when you are angry or furious while driving</u>. There are no right or wrong answers. Do not spend too much time on any one statement.

		Almost Never	Some-times	Often	Almost Always
1.	I give the other driver the finger.	O	O	O	O
2.	I drive right up on the other driver's bumper.	O	O	O	O
3.	I drive a little faster than I was.	O	O	O	O
4.	I try to cut in front of the other driver.	O	O	O	O
5.	I call the other driver names aloud.	O	O	O	O
6.	I make negative comments about the other driver	O	O	O	O
7.	I follow right behind the other driver for a long time.	O	O	O	O
8.	I try to get out of the car and tell the other driver off.	O	O	O	O
9.	I yell questions like "Where did you get your license?"	O	O	O	O
10.	I roll down the window to help communicate my anger.	O	O	O	O
11.	I glare at the other driver.	O	O	O	O
12.	I shake my fist at the other driver.	O	O	O	O
13.	I stick my tongue out at the other driver.	O	O	O	O
14.	I call the other driver names under my breath.	O	O	O	O
15.	I speed up to frustrate the other driver.	O	O	O	O
16.	I purposely block the other driver from doing what he/she wants to do.	O	O	O	O
17.	I bump the other driver's bumper with mine.	O	O	O	O
18.	I go crazy behind the wheel.	O	O	O	O
19.	I leave my brights on in the other driver's rear view mirror.	O	O	O	O
20.	I try to force the other driver to the side of the road.	O	O	O	O
21.	I try to scare the other driver.	O	O	O	O
22.	I do to other drivers what they did to me.	O	O	O	O
23.	I pay even closer attention to being a safe driver.	O	O	O	O
24.	I think about things that distract me from thinking about the other driver.	O	O	O	O
25.	I think things through before I respond.	O	O	O	O

	Almost Never	Some-times	Often	Almost Always
26. I try to think of positive solutions to deal with the situation.	O	O	O	O
27. I drive a lot faster than I was.	O	O	O	O
28. I swear at the other driver aloud.	O	O	O	O
29. I tell myself its not worth getting all mad about.	O	O	O	O
30. I decide not to stoop to their level.	O	O	O	O
31. I swear at the other driver under my breath.	O	O	O	O
32. I turn on the radio or music to calm down.	O	O	O	O
33. I flash my lights at the other driver.	O	O	O	O
34. I make hostile gestures other than giving the finger.	O	O	O	O
35. I try to think of positive things to do.	O	O	O	O
36. I tell myself it's not worth getting involved in.	O	O	O	O
37. I shake my head at the other driver.	O	O	O	O
38. I yell at the other driver.	O	O	O	O
39. I make negative comments about the other driver under my breath.	O	O	O	O
40. I give the other driver a dirty look.	O	O	O	O
41. I try to get out of the car and have a physical fight with the other driver.	O	O	O	O
42. I just try to accept that there are bad drivers on the road.	O	O	O	O
43. I think things like "Where did you get your license?"	O	O	O	O
44. I do things like take deep breaths to calm down.	O	O	O	O
45. I just try and accept that there are frustrating situations while driving.	O	O	O	O
46. I slow down to frustrate the other driver.	O	O	O	O
47. I think about things that distract me from the frustration on the road.	O	O	O	O
48. I tell myself to ignore it.	O	O	O	O
49. I pay even closer attention to other's driving to avoid accidents.	O	O	O	O

Scales involved in the Driving Anger Expression Inventory (DAX):

(1) 12-item *Verbal Aggressive Expression* (α = .88) Items generally involve overt and covert verbal aggression with some nonverbal behaviors such as glares—Items 5, 6, 9, 11, 14, 28, 31, 37, 38, 39, 40, and 43

(2) 11-item *Personal Physical Aggressive Expression* (α = .84) Items generally involve physically aggressive displays or behavior, but not where the person is using the car as an instrument of intimidation, aggression, and frustration—Items 1, 8, 10, 12, 13, 17, 18, 20, 21, 34, and 41

(3) 11-item *Use of the Vehicle to Express Anger* (α = .86) Items generally involve using the vehicle or one's driving behavior to frustrate, intimidate, or express displeasure with the another driver—Items 2, 3, 4, 7, 15, 16, 19, 22, 27, 33, and 46

(4) 15-item *Adaptive/Constructive Expression* (α = .90) Items generally involve cognitive and behavioral strategies for safe driving, problem-solving, distraction and cognitively reframing the situation—Items 23, 24, 25, 26, 29, 30, 32, 35, 36, 42, 44, 45, 47, 48, and 49

(5) 34-item *Aggressive Anger Expression.* This measure is a second order measure which combines Verbal Aggressive Expression, Personal Physical Aggressive Expression, and Use of the Vehicle to Express Anger. It can serve as a general aggressive expression index, if one is desired—sum of Verbal Aggressive Expression, Personal Physical Aggressive Expression, and Use of Vehicle to Express Anger scores.

Driving Anger Scale – Short Form

Reprinted with permission from the author (Deffenbacher, J., et al., 1994)

Directions: Below are several situations you may encounter when you are driving. Try to imagine the incident described is actually happening to you, then indicate the extent to which it would anger or provoke you. Mark your response by filling in the bubble to the right.

	Not at all	A little	Some	Much	Very Much
1. Someone is weaving in and out of traffic	O	O	O	O	O
2. A slow vehicle on a mountain road will not pull over and let people by	O	O	O	O	O
3. Someone backs right out in front of you without looking	O	O	O	O	O
4. You pass a radar speed trap	O	O	O	O	O
5. Someone makes an obscene gesture toward you about your driving	O	O	O	O	O
6. A police officer pulls you over	O	O	O	O	O
7. A truck kicks up sand or gravel on the car you are driving	O	O	O	O	O
8. Someone runs a red light or stop sign	O	O	O	O	O
9. Someone honks at you about your driving	O	O	O	O	O
10. You are driving behind a large truck and cannot see around it	O	O	O	O	O
11. A bicyclist is riding in the middle of the lane and slowing traffic	O	O	O	O	O
12. You are stuck in a traffic jam	O	O	O	O	O
13. Someone speeds up when you try to pass them	O	O	O	O	O
14. Someone is slow in parking and holding up traffic	O	O	O	O	O

Driving Anger Scale

Reprinted with permission from the author (Deffenbacher, J., et al., 1994)

<u>Directions</u>: **Below are several situations <u>you</u> may encounter when you are driving. Try to imagine that the incident described is actually happening to you, then indicate the extent to which it would anger or provoke you. Mark your response by filling in the bubble to the right.**

		<u>Not</u> <u>At All</u>	<u>A</u> <u>Little</u>	<u>Some</u>	<u>Much</u>	<u>Very</u> <u>Much</u>
1.	Someone in front of you does not start up when the light turns green.	O	O	O	O	O
2.	Someone is driving too fast for the road conditions.	O	O	O	O	O
3.	A pedestrian walks slowly across the middle of the street, slowing you.	O	O	O	O	O
4.	Someone is driving too slowly in the passing lane holding up traffic.	O	O	O	O	O
5.	Someone is driving right up on your back bumper.	O	O	O	O	O
6.	Someone is weaving in and out of traffic.	O	O	O	O	O
7.	Someone cuts in front of you on the freeway.	O	O	O	O	O
8.	Someone cuts in and takes the parking spot you have been waiting for.	O	O	O	O	O
9.	Someone is driving slower than reasonable for the traffic flow.	O	O	O	O	O
10.	A slow vehicle on a mountain road will not pull over and let people by.	O	O	O	O	O
11.	You see a police car watching traffic from a hidden position.	O	O	O	O	O
12.	Someone backs right out in front of you without looking.	O	O	O	O	O
13.	Someone runs a red light or stop sign.	O	O	O	O	O
14.	Someone coming toward you at night does not dim their headlights.	O	O	O	O	O
15.	At night someone is driving right behind you with bright lights on.	O	O	O	O	O
16.	You pass a radar speed trap.	O	O	O	O	O
17.	Someone speeds up when you try to pass them.	O	O	O	O	O
18.	Someone is slow in parking and holding up traffic.	O	O	O	O	O
19.	You are stuck in a traffic jam.	O	O	O	O	O
20.	Someone pulls right in front of you when there is no one behind you.	O	O	O	O	O
21.	Someone makes an obscene gesture toward you about your driving.	O	O	O	O	O
22.	You hit a deep pothole that was not marked.	O	O	O	O	O
23.	Someone honks at you about your driving.	O	O	O	O	O
24.	Someone is driving way over the speed limit.	O	O	O	O	O
25.	You are driving behind a truck which has material flapping around in the back.	O	O	O	O	O
26.	Someone yells at you about your driving.	O	O	O	O	O
27.	A police officer pulls you over.	O	O	O	O	O
28.	You are behind a vehicle that is smoking badly or giving off diesel fumes.	O	O	O	O	O
29.	A truck kicks up sand or gravel on the car you are driving.	O	O	O	O	O
30.	You are behind a large truck and cannot see around it.	O	O	O	O	O
31.	You encounter road construction and detours.	O	O	O	O	O
32.	A bicyclist is riding in the middle of the lane and slowing traffic.	O	O	O	O	O
33.	A police car is driving in traffic close to you.	O	O	O	O	O

Domestic Violence Myth Acceptance Scale

Reprinted with permission from the author (Peters, J., 2008)

Domestic Violence Attitudes

The questions below ask about common attitudes toward domestic violence. While we all know the politically or socially correct answer, please answer how you truly think and feel. To answer, put a number on the line before each question indicating how strongly you agree or disagree with each statement

1	2	3	4	5	6	7
Strongly Disagree						Strongly Agree

1. _____ Domestic violence does not affect many people

2. _____ When a man is violent it is because he lost control of his temper.

3. _____ If a woman continues living with a man who beat her, then its her own fault if she is beaten again

4. _____ Making a man jealous is asking for it.

5. _____ Some women unconsciously want their partners to control them.

6. _____ A lot of domestic violence occurs because women keep on arguing about things with their partners.

7. _____ If a woman doesn't like it, she can leave.

8. _____ Most domestic violence involves mutual violence between the partners.

9. _____ Abusive men lose control so much that they don't know what they're doing.

10. _____ I hate to say it, but if a woman stays with the man who abused her, she basically deserves what she gets.

11. _____ Domestic violence rarely happens in my neighborhood

12. _____ Women who flirt are asking for it.

13. _____ Women can avoid physical abuse if they give in occasionally.

14. _____ Many women have an unconscious wish to be dominated by their partners.

15. _____ Domestic violence results from a momentary loss of temper.

16. _____ I don't have much sympathy for a battered woman who keeps going back to the abuser.

17. _____ Women instigate most family violence.

1	2	3	4	5	6	7
Not at all						Entirely

18. _____ If a woman goes back to the abuser, how much is that due to something in her character?

DVMAS Scoring

Add all items and divide by 18 for mean score.

DVMAS Means & reliabilities

Study	Mean, SD	Mean, Males	Mean, Females	Alpha
Peters, 2003	$M = 2.3\ SD = .85$	$M = 2.6, SD = .89$	$M = 2.09, SD = .76$	.88
Peters, ND	$M = 2.5, SD = .84$	$M = 2.8, SD = .82$	$M = 2.3, SD = .79$	.865

Maudsley Violence Questionnaire

M	A

Reprinted with permission from the author (Walker, J., 2005).

MVQ *(Developed at the South London and Maudsley NHS Trust)*

Name: _____   Date: _____   Gender: M ☐ F ☐

*Everyone has ideas about what is right and wrong and what they would do in difficult situations. Below are some statements about various situations and what you would do or what you think is right and wrong. There are no correct or incorrect answers or trick questions; it is your view that is important. Simply tick the box to show whether the statement is true or false – **for you**.*

		True	False
1.	It is shameful to walk away from a fight.		
2.	I tend to just react physically without thinking.		
3.	When you are pushed to your limit, there is nothing you can do except fight.		
4.	You can never face people again if you show you are frightened.		
5.	Most people won't learn unless you physically hurt them.		
6.	I enjoy watching violence on TV or in films.		
7.	It is OK to hit someone who **threatens** to make you look stupid.		
8.	It is OK to hit your partner if they behave unacceptably.		
9.	I expect real men to be violent.		
10.	If you don't stick up for yourself physically you will get trodden on.		
11.	Being violent shows you are a man.		
12.	I am totally against violence.		
13.	Sometimes you have to use violence to get what you want.		
14.	It is OK (or normal) to hit someone if they hit you first.		
15.	You won't survive if you run away from fights and arguments.		
16.	If I am provoked, I can't help but hit the person who provoked me.		
17.	Fighting can make you feel alive and 'fired up'.		
18.	It is OK to hit someone who **threatens** your family.		
19.	If I felt threatened by someone, I would stop them by attacking them first.		
20.	Physical violence is a necessary sign of strength and power.		
21.	Violence is second nature to me.		
22.	People who irritate you deserve to be hit.		
23.	If I get angry, hitting out makes me feel better.		
24.	I just seem to attract violence.		
25.	Fighting can help to sort out most disagreements.		

		True	False
26.	Men who are gentle get walked on.		
27.	It is OK to have violence on TV.		
28.	Sometimes you have to be violent to show that you are a man.		
29.	I hate violence.		
30.	If someone attacked me verbally, I would attack them physically.		
31.	When I can't think of what to say, it's easier to react with my fists.		
32.	If someone cuts you up in traffic, it's OK to swear at them.		
33.	It is OK (or normal) to hit women if you need to teach them a lesson.		
34.	I enjoy watching violent sports (e.g. boxing).		
35.	If I don't show that I'm tough and strong, people will think I'm weak and pathetic.		
36.	It is OK to hit someone who upsets you.		
37.	I wouldn't feel bad about hitting someone if they really deserved it.		
38.	When I have hurt people, I feel bad or even hate myself for it afterwards.		
39.	It is OK to hit someone if they make you look stupid.		
40.	It is OK to have violence in films at the cinema.		
41.	Some people only understand when you show them through physical strength.		
42.	I enjoy fighting.		
43.	Fear is a sign of weakness.		
44.	It is OK to be violent if someone **threatens** to damage your property.		
45.	I believe that if someone annoys you, you have a right to get them back, by whatever means necessary.		
46.	If I were in a potentially violent situation, I would automatically confront the person threatening me.		
47.	I would rather lose a fight and get beaten up than embarrass myself by walking away.		
48.	Being violent shows you are strong.		
49.	It is OK to hit someone who **threatens** your partner.		
50.	Being violent shows that you can assert yourself.		
51.	It is normal for men to want to fight.		
52.	Because anyone can suffer hurt and pain, you should not hit other people.		
53.	I see myself as a violent person.		
54.	'Real men' are not afraid of fighting.		
55.	If you are not willing to fight it means you are weak and pathetic.		
56.	If trouble starts, I wouldn't think about it - I would just get stuck in and fight.		

MVQ – page 2 (of 2)

Maudsley Violence Questionnaire

Reprinted with permission from the author (Walker, J., 2005).

M	A

MVQ *(Developed at the South London and Maudsley NHS Trust)* **MACHISMO**

Name: _____   Date: _____   Gender: M ☐ F ☐

(Photocopy onto OHP slide and overlay onto completed MVQ)

All 'True' answers score one point, except items 12, 29, 38 and 52 which are reverse scored
Items in Italics are 'Acceptance of Violence' Scale (14 items); other items are 'Machismo' Scale (42 items)

		True	False
1.	It is shameful to walk away from a fight.		
2.	I tend to just react physically without thinking.		
3.	When you are pushed to your limit, there is nothing you can do except fight.		
4.	You can never face people again if you show you are frightened.		
5.	Most people won't learn unless you physically hurt them.		
6.	*I enjoy watching violence on TV or in films.*		
7.	It is OK to hit someone who **threatens** to make you look stupid.		
8.	It is OK to hit your partner if they behave unacceptably.		
9.	I expect real men to be violent.		
10.	If you don't stick up for yourself physically you will get trodden on.		
11.	Being violent shows you are a man.		
12.	*I am totally against violence.*		
13.	Sometimes you have to use violence to get what you want.		
14.	*It is OK (or normal) to hit someone if they hit you first.*		
15.	You won't survive if you run away from fights and arguments.		
16.	If I am provoked, I can't help but hit the person who provoked me.		
17.	*Fighting can make you feel alive and 'fired up'.*		
18.	*It is OK to hit someone who **threatens** your family.*		
19.	If I felt threatened by someone, I would stop them by attacking them first.		
20.	Physical violence is a necessary sign of strength and power.		
21.	Violence is second nature to me.		
22.	People who irritate you deserve to be hit.		
23.	If I get angry, hitting out makes me feel better.		
24.	I just seem to attract violence.		
25.	Fighting can help to sort out most disagreements.		

MACHISMO - MVQ – page 1 (of 2)

		True	False
26.	Men who are gentle get walked on.		
27.	*It is OK to have violence on TV.*		
28.	Sometimes you have to be violent to show that you are a man.		
29.	*I hate violence.*		
30.	If someone attacked me verbally, I would attack them physically.		
31.	When I can't think of what to say, it's easier to react with my fists.		
32.	*If someone cuts you up in traffic, it's OK to swear at them.*		
33.	It is OK (or normal) to hit women if you need to teach them a lesson.		
34.	*I enjoy watching violent sports (e.g. boxing).*		
35.	If I don't show that I'm tough and strong, people will think I'm weak and pathetic.		
36.	It is OK to hit someone who upsets you.		
37.	*I wouldn't feel bad about hitting someone if they really deserved it.*		
38.	*When I have hurt people, I feel bad or even hate myself for it afterwards.*		
39.	It is OK to hit someone if they make you look stupid.		
40.	*It is OK to have violence in films at the cinema.*		
41.	Some people only understand when you show them through physical strength.		
42.	I enjoy fighting.		
43.	Fear is a sign of weakness.		
44.	It is OK to be violent if someone **threatens** to damage your property.		
45.	I believe that if someone annoys you, you have a right to get them back, by whatever means necessary.		
46.	If I were in a potentially violent situation, I would automatically confront the person threatening me.		
47.	I would rather lose a fight and get beaten up than embarrass myself by walking away.		
48.	Being violent shows you are strong.		
49.	*It is OK to hit someone who **threatens** your partner.*		
50.	Being violent shows that you can assert yourself.		
51.	It is normal for men to want to fight.		
52.	*Because anyone can suffer hurt and pain, you should not hit other people.*		
53.	I see myself as a violent person.		
54.	'Real men' are not afraid of fighting.		
55.	If you are not willing to fight it means you are weak and pathetic.		
56.	If trouble starts, I wouldn't think about it - I would just get stuck in and fight.		

MACHISMO – MVQ – page 2 (of 2)

Maudsley Violence Questionnaire

Reprinted with permission from the author (Walker, J., 2005).

M	A

MVQ *(Developed at the South London and Maudsley NHS Trust)* **ACCEPTANCE**

Name: _____   Date: _____   Gender: M ☐ F ☐

(Photocopy onto OHP slide and overlay onto completed MVQ)

All 'True' answers score one point, except items 12, 29, 38 and 52 which are reverse scored
Items in Italics are 'Acceptance of Violence' Scale (14 items); other items are 'Machismo' Scale (42 items)

		True	False
1.	It is shameful to walk away from a fight.		
2.	I tend to just react physically without thinking.		
3.	When you are pushed to your limit, there is nothing you can do except fight.		
4.	You can never face people again if you show you are frightened.		
5.	Most people won't learn unless you physically hurt them.		
6.	*I enjoy watching violence on TV or in films.*		
7.	It is OK to hit someone who **threatens** to make you look stupid.		
8.	It is OK to hit your partner if they behave unacceptably.		
9.	I expect real men to be violent.		
10.	If you don't stick up for yourself physically you will get trodden on.		
11.	Being violent shows you are a man.		
12.	*I am totally against violence.*		
13.	Sometimes you have to use violence to get what you want.		
14.	*It is OK (or normal) to hit someone if they hit you first.*		
15.	You won't survive if you run away from fights and arguments.		
16.	If I am provoked, I can't help but hit the person who provoked me.		
17.	*Fighting can make you feel alive and 'fired up'.*		
18.	*It is OK to hit someone who **threatens** your family.*		
19.	If I felt threatened by someone, I would stop them by attacking them first.		
20.	Physical violence is a necessary sign of strength and power.		
21.	Violence is second nature to me.		
22.	People who irritate you deserve to be hit.		
23.	If I get angry, hitting out makes me feel better.		
24.	I just seem to attract violence.		
25.	Fighting can help to sort out most disagreements.		

		True	False
26.	Men who are gentle get walked on.		
27.	*It is OK to have violence on TV.*		
28.	Sometimes you have to be violent to show that you are a man.		
29.	*I hate violence.*		
30.	If someone attacked me verbally, I would attack them physically.		
31.	When I can't think of what to say, it's easier to react with my fists.		
32.	*If someone cuts you up in traffic, it's OK to swear at them.*		
33.	It is OK (or normal) to hit women if you need to teach them a lesson.		
34.	*I enjoy watching violent sports (e.g. boxing).*		
35.	If I don't show that I'm tough and strong, people will think I'm weak and pathetic.		
36.	It is OK to hit someone who upsets you.		
37.	*I wouldn't feel bad about hitting someone if they really deserved it.*		
38.	*When I have hurt people, I feel bad or even hate myself for it afterwards.*		
39.	It is OK to hit someone if they make you look stupid.		
40.	*It is OK to have violence in films at the cinema.*		
41.	Some people only understand when you show them through physical strength.		
42.	I enjoy fighting.		
43.	Fear is a sign of weakness.		
44.	It is OK to be violent if someone **threatens** to damage your property.		
45.	I believe that if someone annoys you, you have a right to get them back, by whatever means necessary.		
46.	If I were in a potentially violent situation, I would automatically confront the person threatening me.		
47.	I would rather lose a fight and get beaten up than embarrass myself by walking away.		
48.	Being violent shows you are strong.		
49.	*It is OK to hit someone who **threatens** your partner.*		
50.	Being violent shows that you can assert yourself.		
51.	It is normal for men to want to fight.		
52.	*Because anyone can suffer hurt and pain, you should not hit other people.*		
53.	I see myself as a violent person.		
54.	'Real men' are not afraid of fighting.		
55.	If you are not willing to fight it means you are weak and pathetic.		
56.	If trouble starts, I wouldn't think about it - I would just get stuck in and fight.		

ACCEPTANCE – MVQ – page 2 (of 2)

Multidimensional Peer-Victimization Scale

Reprinted with permission from the author (Mynard, H., and Joseph, S., 2000)

Below is a list of things that some children do to other children. How often during the last school year has another pupil done these things to you? Please answer by putting a tick in one of the three columns for each of the 16 questions.

		Not at All	Once	More than once
1.	Punched me			
2.	Tried to get me into trouble with my friends			
3.	Called me names			
4.	Took something of mine without permission			
5.	Kicked me			
6.	Tried to make my friends turn against me			
7.	Made fun of me because of my appearance			
8.	Tried to break something of mine			
9.	Hurt me physically in some way			
10.	Refused to talk to me			
11.	Made fun of me for some reason			
12.	Stole something from me			
13.	Beat me up			
14.	Made other people not talk to me			
15.	Swore at me			
16.	Deliberately damaged some property of mine			

Scoring key for the MPVS:

Not at all = 0

Once = 1

More than once = 2

Scores on the total scale have a possible range of 0 to 32, and a possible range of 0 to 8 on each of the four subscales.

Subscales

Items 1 + 5 + 9 + 13 = physical victimisation scale

Items 2 + 6 + 10 + 14 = social manipulation scale

Items 3 + 7 + 11 + 15 = verbal victimization scale

Items 4 + 8 + 12 + 16 = attacks on property scale

Propensity for Abusiveness Scale

Reprinted with permission from the author (Dutton, D., 1995)

PAS

PART 1

For each of the statements below, please circle the number to the right of the statement that most accurately describes how the it applies to you, from 1 (completely undescriptive of you) to 5 (completely descriptive of you).

1	2	3	4	5
completely undescriptive of you	mostly undescriptive of you	partly undescriptive & partly descriptive	mostly descriptive of you	completely descriptive of you

1.   I can make myself angry about something in the past just   1 2 3 4 5
     by thinking about it.

2.   I get so angry, I feel that I might lose control.   1 2 3 4 5

3.   If I let people see the way I feel, I'd be considered a hard 1 2 3 4 5
     person to get along with.

PART 2

For each of the statements below, please indicate how true it is about you by circling the appropriate number.

1	2	3	4	5
never true	seldom true	sometimes true	often true	always true

4.   I see myself in totally different ways at different times.   1 2 3 4 5

5.   I feel empty inside.   1 2 3 4 5

6.   I tend to feel things in a somewhat extreme way,   1 2 3 4 5
     experiencing either great joy or intense despair.

7.   It is hard for me to be sure about what others think of me, 1 2 3 4 5
     even people who have known me very well.

8.   I feel people don't give me the respect I deserve unless I   1 2 3 4 5
     put pressure on them.

9.   Somehow, I never know quite how to conduct myself with   1 2 3 4 5
     people.

PART 3

Please read each of the following statements and rate the extent to which it describes your feelings about <u>romantic relationships</u> by circling the appropriate number. Think about all of your romantic relationships, past and present, and respond in terms of how you <u>generally</u> feel in these relationships.

Not at all like me		Somewhat like me		Very much like me
1	2	3	4	5

10.	I find it difficult to depend on other people.	1 2 3 4 5
11.	I worry that I will be hurt if I allow myself to become too close to others.	1 2 3 4 5
12.	I am somewhat uncomfortable being close to others.	1 2 3 4 5

PART 4

How often have you experienced each of the following in the <u>last two months</u>? Please circle the appropriate number.

0	1	2	3
never	occasionally	fairly often	very often

13.	Insomnia (trouble getting to sleep)	0 1 2 3
14.	Restless sleep	0 1 2 3
15.	Nightmares	0 1 2 3
16.	Anxiety attacks	0 1 2 3
17.	Fear of women	0 1 2 3
18.	Feeling tense all the time	0 1 2 3
19.	Having trouble breathing	0 1 2 3

PART 5

Beside each statement, please circle the number of the response listed below that best describes how often the experience happened to you with your mother (or female guardian) and father (or male guardian) when you were growing up. If you had more than one mother/father figure, please answer for the persons who you feel played the most important role in your upbringing.

1	2	3	4
never occurred	occasionally occurred	often occurred	always occurred

		Father or Guardian	Mother or Guardian
20.	My parent punished me even for small offenses.	1 2 3 4	1 2 3 4
21.	As a child I was physically punished or scolded in the presence of others.	1 2 3 4	1 2 3 4
22.	My parent gave me more corporal (physical) punishment than I deserved.	1 2 3 4	1 2 3 4
23.	I felt my parent thought it was *my* fault when he/she was unhappy.	1 2 3 4	1 2 3 4
24.	I think my parent was mean and grudging toward me.	1 2 3 4	1 2 3 4
25.	I was punished by my parent without having done anything	1 2 3 4	1 2 3 4
26.	My parent criticized me and told me how lazy and useless I was in front of others.	1 2 3 4	1 2 3 4
27.	My parent would punish me hard, even for trifles.	1 2 3 4	1 2 3 4
28.	My parent treated me in such a way that I felt ashamed.	1 2 3 4	1 2 3 4
29.	I was beaten by my parent.	1 2 3 4	1 2 3 4

Proximal Antecedents of Violent Episodes

Reprinted with permission from the author (Babcock, J., et al., 2004).

Final 20 Item Scale

Sometimes there are situations when people are more likely to become

PHYSICALLY aggressive than other times. Sometimes people feel that violence is

justified, given the situation. Please indicate how likely it is that <u>you</u> would be

physically aggressive in each of the following types of situations, if they were to arise.

Please answer as carefully and accurately as you can by circling a number for each of the items below.

How likely are you to be PHYSICALLY AGGRESSIVE in each of the following situations?						
1. My partner does something to offend or "disrespect" me.	Not at all Likely 1 6	Very Unlikely 2	Somewhat Unlikely 3	Somewhat Likely 4	Very Likely 5	Extremely Likely
2. My partner threatens to leave me.	Not at all Likely 1 6	Very Unlikely 2	Somewhat Unlikely 3	Somewhat Likely 4	Very Likely 5	Extremely Likely
3. My partner just won't stop talking or nagging.	Not at all Likely 1 6	Very Unlikely 2	Somewhat Unlikely 3	Somewhat Likely 4	Very Likely 5	Extremely Likely
4. I walk in and catch my partner having sex with someone.	Not at all Likely 1 6	Very Unlikely 2	Somewhat Unlikely 3	Somewhat Likely 4	Very Likely 5	Extremely Likely
5. My partner says "I wish I never married you."	Not at all Likely 1 6	Very Unlikely 2	Somewhat Unlikely 3	Somewhat Likely 4	Very Likely 5	Extremely Likely
6. My partner spends a lot of time with close friends of the opposite sex.	Not at all Likely 1 6	Very Unlikely 2	Somewhat Unlikely 3	Somewhat Likely 4	Very Likely 5	Extremely Likely
7. I find out that my partner has been flirting with someone.	Not at all Likely 1 6	Very Unlikely 2	Somewhat Unlikely 3	Somewhat Likely 4	Very Likely 5	Extremely Likely
8. My partner comes home late.	Not at all Likely 1 6	Very Unlikely 2	Somewhat Unlikely 3	Somewhat Likely 4	Very Likely 5	Extremely Likely
9. My partner spends money without	Not at	Very Unlikely	Somewhat	Somewhat	Very	Extremely

consulting me.	all Likely 1 6		Unlikely 3	Likely 4	Likely 5
10. When my partner and I argue about sex.	Not at all Likely 1 6	Very Unlikely 2	Somewhat Unlikely 3	Somewhat Likely 4	Very Likely	Extremely Likely 5
11. My partner threatens to divorce me.	Not at all Likely 1 6	Very Unlikely 2	Somewhat Unlikely 3	Somewhat Likely 4	Very Likely	Extremely Likely 5
12. My partner ridicules or makes fun of me.	Not at all Likely 1 6	Very Unlikely 2	Somewhat Unlikely 3	Somewhat Likely 4	Very Likely	Extremely Likely 5
13. My partner tells me not to do something that I want to do.	Not at all Likely 1 6	Very Unlikely 2	Somewhat Unlikely 3	Somewhat Likely 4	Very Likely	Extremely Likely 5
14. My partner tries to control me.	Not at all Likely 1 6	Very Unlikely 2	Somewhat Unlikely 3	Somewhat Likely 4	Very Likely	Extremely Likely 5
15. My partner interrupts me when I'm talking.	Not at all Likely 1 6	Very Unlikely 2	Somewhat Unlikely 3	Somewhat Likely 4	Very Likely	Extremely Likely 5

16. My partner does not include me in important decisions.	Not at all Likely 1 6	Very Unlikely 2	Somewhat Unlikely 3	Somewhat Likely 4	Very Likely	Extremely Likely 5
17. My partner ignores me.	Not at all Likely 1 6	Very Unlikely 2	Somewhat Unlikely 3	Somewhat Likely 4	Very Likely	Extremely Likely 5
18. My partner is physically aggressive towards me first.	Not at all Likely 1 6	Very Unlikely 2	Somewhat Unlikely 3	Somewhat Likely 4	Very Likely	Extremely Likely 5
19. My partner tries to leave during an argument.	Not at all Likely 1 6	Very Unlikely 2	Somewhat Unlikely 3	Somewhat Likely 4	Very Likely	Extremely Likely 5
20. My partner blames me for something I didn't do.	Not at all Likely 1 6	Very Unlikely 2	Somewhat Unlikely 3	Somewhat Likely 4	Very Likely	Extremely Likely 5

Scoring Key for Three Subscales:

Violence to Control = Item9 + Item12 + Item13 + Item14 + Item15 + Item16 + Item17 + Item18 + Item19 Item20 .

Violence out of Jealousy = Item5 + Item6 + Item7 + Item8.

Violence following Verbal Abuse = Item1 + Item2 + Item3 + Item5 + Item10 + Item11.

Richardson Conflict Response Questionnaire

Reprinted with permission of the author (Green, L., Richardson, D., and Lago, T., 1996)

Here is a list of things you might do when angry with someone. Please think of what you usually do when you have a conflict or disagreement with your romantic partner. How often have you made each of these responses when angry or upset with your romantic partner? Use the following code:

1 = Never   2 = Seldom   3 = Sometimes   4 = Often   5 = Very Often

_____ 1. Yelled or screamed at them.

_____ 2. Did things to irritate them.

_____ 3. Threatened to hit or throw something at them.

_____ 4. Made up stories to get them in trouble.

_____ 5. Did not show that I was angry.

_____ 6. Cursed at them.

_____ 7. Threw something at them.

_____ 8. Tried to make them look stupid.

_____ 9. Stomped out of the room.

_____ 10. Made negative comments about their appearance to someone else.

_____ 11. Hit (or tried to hit) them with something hard.

_____ 12. Insulted them or called them names to their face.

_____ 13. Talked the matter over.

_____ 14. Spread rumors about them.

_____ 15. Sulked and refused to talk about it.

_____ 16. Kicked (or tried to kick) the other person.

_____ 17. Dropped the matter entirely.

_____ 18. Took something that belonged to them.

_____ 19. Hit (or tried to hit) the other person but not with anything.

_____ 20. Gossiped about them behind their back.

_____ 21. Pushed, grabbed or shoved them.

_____ 22. Called them names behind their back.

_____ 23. Told others not to associate with them.

_____ 24. Waited until I calmed down and then discussed the problem.

_____ 25. Told others about the matter.

_____ 26. Threw something (but not at the other) or smashed something.

_____   27. Destroyed or damaged something that belonged to them.

_____   28. Gathered other friends to my side.

Background Information

Gender: M F   Age: _____   Gender of Romantic Partner: M   F

Year in College: Freshman   Sophomore   Junior   Senior

Severity of Violence Against Men Scale (SVAMS)

Reprinted with permission from the author (Marshall, L., 1992).

How often did you...

shake a finger at him	[threats - mild violence]
make threatening gestures or faces at him	
shake a fist at him	
act like a bully toward him	
grab him suddenly or forcefully	
hit or kick a wall, door or furniture	[threats - moderate violence]
threaten to harm/damage things he cares about	
destroy something belonging to him	
throw, smash or break an object	
threaten to destroy property	
drive dangerously with him in the car	
throw an object at him	
threaten to hurt him	[threats - serious violence]
threaten to kill yourself	
threaten someone he cares about	
threaten to kill him	
act like you wanted to kill him	
threaten him with a club-like object	
threaten him with a weapon	
threaten him with a knife or gun	
hold him down pinning him in place	[acts - minor violence]
push or shove him	
shake or roughly handle him	
spank him	
twist his arm	[acts - mild violence]
pull his hair	
scratch him	
bite him	
kick him	
slap him with the palm of your hand	[acts - moderate violence]
slap him with the back of your hand	
punch him	
slap him repeatedly around his face and head	
hit him with an object	[acts severe violence]
stomp on him	
choke him	
beat him up	
burn him with something	
use a club-like object on him	
use a knife or gun on him	
demand sex whether he wanted it or not	[sexual aggression]

make him have sexual intercourse against his will
make him have oral (mouth) sex against his will
physically force him to have sex
make him have anal (bottom) sex against his will
use an object on him in a sexual way

Severity of Violence Against Women Scale (SVAWS)

Reprinted with permission from the author (Marshall, L., 1992).

How often did he...

hit or kick a wall, door or furniture	[threats - symbolic violence]
throw, smash or break an object	
drive dangerously with you in the car	
throw an object at you	
shake a finger at you	[threats - mild violence]
make threatening gestures or faces at you	
shake a fist at you	
act like a bully toward you	
destroy something belonging to you	[threats - moderate violence]
threaten to harm or damage things you care about	
threaten to destroy property	
threaten someone you care about	
threaten to hurt you	[threats - serious violence]
threaten to kill himself	
threaten to kill you	
threaten you with a weapon	
threaten you with a club-like object	
act like he wanted to kill you	
threaten you with a knife or gun	
hold you down pinning you in place	[acts - mild violence]
push or shove you	
grab you suddenly or forcefully	
shake or roughly handle you	
scratch you	[acts - minor violence]
pull your hair	
twist your arm	
spank you	
bite you	
slap you with the palm of his hand	[acts - moderate violence]
slap you with the back of his hand	
slap you around your face and head	
hit you with an object	[acts - serious violence]
punch you	
kick you	
stomp on you	
choke you	
burn you with something	
use a club-like object on you	
beat you up	
use a knife or gun on you	
demand sex whether you wanted it or not	[sexual aggression]

make you have oral (mouth) sex against your will
make you have sexual intercourse against your will
physically force you to have sex
make you have anal (bottom) sex against your will
use an object on you in a sexual way

Sexual Experiences Survey – Short Form Perpetration

Reprinted with permission from the author (Koss, M., and the SES Collaborative, 2006)

SES-SFP

The following questions concern sexual experiences. We know these are personal questions, so we do not ask your name or other identifying information. Your information is completely confidential. We hope this helps you to feel comfortable answering each question honestly. Place a check mark in the box ☐ showing the number of times each experience has happened. If several experiences occurred on the same occasion--for example, if one night you told some lies and had sex with someone who was drunk, you would check both boxes a and c. The past 12 months refers to the past year going back from today. Since age 14 refers to your life starting on your 14th birthday and stopping one year ago from today.

Sexual Experiences		How many times in the past 12 months?	How many times since age 14?
1.	I fondled, kissed, or rubbed up against the private areas of someone's body (lips, breast/chest, crotch or butt) or removed some of their clothes without their consent *(but did not attempt sexual penetration)* by:	0 1 2 3+	0 1 2 3+
	a. Telling lies, threatening to end the relationship, threatening to spread rumors about them, making promises about the future I knew were untrue, or continually verbally pressuring them after they said they didn't want to.	☐ ☐ ☐ ☐	☐ ☐ ☐ ☐
	b. Showing displeasure, criticizing their sexuality or attractiveness, getting angry but not using physical force after they said they didn't want to.	☐ ☐ ☐ ☐	☐ ☐ ☐ ☐
	c. Taking advantage when they were too drunk or out of it to stop what was happening.	☐ ☐ ☐ ☐	☐ ☐ ☐ ☐
	d. Threatening to physically harm them or someone close to them.	☐ ☐ ☐ ☐	☐ ☐ ☐ ☐
	e. Using force, for example holding them down with my body weight, pinning their arms, or having a weapon.	☐ ☐ ☐ ☐	☐ ☐ ☐ ☐
2.	I had oral sex with someone or had someone perform oral sex on me without their consent by:	0 1 2 3+	0 1 2 3+
	a. Telling lies, threatening to end the relationship, threatening to spread rumors about them, making promises about the future I knew were untrue, or continually verbally pressuring them after they said they didn't want to.	☐ ☐ ☐ ☐	☐ ☐ ☐ ☐
	b. Showing displeasure, criticizing their sexuality or attractiveness, getting angry but not using physical force after they said they didn't want to.	☐ ☐ ☐ ☐	☐ ☐ ☐ ☐
	c. Taking advantage when they were too drunk or out of it to stop what was happening.	☐ ☐ ☐ ☐	☐ ☐ ☐ ☐

		How many times in the past 12 months?	How many times since age 14?
	d. Threatening to physically harm them or someone close to them.	☐ ☐ ☐ ☐	☐ ☐ ☐ ☐
	e. Using force, for example holding them down with my body weight, pinning their arms, or having a weapon.	☐ ☐ ☐ ☐	☐ ☐ ☐ ☐
3.	**I put my penis (men only) or I put my fingers or objects (all respondents) into a woman's vagina without her consent by:**	0 1 2 3+	0 1 2 3+
	a. Telling lies, threatening to end the relationship, threatening to spread rumors about them, making promises about the future I knew were untrue, or continually verbally pressuring them after they said they didn't want to.	☐ ☐ ☐ ☐	☐ ☐ ☐ ☐
	b. Showing displeasure, criticizing their sexuality or attractiveness, getting angry but not using physical force after they said they didn't want to.	☐ ☐ ☐ ☐	☐ ☐ ☐ ☐
	c. Taking advantage when they were too drunk or out of it to stop what was happening.	☐ ☐ ☐ ☐	☐ ☐ ☐ ☐
	d. Threatening to physically harm them or someone close to them.	☐ ☐ ☐ ☐	☐ ☐ ☐ ☐
	e. Using force, for example holding them down with my body weight, pinning their arms, or having a weapon.	☐ ☐ ☐ ☐	☐ ☐ ☐ ☐
4.	**I put in my penis (men only) or I put my fingers or objects (all respondents) into someone's butt without their consent by:**	0 1 2 3+	0 1 2 3+
	a. Telling lies, threatening to end the relationship, threatening to spread rumors about them, making promises about the future I knew were untrue, or continually verbally pressuring them after they said they didn't want to.	☐ ☐ ☐ ☐	☐ ☐ ☐ ☐
	b. Showing displeasure, criticizing their sexuality or attractiveness, getting angry but not using physical force after they said they didn't want to.	☐ ☐ ☐ ☐	☐ ☐ ☐ ☐
	c. Taking advantage when they were too drunk or out of it to stop what was happening.	☐ ☐ ☐ ☐	☐ ☐ ☐ ☐
	d. Threatening to physically harm them or someone close to them.	☐ ☐ ☐ ☐	☐ ☐ ☐ ☐
	e. Using force, for example holding them down with my body weight, pinning their arms, or having a weapon.	☐ ☐ ☐ ☐	☐ ☐ ☐ ☐
5.	**Even though it did not happen, I TRIED to have oral sex with someone or make them have oral sex with me without their consent by:**	0 1 2 3+	0 1 2 3+
	a. Telling lies, threatening to end the relationship, threatening to spread rumors about them, making promises about the future I knew were untrue, or continually verbally pressuring them after they said they didn't want to.	☐ ☐ ☐ ☐	☐ ☐ ☐ ☐
	b. Showing displeasure, criticizing their sexuality or attractiveness, getting angry but not using physical force after they said they didn't want to.	☐ ☐ ☐ ☐	☐ ☐ ☐ ☐
	c. Taking advantage when they were too drunk or out of it to stop what was happening.	☐ ☐ ☐ ☐	☐ ☐ ☐ ☐

		How many times in the past 12 months?				How many times since age 14?			
d.	Threatening to physically harm them or someone close to them.	☐	☐	☐	☐	☐	☐	☐	☐
e.	Using force, for example holding them down with my body weight, pinning their arms, or having a weapon.	☐	☐	☐	☐	☐	☐	☐	☐

		How many times in the past 12 months?				How many times since age 14?			
6.	**Even though it did not happen, I TRIED put in my penis (men only) or I tried to put my fingers or objects (all respondents) into a woman's vagina without their consent by:**	0	1	2	3+	0	1	2	3+
a.	Telling lies, threatening to end the relationship, threatening to spread rumors about them, making promises about the future I knew were untrue, or continually verbally pressuring them after they said they didn't want to.	☐	☐	☐	☐	☐	☐	☐	☐
b.	Showing displeasure, criticizing their sexuality or attractiveness, getting angry but not using physical force after they said they didn't want to.	☐	☐	☐	☐	☐	☐	☐	☐
c.	Taking advantage when they were too drunk or out of it to stop what was happening.	☐	☐	☐	☐	☐	☐	☐	☐
d.	Threatening to physically harm them or someone close to them.	☐	☐	☐	☐	☐	☐	☐	☐
e.	Using force, for example holding them down with my body weight, pinning their arms, or having a weapon.	☐	☐	☐	☐	☐	☐	☐	☐
7.	**Even though it did not happen, I TRIED to put in my penis (men only) or I tried to put my fingers or objects (all respondents) into someone's butt without their consent by:**	0	1	2	3+	0	1	2	3+
a.	Telling lies, threatening to end the relationship, threatening to spread rumors about them, making promises about the future I knew were untrue, or continually verbally pressuring them after they said they didn't want to.	☐	☐	☐	☐	☐	☐	☐	☐
b.	Showing displeasure, criticizing their sexuality or attractiveness, getting angry but not using physical force after they said they didn't want to.	☐	☐	☐	☐	☐	☐	☐	☐
c.	Taking advantage when they were too drunk or out of it to stop what was happening.	☐	☐	☐	☐	☐	☐	☐	☐
d.	Threatening to physically harm them or someone close to them.	☐	☐	☐	☐	☐	☐	☐	☐
e.	Using force, for example holding them down with my body weight, pinning their arms, or having a weapon.	☐	☐	☐	☐	☐	☐	☐	☐

8. I am: Female ☐   Male ☐   My age is _____ years and
   _____ months.

9. Did you do any of the acts described in this survey 1 or more times?   Yes ☐   No ☐
   If yes, what was the sex of the person or persons to whom you did them?

   Female only   ☐
   Male only   ☐
   Both females and males   ☐

   I reported no experiences   ☐

10. Do you think you may have you ever raped someone?   Yes ☐   No ☐

Sexual Experiences Survey – Short Form Victimization

Reprinted with permission from the author (Koss, M., and the SES Collaborative, 2006).

SES-SFV

The following questions concern sexual experiences that you may have had that were unwanted. We know that these are personal questions, so we do not ask your name or other identifying information. Your information is completely confidential. We hope that this helps you to feel comfortable answering each question honestly. Place a check mark in the box ☐ showing the number of times each experience has happened to you. If several experiences occurred on the same occasion--for example, if one night someone told you some lies and had sex with you when you were drunk, you would check both boxes a and c. The past 12 months refers to the past year going back from today. Since age 14 refers to your life starting on your 14th birthday and stopping one year ago from today.

Sexual Experiences	How many times in the past 12 months?	How many times since age 14?
1. Someone fondled, kissed, or rubbed up against the private areas of my body (lips, breast/chest, crotch or butt) or removed some of my clothes without my consent *(but did not attempt sexual penetration)* by:	0 1 2 3+	0 1 2 3+
a. Telling lies, threatening to end the relationship, threatening to spread rumors about me, making promises I knew were untrue, or continually verbally pressuring me after I said I didn't want to.	☐ ☐ ☐ ☐	☐ ☐ ☐ ☐
b. Showing displeasure, criticizing my sexuality or attractiveness, getting angry but not using physical force, after I said I didn't want to.	☐ ☐ ☐ ☐	☐ ☐ ☐ ☐
c. Taking advantage of me when I was too drunk or out of it to stop what was happening.	☐ ☐ ☐ ☐	☐ ☐ ☐ ☐
d. Threatening to physically harm me or someone close to me.	☐ ☐ ☐ ☐	☐ ☐ ☐ ☐
e. Using force, for example holding me down with their body weight, pinning my arms, or having a weapon.	☐ ☐ ☐ ☐	☐ ☐ ☐ ☐
2. Someone had oral sex with me or made me have oral sex with them without my consent by:	0 1 2 3+	0 1 2 3+
a. Telling lies, threatening to end the relationship, threatening to spread rumors about me, making promises I knew were untrue, or continually verbally pressuring me after I said I didn't want to.	☐ ☐ ☐ ☐	☐ ☐ ☐ ☐
b. Showing displeasure, criticizing my sexuality or attractiveness, getting angry but not using physical force, after I said I didn't want to.	☐ ☐ ☐ ☐	☐ ☐ ☐ ☐
c. Taking advantage of me when I was too drunk or out of it to stop what was happening.	☐ ☐ ☐ ☐	☐ ☐ ☐ ☐
d. Threatening to physically harm me or someone close to me.	☐ ☐ ☐ ☐	☐ ☐ ☐ ☐

			How many times in the past 12 months?				How many times since age 14?			
	e.	Using force, for example holding me down with their body weight, pinning my arms, or having a weapon.	□	□	□	□	□	□	□	□
3.	**If you are a male, check box and skip to item 4** □ **A man put his penis into my vagina, or someone inserted fingers or objects without my consent by:**		0	1	2	3+	0	1	2	3+
	a.	Telling lies, threatening to end the relationship, threatening to spread rumors about me, making promises I knew were untrue, or continually verbally pressuring me after I said I didn't want to.	□	□	□	□	□	□	□	□
	b.	Showing displeasure, criticizing my sexuality or attractiveness, getting angry but not using physical force, after I said I didn't want to.	□	□	□	□	□	□	□	□
	c.	Taking advantage of me when I was too drunk or out of it to stop what was happening.	□	□	□	□	□	□	□	□
	d.	Threatening to physically harm me or someone close to me.	□	□	□	□	□	□	□	□
	e.	Using force, for example holding me down with their body weight, pinning my arms, or having a weapon.	□	□	□	□	□	□	□	□
4.	**A man put his penis into my butt, or someone inserted fingers or objects without my consent by:**		0	1	2	3+	0	1	2	3+
	a.	Telling lies, threatening to end the relationship, threatening to spread rumors about me, making promises I knew were untrue, or continually verbally pressuring me after I said I didn't want to.	□	□	□	□	□	□	□	□
	b.	Showing displeasure, criticizing my sexuality or attractiveness, getting angry but not using physical force, after I said I didn't want to.	□	□	□	□	□	□	□	□
	c.	Taking advantage of me when I was too drunk or out of it to stop what was happening.	□	□	□	□	□	□	□	□
	d.	Threatening to physically harm me or someone close to me.	□	□	□	□	□	□	□	□
	e.	Using force, for example holding me down with their body weight, pinning my arms, or having a weapon.	□	□	□	□	□	□	□	□
5.	**Even though it didn't happen, someone TRIED to have oral sex with me, or make me have oral sex with them without my consent by:**		0	1	2	3+	0	1	2	3+
	a.	Telling lies, threatening to end the relationship, threatening to spread rumors about me, making promises I knew were untrue, or continually verbally pressuring me after I said I didn't want to.	□	□	□	□	□	□	□	□
	b.	Showing displeasure, criticizing my sexuality or attractiveness, getting angry but not using physical force, after I said I didn't want to.	□	□	□	□	□	□	□	□
	c.	Taking advantage of me when I was too drunk or out of it to stop what was happening.	□	□	□	□	□	□	□	□
	d.	Threatening to physically harm me or someone close to me.	□	□	□	□	□	□	□	□

		How many times in the past 12 months?	How many times since age 14?
	e. Using force, for example holding me down with their body weight, pinning my arms, or having a weapon.	☐ ☐ ☐ ☐	☐ ☐ ☐ ☐

6.	**If you are male, check this box and skip to item 7.** ☐ **Even though it didn't happen, a man TRIED to put his penis into my vagina, or someone tried to stick in fingers or objects without my consent by:**	0 1 2 3+	0 1 2 3+
	a. Telling lies, threatening to end the relationship, threatening to spread rumors about me, making promises I knew were untrue, or continually verbally pressuring me after I said I didn't want to.	☐ ☐ ☐ ☐	☐ ☐ ☐ ☐
	b. Showing displeasure, criticizing my sexuality or attractiveness, getting angry but not using physical force, after I said I didn't want to.	☐ ☐ ☐ ☐	☐ ☐ ☐ ☐
	c. Taking advantage of me when I was too drunk or out of it to stop what was happening.	☐ ☐ ☐ ☐	☐ ☐ ☐ ☐
	d. Threatening to physically harm me or someone close to me.	☐ ☐ ☐ ☐	☐ ☐ ☐ ☐
	e. Using force, for example holding me down with their body weight, pinning my arms, or having a weapon.	☐ ☐ ☐ ☐	☐ ☐ ☐ ☐

7.	**Even though it didn't happen, a man TRIED to put his penis into my butt, or someone tried to stick in objects or fingers without my consent by:**	0 1 2 3+	0 1 2 3+
	a. Telling lies, threatening to end the relationship, threatening to spread rumors about me, making promises I knew were untrue, or continually verbally pressuring me after I said I didn't want to.	☐ ☐ ☐ ☐	☐ ☐ ☐ ☐
	b. Showing displeasure, criticizing my sexuality or attractiveness, getting angry but not using physical force, after I said I didn't want to.	☐ ☐ ☐ ☐	☐ ☐ ☐ ☐
	c. Taking advantage of me when I was too drunk or out of it to stop what was happening.	☐ ☐ ☐ ☐	☐ ☐ ☐ ☐
	d. Threatening to physically harm me or someone close to me.	☐ ☐ ☐ ☐	☐ ☐ ☐ ☐
	e. Using force, for example holding me down with their body weight, pinning my arms, or having a weapon.	☐ ☐ ☐ ☐	☐ ☐ ☐ ☐

8. I am: Female ☐   Male ☐ My age is _____ years and
_____months.

9. Did any of the experiences described in this survey happen to you 1 or more times? Yes ☐
No ☐
What was the sex of the person or persons who did them to you?
            Female only   ☐
            Male only   ☐
            Both females and males   ☐
            I reported no experiences ☐
10. Have you ever been raped? Yes ☐   No ☐

Scoring of SES Short Forms
Koss, M.P. and the SES Collaboration*
September 5, 2008

*Members include Antonia Abbey (Wayne State University), Rebecca Campbell (Michigan State University), Sarah Cook (Georgia State University), Mary Koss (University of Arizona), Jeanette Norris (University of Washington), Maria Testa (The University at Buffalo), Sarah Ullman (University of Illinois at Chicago), Carolyn West (University of Washington at Takoma), and Jacquelyn White (University of North Carolina at Greensboro).

All versions of the revised SES measure behavior that meets legal definitions of various sex crimes, with the exception of acts accomplished by verbal coercion not involving threats of physical harm. The acts accomplished by coercion are certainly on the sexual assault spectrum and they are of interest in many fields and settings, but it is important to clearly understand that they are not crimes. Feminist legal scholars argue that these acts should be forms of attempted rape and rape and recommend changing statutory definitions of rape as a goal for advocate policy reform.

Scoring of the SES—Short Form Perpetration

Scoring based on individual items
        To estimate the frequency of each type of unwanted sex act and/or the rate of each tactic to compel unwanted sex, calculate the percentage of respondents who respond yes to each choice a through e for each item 1 through 7.

Ordinal Scoring

Reporting prevalence by category
To score prevalence of each category, use the following instructions. Note that this set of scoring rules will result in percentages that exceed 100% because respondents could have perpetrated more than one type of incident. The procedures for mutually exclusive scoring when the goal is to count people only once according to the most severe act perpetrated follow this section.

1. Non-perpetrator: responds 0 times to all items
2. Sexual Contact: any number of times >0 to item 1 for any strategy a through e
3. Attempted coercion: any number of times >0 to strategy a or strategy b for items 5, 6, or 7
4. Coercion: any number of times >0 to strategy a or strategy b for items 2, 3, or 4
5. Attempted rape: any number of times >0 to strategies c, d, or e on items 5, 6 or 7
6. Rape: any number of times >0 to strategies c, d, or e on items 2, 3, or 4

Scoring Mutually Exclusive Categories
To create non-redundant scores, use the following instructions to place each person into the category of their most severe experience. These scoring rules result in category percentages that add to 100%.

1. Non-perpetrator: all 7 items checked 0 times on a, b, c, d, e
2. Sexual Contact: any number of times >0 to item 1 for any strategy a through e and no to all other items
3. Attempted Coercion: any number of times >0 for strategy a or strategy b for items 5, 6, or 7 and 0 times to strategies c, d, & e on all items
4. Coercion—any number of times >0 for strategy a or strategy b for items 2, 3, or 4 and 0 times to strategies c, d, & e on all items
5. Attempted rape—any number of times >0 for strategies c, d, & e on items 5, 6, or 7 and reported 0 times to strategies c, d, & e on items 2, 3, and 4, regardless of responses to strategies a & b for any item.
6. Rape—any number of times >0 to strategies c, d, & e on items 2, 3, and 4, regardless of responses to any other items (including responses to strategies a and b for any item)

Scoring of the SES—Short Form Victimization

Scoring based on individual items
To estimate the frequency of each type of unwanted sexual victimization and/or the rate of each tactic used to compel unwanted sex, calculate the percentage of respondents who respond yes to each choice a through e for each item 1 through 7.

Ordinal scoring

Reporting prevalence by category
To score prevalence of each category, use the following instructions. Note that this set of scoring rules will result in percentages that exceed 100% because respondents could have had more than one type of incident. The procedures for mutually exclusive scoring when the goal is to count people only once according to the most severe act experienced follow this section.

1. Non-victim: responds 0 times to all items
2. Sexual Contact: any number of times >0 to item 1 for any strategy a through e
3. Attempted coercion: any number of times >0 to strategy a or strategy b for items 5, 6, or 7
4. Coercion: any number of times >0 to strategy a or strategy b for items 2, 3, or 4
5. Attempted rape: any number of times >0 to strategies c, d, or e on items 5, 6 or 7
6. Rape: any number of times >0 to strategies c, d, or e on items 2, 3, or 4

Scoring Mutually Exclusive Categories
To create non-redundant scores, use the following instructions to place each person into the category of their most severe experience. These scoring rules result in category percentages that add to 100%.

1. Non-victim: all 7 items checked 0 times on a, b, c, d, e
2. Sexual Contact: any number of times >0 to item 1 for any strategy a through e and no to all other items
3. Attempted Coercion: any number of times >0 for strategy a or strategy b for items 5, 6, or 7 and 0 times to strategies c, d, & e on all items
4. Coercion—any number of times >0 for strategy a or strategy b for items 2, 3, or 4 and 0 times to strategies c, d, & e on all items
5. Attempted rape—any number of times >0 for strategies c, d, & e on items 5, 6, or 7 and reported 0 times to strategies c, d, & e on items 2, 3, and 4, regardless of responses to strategies a & b for any item.
6. Rape—any number of times >0 to strategies c, d, & e on items 2, 3, and 4, regardless of responses to any other items (including responses to strategies a and b for any item)

Citation for the SES: Koss, M.P., Abbey, A., Campbell, R., Cook, S; Norris, J., Testa, C., Ullman, S., West, C., & White, J. (2007). Revising the SES: A collaborative process to improve assessment of sexual aggression and victimization. *Psychology of Women Quarterly, 31,* 357-370.

Contact Information:
Mary P. Koss, Ph.D., Regents' Professor
Mel and Enid Zuckerman College of Public Health
University of Arizona
1295 N. Martin Street
Tucson, Arizona 85724
mpk@u.arizona.edu
(520)-626-3998 (voice)
(520) 626-8716 (fax)

Subtle and Overt Psychological Abuse of Women Scale (SOPAS)

Reprinted with permission from the author (Marshall, L., 2000)

Most of these things happen in all relationships. These are things your partner may do in a loving, joking or serious way. Choose a number from the above scale to show how often he does each thing.

HOW OFTEN DOES HE...

_____ play games with your head

_____ act like he knows what you did when he wasn't around

_____ blame you for him being angry or upset

_____ change his mind but not tell you until it's too late

_____ discourage you from having interests that he isn't part of

_____ do or say something that harms your self-respect or your pride in yourself

_____ encourage you to do something then somehow make it difficult to do it

_____ belittle, find fault or put down something you were pleased with or felt good about

_____ get more upset than you are when you tell him how you feel

_____ make you feel bad when you did something he didn't want you to do

_____ make you feel like nothing you say will have an effect on him

_____ make you choose between something he wants and something you want or need

_____ say or do something that makes you feel unloved or unlovable

_____ make you worry about whether you could take care of yourself

_____ make you feel guilty about something you have done or have not done

IN A LOVING, JOKING OR SERIOUS WAY, HOW OFTEN DOES HE...

_____ use things you've said against you, like if you say you made a mistake, how often does he use that against you later

_____ make you worry about your emotional health and well-being

_____ make you feel like you have to fix something he did that turned out badly

_____ put himself first, not seeming to care what you want

_____ get you to question yourself, making you feel insecure or less confident

_____ remind you of times he was right and you were wrong

_____ say his actions, which hurt you, are good for you or will make you a better person

_____ say something that makes you worry about whether you're going crazy

_____ act like he owns you

_____ somehow make you feel worried or scared even if you're not sure why

_____ somehow make it difficult for you to go somewhere or talk to someone

_____ somehow keep you from having time for yourself

_____ act like you over-react or get too upset

_____ get upset when you did something he didn't know about

_____ tell you the problems in your relationship are your fault

_____ interrupt or sidetrack you when you're doing something important

_____ blame you for his problems

_____ try to keep you from showing what you feel

_____ try to keep you from doing something you want to do or have to do

_____ try to convince you something was like he said when you know that isn't true

Index

G.F. Ronan et al., *Practitioner's Guide to Empirically Supported Measures of Anger, Aggression,*
and Violence, ABCT Clinical Assessment Series, DOI 10.1007/978-3-319-00245-3,
© Springer International Publishing Switzerland 2014

CPSIA information can be obtained at www.ICGtesting.com
Printed in the USA
LVOW02s2218071013

355896LV00004B/57/P